Nomenclature and Criteria for Diagnosis of the Heart and G:

D0292422

Nomenclature and Criteria for Diagnosis of Diseases of the Heart and Great Vessels

Ninth Edition

The Criteria Committee of the New York Heart Association

Editor
Martin Dolgin, M.D.

Associate Editors
Arthur C. Fox, M.D.
Richard Gorlin, M.D.
Richard I. Levin, M.D.

Criteria Committee
Richard B. Devereaux, M.D.
Martin Dolgin, M.D.
Stephen M. Factor, M.D.
John D. Fisher, M.D.
Arthur C. Fox, M.D.
Seymour Furman, M.D.
Richard Gorlin, M.D.
O. Wayne Isom, M.D.
Itzhak Kronzon, M.D.
Richard I. Levin, M.D.
Mariano J. Rey, M.D.
Samuel B. Ritter, M.D.
Clive Rosendorff, M.D.
Joseph J. Sanger, M.D.
Edmund H. Sonnenblick, M.D.
Paul A. Tunick, M.D.
Jeffrey C. Weinreb, M.D.

Little, Brown and Company
Boston/New York/Toronto/London

Library of Congress Cataloging-in-Publication Data

Nomenclature and criteria for diagnosis of diseases of the heart and
    great vessels / the Criteria Committee of the New York Heart
    Association. — 9th ed. / editor, Martin Dolgin ; associate editors,
    Arthur C. Fox, Richard Gorlin, Richard I. Levin ; Criteria
    Committee, Richard B. Devereaux . . . [et al.]
        p.   cm.
    Includes bibliographical references and index.
    ISBN 0-316-60538-7
    1. Cardiovascular system—Diseases—Diagnosis. I. Dolgin,
Martin. II. New York Heart Association. Criteria Committee.
    [DNLM: 1. Cardiovascular Diseases—diagnosis. 2. Cardiovascular
Diseases—nomenclature. 3. Cardiovascular Diseases—classification.
WG 141 N799 1994]
RC683.N37   1994
616.1'075—dc20
DNLM/DLC
for Library of Congress   93-43623
                                                                    CIP
Printed in the United States of America

RRD-VA

Sixth Edition, 1964
    Diseases of the Heart and Blood Vessels:
    Nomenclature and Criteria for Diagnosis
Fifth Edition, 1953
    Nomenclature and Criteria for Diagnosis
    of Diseases of the Heart and Blood Vessels
Fourth Edition, 1939
    Nomenclature and Criteria for Diagnosis of Diseases of the Heart
Third Edition, 1932
Second Edition, 1929
First Edition, 1928
    Criteria for the Classification and Diagnosis of Heart Disease

Editorial: Nancy Megley
Production Editor: Anne Holm
Copyeditor: Debra Corman
Indexer: Nancy Newman
Production Supervisor: Michael A. Granger
Cover Designer: Michael A. Granger

To the volunteers, past and present, of the New York Heart Association, who have sustained the Association in its efforts to reduce disability and death from diseases of the heart and blood vessels through research, education, and community programs

Contents

Preface

During the early decades of this century, physicians involved in the establishment of cardiac clinics at Bellevue and then other hospitals in New York City perceived the need to standardize not only clinic procedures and care but also cardiovascular nomenclature and diagnostic criteria. Responding to this need, the New York Heart Association published in 1928 a detailed set of criteria titled *Criteria for Classification and Diagnosis of Heart Disease*. In the subsequent 50 years, seven revisions were issued. While the title and content of the book changed as the theory and practice of cardiology evolved, the primary objective remained the same: to provide readers with concise descriptions of the principal causes and manifestations of cardiovascular diseases and the specific criteria for their diagnosis. Generations of medical students, physicians, and nurses have found the book a useful learning resource that complements traditional cardiology textbooks.

Two objectives guided the preparation of the Ninth Edition of *Nomenclature and Criteria for Diagnosis of Diseases of the Heart and Great Vessels*. This edition should reflect the important advances in knowledge of the general biology of cardiovascular diseases, and the development of newer diagnostic methods and their clinical application, that have occurred since publication of the Eighth Edition in 1979. The Ninth Edition should retain the general principles, format, and tenor of the Eighth.

The special literary challenge has been to incorporate new data and yet preserve the relatively small size of the book and prevent its transformation from a manual of cardiovascular diagnosis to a formal textbook of cardiology. While much of the Eighth Edition text has been retained, significant deletions, additions, and other modifications have been made. Numerical classification of diagnoses has been discontinued. Illustrative materials have been judged inappropriate for a book of this type and, except for five tables, have been omitted. The major cardiovascular diagnostic technologies that became preeminent in the last 15 years—echocardiography, intracardiac electrography, computed tomography, magnetic resonance imaging, and stress physiology with specialized radionuclide methods—are recognized by separate, more general descriptions as well as by selective inclusion in the review of specific diagnostic entities. The five-component complete cardiac diagnosis has been retained, but the evaluative terms *Status* and *Prognosis* have been replaced by *Functional Capacity* and *Objective Assessment*.

It is hoped that the Ninth Edition continues the tradition, so successfully established in previous editions, of providing brief, sophisticated descriptions of circulatory diseases and criteria for their diagnosis. The present Criteria Committee acknowledges its indebtedness to its predecessors.

Criteria Committee

Introduction: The Complete Cardiac Diagnosis

In this handbook of cardiovascular diagnosis, descriptions of disease and diagnostic criteria are organized into separate categories—etiologic, anatomic, and physiologic. These categories identify the principal characteristics of diseases of the heart and great vessels that are of clinical importance. It is proposed that a complete cardiac diagnosis should contain five components (see Section 4): the Etiologic, Anatomic, and Physiologic Diagnoses and the summary overall evaluation of the patient's cardiovascular status, Functional Capacity and Objective Assessment. This structured format expresses all the important elements of a cardiac diagnosis, which should prevent incomplete diagnostic statements that may result in inappropriate medical management.

The lists of etiologic, anatomic, and physiologic diagnoses given in Sections 1, 2, and 3 include most of the important diseases but are not meant to be exhaustive in scope. Additional entities may be used when appropriate.

Identification of correct diagnoses will require investigative studies of varying degrees of sophistication ranging from relatively simple but rigorous clinical observations to complex hemodynamic, radiologic, echocardiographic, electrophysiologic, or biochemical studies. Not infrequently, exact diagnoses are not established or cannot be established despite extensive study. This kind of uncertainty can be indicated in the diagnostic formulation by placing question marks before the items in the differential diagnosis. The complete cardiac diagnosis should be kept current and revised as new diagnostic information is acquired.

Criteria for anatomic and physiologic diagnoses have been made more detailed and precise in this edition. This reflects advances in imaging techniques that permit more accurate recognition of anatomic abnormalities and their physiologic consequences. The increased sensitivity of these techniques allows detection of some mild structural abnormalities before they have caused any functional disorder.

Wherever appropriate, the specific criteria for diagnosis listed at the end of each disease description have been divided into two groups: Initial Diagnosis and Definitive Diagnosis. This system conforms to the actual decision-making process used by physicians in clinical practice. It is not meant to rank criteria in their order of predictive accuracy, and it is not to be used to characterize the diseases listed in the complete cardiac diagnosis. Criteria for the Initial Diagnosis are based on data obtained from the history, physical examination, electrocardiogram, chest x-ray, and other readily available laboratory data. The Initial Diagnosis is the "working" diagnosis and is often highly accurate. It is used not only to initiate treatment but also to select investigative studies required to establish the Definitive Diagnosis. Criteria for the Definitive Diagnosis are based on data obtained from diagnostic procedures that attempt to delineate the precise anatomic and physiologic characteristics of the disease. Such procedures may include echocardiography, cardiac catheterization, contrast angiography and ventriculography, electrophysiologic tests, nuclear imaging, computed tomography, magnetic resonance imaging, endomyocardial biopsy, and specific biochemical analyses.

Certain patients may have symptoms or abnormal physical signs that are referable to the heart but, after detailed study, cannot be ascribed with certainty to structural or functional cardiac disease. In such cases, the diagnosis should be No Heart Disease, Unexplained Manifestation. Patients who have a disease that may involve the heart but has not done so by the time of observation are to be designated as having No Heart Disease, Predisposing Etiologic Factor (see Section 5).

The use of the five-component complete cardiac diagnosis is illustrated in the following examples.

A Patient with Acute Myocardial Infarction

Cardiac Diagnosis on Admission

Etiologic Diagnosis
   Atherosclerosis
   Hypertension
Anatomic Diagnosis
   Coronary Atherosclerosis
   Myocardial Fibrosis
   Thromboses of Left Coronary Artery
   Acute Anteroseptal Myocardial Infarction
   Left Ventricular Hypertrophy

Physiologic Diagnosis
    Sinus Tachycardia
    Sustained Ventricular Tachycardia
    Left Ventricular Failure

Functional Capacity   IV
Objective Assessment   D

Cardiac Diagnosis at Discharge

Etiologic Diagnosis
    Atherosclerosis
    Hypertension
Anatomic Diagnosis
    Atherosclerosis of Left Anterior Descending Coronary
        Artery, Right Coronary Artery, Left Circumflex Cor-
        onary Artery
    Thrombosis of Left Anterior Descending Coronary Ar-
        tery
    Anterior Wall Myocardial Infarction
    Ventricular Aneurysm
    Left Ventricular Hypertrophy
Physiologic Diagnosis
    Normal Sinus Rhythm
    Multifocal Ventricular Premature Depolarizations
    Reversible Myocardial Ischemia
    Left Ventricular Systolic and Diastolic Dysfunction

Functional Capacity   II
Objective Assessment   C

A Patient with Paroxysmal Tachycardia

Cardiac Diagnosis

Etiologic Diagnosis
    Unknown
    ? Congenital Anomaly
Anatomic Diagnosis
    Unknown
    ?Accessory Atrioventricular Conduction Pathway
Physiologic Diagnosis
    Paroxysmal Supraventricular Tachycardia
    ? Ventricular Preexcitation

Functional Capacity   II
Objective Assessment   Undetermined

A Patient with Rheumatic Heart Disease

Cardiac Diagnosis

Etiologic Diagnosis
   Rheumatic Fever—Inactive
Anatomic Diagnosis
   Enlarged Left Atrium, Left Ventricle, Pulmonary Artery and Right Ventricle
   Mitral Valve Deformity (calcified immobile leaflets)
Physiologic Diagnosis
   Atrial Fibrillation, Mitral Stenosis, Mitral Regurgitation, Pulmonary Hypertension

Functional Capacity   III
Objective Assessment   C

A Patient with Anginal Syndrome

Cardiac Diagnosis

Etiologic Diagnosis
   Unknown
Anatomic Diagnosis
   Unknown
Physiologic Diagnosis
   Normal Sinus Rhythm
   Anginal Syndrome
   ? Reduced Coronary Reserve

Functional Capacity   II
Objective Assessment   A

Nomenclature and Criteria for Diagnosis of Diseases of the Heart and Great Vessels

Notice

The indications and dosages of all drugs in this book have been recommended in the medical literature and conform to the practices of the general medical community. The medications described do not necessarily have specific approval by the Food and Drug Administration for use in the diseases and dosages for which they are recommended. The package insert for each drug should be consulted for use and dosage as approved by the FDA. Because standards for usage change, it is advisable to keep abreast of revised recommendations, particularly those concerning new drugs.

The Etiologic Cardiac Diagnosis

NOMENCLATURE

Acromegaly
Aging
Alcoholism
Amyloidosis
Anemia
Ankylosing Spondylitis
Atherosclerosis
Carcinoid Tumor
Congenital Anomaly
Friedreich's Ataxia
Hemochromatosis
Homocystinuria
Hypertension
Hyperthyroidism
Hypothyroidism
Infection
Intervention
Kawasaki Disease (Mucocutaneous Lymph Node Syndrome)
Lysosomal Storage Diseases
Marfan's Syndrome
Neoplasms
Obesity
Paget's Disease of Bone (Osteitis Deformans)
Pheochromocytoma
Polyarteritis Nodosa
Pregnancy (Peripartum Cardiomyopathy)
Progressive Muscular Dystrophy (Duchenne Type)
Progressive Systemic Sclerosis (Scleroderma)
Pulmonary Disease (Cor Pulmonale)
Radiation
Reiter's Syndrome
Rheumatic Fever/Rheumatic Heart Disease
Rheumatoid Arthritis
Sarcoidosis
Systemic Arteriovenous Fistula
Systemic Lupus Erythematosus
Toxic Agent
Transplantation
Trauma

Unknown Etiology
Uremia

ACROMEGALY

The Disease

Acromegaly is characterized by progressive swelling of tissues and organs due to the anabolic actions of excessive growth hormone, with variable manifestations based on both tissue overgrowth and direct hormonal stimulation.

Molecular and Cellular Biology

Manifestations are caused by the unregulated oversecretion of growth hormone or somatotropin, a 191–amino acid protein secreted by the anterior pituitary. The oversecretion is almost always due to a pituitary adenoma. Growth hormone stimulates the synthesis of insulin-like growth factors that, in combination with growth hormone itself, induce anabolic changes throughout the body. The exact mechanism of the growth hormone effect is unknown. A digitalis-like factor in the plasma of patients with acromegaly has been described.

Cardiac Involvement

The heart is hypertrophied, often out of proportion to the other organs. Existence of a specific "acromegalic cardiomyopathy" is controversial, but there are direct effects of growth hormone on cardiac function. There may be concomitant hypertension and atherosclerotic coronary artery disease, related or unrelated to acromegaly. Dyspnea, fatigue, peripheral edema, and syncope may be the presenting symptoms.

THE FOLLOWING CRITERIA ARE REQUIRED FOR THE DIAGNOSIS OF HEART DISEASE DUE TO ACROMEGALY.

Cardiac enlargement with or without ventricular failure, in the presence of clinical and biochemical evidence for acromegaly and in the absence of coronary atherosclerosis and systemic hypertension.

AGING

The Disease

Aging is not a disease, and whether aging alone is associated with a specific set of changes in the cardiovascular system is controversial.

Molecular and Cellular Biology

The mechanism of aging is unknown. Cultured human cells exhibit finite proliferative life spans that are related directly to the age of the donor, suggesting that each cell type maintains a biologic clock that controls both senescence and apoptosis, or programmed cell death in the absence of injury from without. Alternatively, aging may be the sum of metabolic alterations of cells that are not repaired, such as oxidation, cross-linking, and glycation of proteins and DNA.

Cardiac Involvement

Many of the diseases affecting the heart and vasculature are more common with advanced age. However, it is not clear whether aging directly alters the cardiovascular system in physiologically important ways or whether many of the observed changes are due to deconditioning. In general, changes ascribed to aging include loss of arterial compliance, hypertrophy of the left ventricle, prolongation of contraction and relaxation, a decline in beta-adrenergic responsiveness, and a decline in pericardial compliance.

THE FOLLOWING CRITERIA ARE REQUIRED FOR THE DIAGNOSIS OF HEART DISEASE DUE TO AGING.

Changes of the heart or vasculature known to occur with aging in the absence of any other known etiology.

ALCOHOLISM

The Disease

Alcohol is the most commonly used psychoactive agent, and alcoholism, or the chronic abuse of and dependence on alcohol, may be present in 10 percent of Western populations. Alcoholism is characterized by genetic predisposition, addiction to alcohol that may begin in adolescence, and a series of complications including acute hepatitis, fatty degeneration and cirrhosis of the liver, anemia, dementia, and cardiomyopathy.

Molecular and Cellular Biology

It is now accepted that alcoholism is a heritable trait. Two clinical types have been described, with the onset of type 1 generally after 25 years of age and the onset of type 2 before. Abnormalities in the activities of the platelet enzymes monoamine oxidase and adenylate cyclase have been described in alcoholics; based on the observation of a series of neurochemical defects in inbred "alcoholic" rats, it has been speculated that the platelet enzyme abnormalities may be part of the underlying biochemical trait. Most of the organ pathology in alcoholism is due to the toxicity of ethanol, its metabolites, and the generation of acetaldehyde from ethanol by oxidation. Toxicity is mediated by the generation of NADH by alcohol dehydrogenase, the induction of microsomal oxidizing enzymes including the novel and specific P450IIE1, which may generate highly toxic metabolites of common drugs and environmental compounds.

Cardiac Involvement

Acute exposure to alcohol decreases systolic function. Chronic exposure results in a dilated cardiomyopathy, primarily due to the toxicities described above rather than to nutritional deprivation. The symptoms are those of congestive heart failure related to the cardiomyopathy: dyspnea, orthopnea, paroxysmal nocturnal dyspnea, and so on. Atrial fibrillation, marked sinus tachycardia, and ventricular premature depolarizations may occur. Treatment requires absolute abstinence from alcohol intake and may reverse the process dramatically.

THE FOLLOWING CRITERIA ARE REQUIRED FOR THE DIAGNOSIS OF HEART DISEASE DUE TO ALCOHOLISM.

The appearance of arrhythmias, cardiac enlargement, or ventricular failure in the course of chronic alcoholism, in the absence of other causes of heart disease.

AMYLOIDOSIS

The Disease

Amyloidosis is a group of diseases caused by abnormal deposition of a widely heterogeneous group of proteins in multiple organs. There are hereditary and sporadic forms and a relationship with chronic illnesses such as rheumatoid arthritis and the dysproteinemias. The proteins, when stained with Congo red, exhibit apple-green birefringence under polarized light, and this finding on microscopic analysis of a biopsy specimen is the criterion for diagnosis. The accumulation of amyloid fibrils results in dysfunction of the affected organ and may result in death. The older classification of "isolated" or "senile," "familial," and "secondary" or "systemic" has been supplanted by specific categorizations based on an understanding of the underlying molecular disorder.

Molecular and Cellular Biology

The fibrillar deposits of amyloid are composed of immunoglobulin light chains (AL), amyloid A protein (AA, the serum component of which is an apolipoprotein), variously point-mutated transthyretin (a thyroxin- and retinol-binding protein previously called prealbumin), gelsolin, apolipoprotein A1, and others. A pentagonal protein of a curious family called "pentraxins" is associated with the systemic forms of amyloidosis. It is called the amyloid P component (AP) and is distinct from the fibrillar proteins. Point mutations in the fibrillar proteins may result in instability or affinity for particular structures and have been described in familial disorders characterized by polyneuropathy, kidney disease, cardiac dysfunction, and others.

Cardiac Involvement

The cardiac amyloid deposition seen as a feature of primary (familial) amyloidosis becomes manifest in the fourth or fifth decade and is usually accompanied by evidence of involvement of the peripheral nerves and the kidneys. Extensive infiltration of the heart by amyloid can lead to cardiomegaly, atrial arrhythmias, especially atrial fibrillation, conduction defects, low voltage of QRS–T, and a reduction in myocardial compliance, with consequent interference with diastolic filling. Diastolic and systolic dysfunction result in symptoms of congestive heart failure and may ultimately cause death.

THE FOLLOWING CRITERIA ARE REQUIRED FOR THE DIAGNOSIS OF HEART DISEASE DUE TO AMYLOIDOSIS.

Initial
Cardiac enlargement, evidence of diminished ventricular compliance, atrial arrest or arrhythmias, conduction defects, or low QRS–T voltage in the absence of other known causes of these findings.

Definitive
Evidence of amyloid in a biopsy specimen.

ANEMIA

The Disease

Anemia is a state of inadequate oxygen carriage by the blood due to decreased hemoglobin and may be associated with a diminished number or size of erythrocytes. The causes and manifestations are many.

Molecular and Cellular Biology

The causes of anemia range from hemorrhage and hemolysis to vitamin deficiency (B_{12}, folate), to substrate deficiency (iron), to mutations of hemoglobin (sickle cell disease due to the mutation: alpha-2, beta-$2^{6glu \rightarrow val}$) and other proteins (hereditary spherocytosis). The manifestations of the anemia are related not only to the level of hemoglobin but also to secondary complications related to the specific blood cell anomaly.

Cardiac Involvement

Regardless of cause, as the anemia and associated hypoxemia worsen and blood viscosity declines, peripheral resistance falls and cardiac output rises. Chronic, severe anemia is generally associated with eccentric cardiac hypertrophy and dilatation as seen in volume overload states. Dyspnea can result from anemia alone and does not necessarily indicate the presence of pulmonary congestion. Other symptoms attributable to anemia are fatigue, malaise, palpitations, weakness, and dizzy spells. Angina may be a prominent symptom but almost always reflects underlying coronary artery disease. Systolic and diastolic murmurs of any variety can occur. Heart disease due to anemia is reversible with successful treatment of the anemia; the signs and symptoms of congestion and cardiac dilatation disappear, and the cardiac output falls. In hereditary forms of chronic anemia, additional factors predispose to the development of heart disease. In thalassemia major, multiple blood transfusions result in myocardial hemosiderosis. In sickle cell disease, pulmonary thromboses during crises promote the development of pulmonary hypertension, and coronary thromboses produce myocardial necrosis with ischemic cardiomyopathy.

THE FOLLOWING CRITERIA ARE REQUIRED FOR THE DIAGNOSIS OF HEART DISEASE DUE TO ANEMIA.

Dilatation of the heart with or without congestion of the circulation in the presence of marked anemia.

ANKYLOSING SPONDYLITIS

The Disease

This is the major illness of a group of disorders known as seronegative arthritis. It is characterized by sacroiliitis and peripheral inflammatory arthropathy with a predilection for the insertions of ligaments into bone known as the "entheses," affects men more than women, usually begins at about the age of 20, appears to have a hereditary component, and is not associated with rheumatoid factor.

Molecular and Cellular Biology

Almost all patients with ankylosing spondylitis are HLA-B27 positive, and approximately 20 percent of all HLA-B27-positive individuals have ankylosing spondylitis. It is assumed that exposure to an environmental factor triggers expression of the syndrome. While much attention has focused on the potential pathogenicity of the B27 molecule, restriction fragment length polymorphism analysis in patients and controls has not demonstrated an allelic relationship, and experiments with transgenic mice have not proved the hypothesis. Antigenic microbial cross-reactivity with B27, especially with *Klebsiella* and *Shigella*, has also been suggested to play a role.

Cardiac Involvement

Cardiac involvement increases with duration of the arthritis. Inflammation and scarring of the ascending aorta and valve cusps and dilation of the valve ring can produce aortic regurgitation. Myocarditis and cardiomyopathy may precede or follow the development of aortic regurgitation.

THE FOLLOWING CRITERIA ARE REQUIRED FOR THE DIAGNOSIS OF HEART DISEASE DUE TO ANKYLOSING SPONDYLITIS.

Aortic regurgitation, myocarditis, or cardiomyopathy in the presence of ankylosing spondylitis and the absence of other known causes.

ATHEROSCLEROSIS

The Disease

Progressive narrowing of arteries due to the development of intimal plaques consisting of variable proportions of smooth muscle cells, macrophages, fibroblasts, lipids, and noncellular components.

Molecular and Cellular Biology

The precise etiology is unknown. Hereditary and environmental factors modify the likelihood of occurrence. These include family history, hypercholesterolemia, diabetes mellitus, hypertension, smoking, a sedentary lifestyle, obesity, and the type A personality. Of lipid components, excesses of low-density lipoprotein (LDL) and lipoprotein (a) [Lp(a)] enhance, while an excess of high-density lipoprotein (HDL) inhibits the development of atherosclerosis. An interplay between an abnormal plasma environment, platelets, monocytes, and lymphocytes with the endothelium initiates the process, which continues over decades. Recruitment of leukocytes and smooth muscle cells to the subendothelial space, where they may proliferate, is under complex control involving the synthesis and release of mitogens and cytokines, the most prominent of which is platelet-derived growth factor (PDGF). These molecules are synthesized and released inappropriately and in abnormal quantities by the "activation" of one or more of the cells listed above. Current theories of atherogenesis include the response-to-injury hypothesis, in which endothelial damage (or dysfunction) is the primary event; the clonal theory, in which the slow, neoplastic growth of a clone of smooth muscle cells is the primary event; and the infectious theory, in which infection of the vascular wall with one or more viruses is the primary event. The most substantial evidence relates the development of plaque to elevated levels of cholesterol, lipoproteins, and their oxidized forms, which are injurious to the vascular wall directly and through activation of monocytes. Secondary calcification is common.

Cardiac Involvement

The degree of obstruction of the coronary arteries increases slowly over decades, but the process is punctuated by sudden increases in plaque size due to growth and thrombosis. Luminal diameter is narrowed not only by bulk obstruction but also dynamically by the loss of normal endothelium-dependent vasorelaxation, due to abnormalities in synthesis or activity of nitric oxide (endothelium-derived relaxing factor [EDRF]). Regional ischemia due to inadequate coronary arterial flow can occur spontaneously or upon exertion and can result in a variety of physiologic abnormalities including anginal syndromes, silent ischemia, arrhythmias, conduction disturbances, papillary muscle dysfunction, ventricular dyssynergy, stunning or hibernation, ventricular failure, and sudden death. Thrombotic occlusion of a coronary artery due to plaque disruption can result in unstable angina, myocardial infarction, or sudden death.

ONE OF THE FOLLOWING CRITERIA IS REQUIRED FOR THE DIAGNOSIS OF HEART DISEASE DUE TO CORONARY ATHEROSCLEROSIS.

1. Classic anginal syndrome in the absence of other known causes.
2. Myocardial infarction in the absence of other known causes.
3. Demonstration by coronary angiography, angioscopy, intravascular echocardiography, computed tomography (CT), or magnetic resonance imaging (MRI) of obstructive coronary disease.
4. Anginal syndrome in the presence of evidence of reversible myocardial ischemia by a noninvasive method.

CARCINOID TUMOR

The Disease

Malignant carcinoid tumor occurs most commonly in the gastrointestinal tract. These tumors originate from enterochromaffin cells, which can produce biologically active molecules. When the levels of these molecules are sufficiently high in the systemic circulation, due in most cases to metastasis of tumor to the liver, the malignant carcinoid syndrome of flushing with or without diarrhea, wheezing, and cardiac manifestations occurs.

Molecular and Cellular Biology

While carcinoid tumors are most common in the appendix and rectum, the carcinoid syndrome is more commonly associated with tumors in the ileum. The manifestations of carcinoid are related to the release of bioactive substances from the tumor, the hallmark of which is serotonin (5-hydroxytryptamine). Increased levels of urinary 5-hydroxyindoleacetic acid (5-HIAA), the major metabolite of serotonin, confirm a diagnosis of carcinoid. The molecular basis of flushing remains unknown; however, in addition to serotonin, the biologically active molecules bradykinin, histamine, neuropeptide K, sub-stance P, and prostaglandins may be produced by carci-noid tumors.

Cardiac Involvement

Serotonin secreted by metastases in the liver into the hepatic vein is the source of high blood levels of the tumor substances in the circulating blood. In an unknown fash-ion, the serotonin or some other circulating factor in-duces the formation of endocardial lesions involving the tricuspid and pulmonic valves and the inner surfaces of the right heart chambers. These lesions are fibrotic plaques characterized by increased numbers of smooth muscle cells, fibroblasts, and their secreted matrix. Trans-forming growth factor beta, which stimulates fibroblasts to secrete extracellular matrix, can be found in increased levels in carcinoid heart lesions. Echocardiographic ab-normalities can be found in approximately 70 percent of patients with midgut carcinoids. The fibrosis of the valves and chordae tendineae can cause pulmonic obstruction or regurgitation and tricuspid regurgitation or obstruction. Endocardial fibrosis can limit ventricular filling. Se-rotonin is partly inactivated in the lung by monoamine oxidase. On this basis, or some other as yet undefined, left-sided heart disease is rare. Clinical manifestations include murmurs of pulmonic and tricuspid regurgitation and symptoms and signs of right-sided congestive heart failure. When systemic vasodilation is prominent, high-output failure may ensue.

THE FOLLOWING CRITERIA ARE REQUIRED FOR THE DIAGNOSIS OF HEART DISEASE DUE TO CARCINOID TUMOR.

Structural lesions of the pulmonic or tricuspid valves and evidence of carcinoid tumor, generally metastatic to the liver.

CONGENITAL ANOMALY

The Disease

Congenital cardiovascular defects result when genetic or environmental factors (intrauterine infection, metabolic disorders, drugs, irradiation, others) interfere with nor-mal development of the heart and great vessels, largely in the first 2 months of gestation. A conservative esti-mate of cardiovascular defects present as a percentage of live births is 0.8 percent, with ventricular septal defect, atrial septal defect, and patent ductus arteriosus the most common, in that order.

Molecular and Cellular Biology

The causes of congenital anomalies are manifold and include single-gene defects, gene deletions, and chromosomal aberrations as well as many environmental factors. Familial aggregations of defects without currently identified genetic errors can also occur.

Cardiac Involvement

Virtually any region of the heart and great vessels may be involved in congenital disease.

THE FOLLOWING CRITERIA ARE REQUIRED FOR THE DIAGNOSIS OF HEART DISEASE DUE TO CONGENITAL ANOMALY.

Initial

Clinical, electrocardiographic (ECG), and radiographic evidence for the specific anomaly present or presumed present at birth.

Definitive

Demonstration of the specific anatomic and physiologic abnormalities of a specific congenital anomaly by echocardiography, angiography, or other techniques.

FRIEDREICH'S ATAXIA

The Disease

Friedreich's ataxia is the most common of the spinocerebellar degenerations and is inherited in an autosomal recessive pattern. It is characterized by progressive degeneration of the posterior columns and the spinocerebellar and pyramidal tracts of the spinal cord, resulting in unsteadiness of gait and hyporeflexia; pes cavus and scoliosis are frequent.

Molecular and Cellular Biology

The genetic defect of Friedreich's ataxia has been localized to chromosome 9q. Recently, a unique, membrane-spanning protein from this chromosomal location has been cloned and shown to be expressed in neuronal but not other tissues.

Cardiac Involvement

Cardiac involvement is probably universal and documented in approximately 90 percent of patients. Generally, the neurologic manifestations occur first and predominate, but occasionally the discovery of a systolic murmur along the upper left sternal border or the appearance of ventricular failure can be the first indication of disease. ECG abnormalities are usually the earliest sign of cardiac involvement; S–T changes and T-wave inversion are prominent and arrhythmias are common in the advanced stages. Two types of myopathy are described. Most common is a concentric, hypertrophic cardiomyopathy without the septal disarray characteristic of familial hypertrophic cardiomyopathy. A much less common dilated cardiomyopathy has also been described.

THE FOLLOWING CRITERIA ARE REQUIRED FOR THE DIAGNOSIS OF HEART DISEASE DUE TO FRIEDREICH'S ATAXIA.

Typical ECG abnormalities or echocardiographic findings consistent with hypertrophic or dilated cardiomyopathy in the presence of Friedreich's ataxia.

HEMOCHROMATOSIS

The Disease

Hemochromatosis is a disease marked by excessive iron deposition in multiple organs including the heart, resulting in a variety of dysfunctions. There is a genetic type and a secondary form related to markedly elevated iron intake as in numerous blood transfusions, especially in children with beta-thalassemia major.

Molecular and Cellular Biology

The familial form is autosomal recessive. The gene is remarkably common, with 10 percent of the population heterozygous for the mutation. The gene (HFE) has not been isolated but has been mapped to chromosome 6p21.3, very close to the HLA-A class I region. In the familial form, the disease is characterized by unregulated absorption of iron. Increased levels of serum iron and ferritin and saturation of transferrin are present. The deposition of iron may cause extensive regional fibrosis by production of superoxides.

Cardiac Involvement

Heart disease, a cardiomyopathy with both dilated and restrictive features, results from excess deposition of iron in the myocardium, with consequent fibrosis. Cardiac enlargement, disturbances in ventricular filling, and ECG abnormalities including low QRS voltage and conduction disturbances may be present. Manifestations of the disease may be prevented by repeated phlebotomy before organ damage has occurred.

THE FOLLOWING CRITERIA ARE REQUIRED FOR THE DIAGNOSIS OF HEART DISEASE DUE TO HEMOCHROMATOSIS.

Dilated or restrictive cardiomyopathy and the demonstration of abnormalities in iron metabolism or a history of a large number of blood transfusions.

HOMOCYSTINURIA

The Disease

Homocystinuria is inherited as an autosomal recessive trait and is characterized by long extremities, ectopia lentis, osteoporosis, emotional disturbances, and vascular thromboses at an early age.

Molecular and Cellular Biology

The disease is usually due to a deficiency of cystathionine beta-synthase, which has its genetic locus on the q21 region of chromosome 21. The enzyme is responsible for converting homocystine to cystathionine. As a result of the deficiency, the sulfur amino acids accumulate. Homocystinemia may also occur in other enzyme deficiency states, such as 5,10-methylene tetrahydrofolate reductase. Homocystine interferes with formation of cross-linkages in collagen, perhaps producing the skeletal and ocular manifestations of the syndrome. It also induces a thrombotic-atherogenic diathesis by injuring endothelium, enhancing platelet adhesiveness, and increasing the binding of lipoprotein (a) to fibrin.

Cardiac Involvement

Homozygotes have a high incidence of thrombosis of coronary, renal, peripheral, and cerebral arteries, with early death. Heterozygote carriers may be more susceptible to coronary artery disease than the general population.

THE FOLLOWING CRITERIA ARE REQUIRED FOR THE DIAGNOSIS OF HEART DISEASE DUE TO HOMOCYSTINURIA.
Myocardial infarction due to coronary thrombosis in an individual with at least two of the phenotypic characteristics of the syndrome of homocystinuria and biochemical evidence of absent or decreased activity of cystathionine beta-synthase.

HYPERTENSION

The Disease

Hypertension is a sustained elevation of systolic or diastolic blood pressure or both and is classified as either "primary, essential, or idiopathic" or "secondary." Secondary causes include renal disease, endocrinopathies, tumors, and drugs. Depending on the definition of abnormal, hypertension is one of the most prevalent conditions in the United States and is one of the most important risk factors for cardiac disease, cerebrovascular disease, and renal failure.

Molecular and Cellular Biology

Secondary hypertension is caused by the presence of a specific vasopressor due to a definable disease. "Essential" hypertension is related to the interplay of polygenic and environmental factors. Abnormalities of molecules and systems that may lead to human hypertension include renin-angiotensin; angiotensinogen; angiotensin-converting enzyme; Na^+-K^+-ATPase; sodium, calcium, and potassium channels; insulin resistance, dyslipidemia, EDRF, endothelin, and many others. Hypertension in experimental animals has been linked to genetic loci that code for several of the molecules implicated in essential human hypertension.

Cardiac Involvement

Arterial hypertension of either the primary or secondary form can lead to systolic and diastolic left ventricular dysfunction, which may precede left ventricular hypertrophy and subsequent congestive heart failure. Hypertension can also induce atherogenesis and coronary artery disease, leading to myocardial ischemia and infarction; left ventricular failure and arrhythmias can ensue.

THE FOLLOWING CRITERIA ARE REQUIRED FOR THE DIAGNOSIS OF HEART DISEASE DUE TO HYPERTENSION.

Evidence of left ventricular hypertrophy or failure in the presence of sustained systemic arterial systolic and diastolic hypertension.

HYPERTHYROIDISM

The Disease

Hyperthyroidism is a result of excessive circulating amounts of thyroxine (T_4) and triiodothyronine (T_3). It is most commonly caused by stimulation of thyroid-stimulating hormone (TSH) receptors by autoimmune IgG (Graves' disease) but can also be due to autonomous thyroid nodules, thyroiditis, excessive production of pituitary TSH, and ingestion of excess T_4 or T_3. Weight loss, tremor, exophthalmos, and other signs of thyrotoxicosis are usually but not necessarily present.

Molecular and Cellular Biology

Thyroid hormones regulate cell membrane transport, genetic control of protein synthesis, and mitochondrial oxidative phosphorylation. Hyperthyroidism affects the heart by three routes:

1. Direct effects of increased T_4 and T_3 binding to nuclear receptors on cardiac gene transcription. This can result in an increased relative synthesis of alpha-myosin heavy chains, which have faster ATPase activity than beta-myosin heavy chains, and may also lead to alterations in calcium channels and in the sarcoplasmic reticulum. Such changes in protein synthesis within the heart may cause increased velocities of myocardial contraction and relaxation.
2. Indirect effects mediated by augmented sympatho-adrenal activity and up-regulation of cardiac beta-adrenoreceptors, with increased cardiac rate and contractility.
3. Indirect effects from an increased cardiac work load secondary to the action on peripheral tissues of excess T_4 and T_3.

Cardiac Involvement

Paroxysmal or sustained atrial arrhythmias, especially atrial fibrillation and less commonly atrial tachycardia and flutter, are frequent and may be the sole manifestation; ventricular premature beats can also occur. Cardiac enlargement, ventricular failure, and anginal syndrome are most frequent in patients with preexisting valvular or atherosclerotic heart disease and thus occur more often in patients over 40. However, arrhythmias, cardiac enlargement, and ventricular failure can sometimes appear in previously normal hearts, and angina can result from spasm of normal coronary arteries. Cardiac abnormalities due to hyperthyroidism usually disappear after successful treatment of the metabolic abnormality.

THE FOLLOWING CRITERIA ARE REQUIRED FOR THE DIAGNOSIS OF HEART DISEASE DUE TO HYPERTHYROIDISM.

Initial
Atrial arrhythmias (tachycardia, flutter, or fibrillation), ventricular ectopy, cardiac enlargement, ventricular failure, or angina plus the clinical suspicion of hyperthyroidism.

Definitive
The clinical findings as described plus biochemical evidence of hyperthyroidism and reversal of the clinical findings following specific treatment.

HYPOTHYROIDISM

The Disease
Hypothyroidism results from deficient levels of circulating T_4 and T_3. It is most often due to atrophy following Hashimoto's lymphocytic thyroiditis and is associated with antimicrosomal and TSH-blocking antibodies. It can also follow treatment of thyroid disease with surgery or radioiodine and can be associated with goiter due to iodine deficiency or disorders in synthesis of thyroid hormones, because of congenital enzyme deficiencies or drugs such as lithium or amiodarone. Manifestations include lethargy, cold intolerance, hoarseness, dry skin, weight gain, dementia, and a generalized increase in capillary permeability, with localized myxedema, pleural, pericardial, and peritoneal effusions. Dilutional hyponatremia, hypercholesterolemia, and hypertriglyceridemia are frequent.

Molecular and Cellular Biology
Hypothyroidism is due to deficiency in T_4 and T_3 at the cellular level. The effects are generally the converse of

those identified with hyperthyroidism. Decreased binding of T_4 and T_3 to nuclear receptors may lead to a relative increase in synthesis of beta-myosin heavy chains, with a slower ATPase activity, and to changes in the sarcoplasmic reticulum; these may contribute to a decreased velocity of contraction and a slower sinus rate. There may also be down-regulation of cardiac beta-receptors.

Cardiac Involvement

Despite these intrinsic cardiac changes, much of the decrease in cardiac output observed in myxedema is secondary to decreased cardiac work load secondary to decreased total body oxygen demands. Pericardial effusions are frequent but accumulate slowly and rarely cause cardiac tamponade; they are best identified and followed by echocardiography. In severe hypothyroidism superimposed on normal hearts, there can be chamber dilatation and recognizable slowing in velocity of the ventricular preejection period, which reflects the decreased rate of tension development. Sinus bradycardia is marked and the Q–T interval can be prolonged. These changes can revert completely to normal with replacement of T_4 and T_3. When congestive heart failure is associated with hypothyroidism, it connotes underlying valvular or myocardial disease.

THE FOLLOWING CRITERIA ARE REQUIRED FOR THE DIAGNOSIS OF HEART DISEASE DUE TO HYPOTHYROIDISM.

Initial

Pericardial effusion, enlargement of or decreased contractile performance of the heart, plus the clinical suspicion of hypothyroidism.

Definitive

The clinical findings as described plus biochemical evidence of hypothyroidism and reversal of the cardiac abnormalities after treatment with T_4 or T_3.

INFECTION

The Disease

Any part of the heart may be involved by infection, but the valvular endothelium is most frequently affected. Infective endocarditis is especially common when structural abnormalities exist because of valvular heart disease, congenital anomalies, previous infection, surgical repair of valves, or insertion of a valve prosthesis. It can occur after *Streptococcus viridans* or enterococci enter the blood during minor infections or dental, genitourinary, or gastrointestinal procedures. Valves that are normal or minimally damaged can be infected by staphylococci, pneumococci, gram-negative organisms, or fungi such as *Aspergillus* or *Candida* when host defenses are impaired by age, neoplasms, chemotherapy, or acquired immunodeficiency syndrome (AIDS), or are overwhelmed in addicts who inject drugs without sterile precautions. Myocarditis and pericarditis are most commonly due to viruses such as Coxsackie, ECHO, cytomegalovirus, and human immunodeficiency virus (HIV), though any systemic viremia, including the common exanthemata, may involve the myocardium. Bacterial myocarditis and pericarditis can complicate endocarditis or can be manifest as the predominant infection, as in tuberculous pericarditis. Spirochetes can cause myocarditis, as in Lyme disease, or aortitis, as in syphilis. Parasites such as *Trichinella* and *Trypanosoma* can cause myocardial disease; schistosomiasis can lead secondarily to pulmonary heart disease.

Molecular and Cellular Biology

Valvular and congenital heart disease can disrupt the protective endothelium by turbulent blood flow, Venturi or jet effects; some infectious agents can directly invade endothelial cells. This exposes collagen, which activates platelets and leads to local deposition of fibrin and blood cells; bacteria adhere to this nidus with mediation by endothelial-derived fibronectins. The resulting vegetation overwhelms local host defenses, permitting growth of bacteria, which can destroy valve components, are a source of emboli, and initiate formation of immune complexes that can produce glomerulonephritis and vasculitis. Early infection of prosthetic valves, before they are covered with endothelium, is predominately by *Staphylococcus epidermidis*, *Staphylococcus aureus*, and gram-negative organisms; late infections involve *S. viridans*, enterococci, and staphylococci.

Cardiac Involvement

Endocarditis can lead to heart failure by destruction of valve tissue and to septal abscesses by contiguous spread from infected native valves or the sewing rings of prostheses. Clinical evidence of acute sepsis, with fever and rigors, can predominate, or there can be a subacute course with low-grade fever, malaise, weight loss, splenomegaly, splinter hemorrhages, and systemic embolization to the brain, spleen, or extremities. Viral myocarditis may cause only fever and changes in repolarization in the ECG or can produce ventricular dilatation and abnormalities in wall movement, congestive heart failure, and arrhythmias. In some patients, there may be progression to dilated cardiomyopathy. Lyme disease and Chagas' disease can cause arrhythmias, heart block, and heart failure. Viral pericarditis is typically associated with fever, chest pain, a pericardial rub, and ECG changes; pericardial effusion can develop. It can follow a chronic and relapsing course and may lead to constrictive pericarditis.

ONE OF THE FOLLOWING CRITERIA IS REQUIRED FOR THE DIAGNOSIS OF INFECTION OF THE HEART.

1. Clinical evidence of endocarditis, myocarditis, or pericarditis plus demonstration of pathogenic organisms (bacterium, virus, fungus, or parasite) by culture or smear from the blood, pericardial fluid, or tissue specimen, or evidence of infection by serologic methods or histologic changes.
2. In the presence of cardiac valve disease, a congenital malformation, a valve prosthesis, or in an immunologically compromised host, new or changing murmurs associated with sustained fever, embolic phenomena, anemia, and splenomegaly.
3. Demonstration by echocardiography or other imaging techniques of a structure consistent with a vegetation due to bacterial infection, plus a clinical picture consistent with endocarditis.

INTERVENTION

A wide variety of surgical and other physical therapeutic interventions may significantly alter existing cardiac disease. When these alterations are relevant to the current cardiac diagnosis, the specific intervention should be cited after noting the etiology of the original heart disease for which the intervention was made—for example, "Atherosclerosis; Intervention: Coronary artery bypass surgery." Further description of the intervention should follow as appropriate in the Anatomy or Physiology categories.

Major categories of such interventions and some examples are

1. Surgery: Aneurysmectomy; Antiarrhythmia device (AICD) implantation; Aortic repair; Aortic resection; Atherectomy; Coronary bypass surgery; Endocardial ablation or resection; Pacemaker implantation; Pericardial window; Pericardiectomy; Repair of Congenital defect; Septal myomectomy; Valve repair; Valve replacement.
2. Interventional cardiology:
   a. Coronary: Atherectomy; Balloon angioplasty; Stent insertion; Thrombolysis (intravenous, intracoronary).
   b. Valvular: Balloon valvuloplasty.
   c. Electrophysiologic: Antiarrhythmia device (AICD); Pacemaker insertion (temporary, permanent); Radiofrequency ablation.

THE FOLLOWING CRITERION IS REQUIRED FOR THE DIAGNOSIS OF INTERVENTION.

Specific evidence for the type of intervention employed.

KAWASAKI DISEASE (MUCOCUTANEOUS LYMPH NODE SYNDROME)

The Disease

Kawasaki disease is of unknown etiology. It begins as a febrile illness in children, initially involves the skin and mucous membranes, and can ultimately involve many organ systems.

Molecular and Cellular Biology

Although a variety of immunologic abnormalities have been described in this disease, the precise pathogenetic mechanisms are unknown.

Cardiac Involvement

Cardiac involvement begins with an arteritis of the vasa vasorum and inflammatory involvement of the heart and pericardium. In later stages, the major coronary arteries are involved throughout their depth and may thrombose or develop aneurysms acutely. These aneurysms can be visualized angiographically or with transesophageal echocardiography and may disappear spontaneously. The myocardium may be permanently damaged by the effects of coronary occlusions.

THE FOLLOWING CRITERIA ARE REQUIRED FOR THE DIAGNOSIS OF HEART DISEASE DUE TO KAWASAKI DISEASE.
Demonstration of coronary artery aneurysms by echocardiography or angiography or of myocardial infarction during or after the course of the clinical syndrome of Kawasaki disease.

LYSOSOMAL STORAGE DISEASES

The Disease

Lysosomal storage diseases are clinical syndromes characterized by abnormal deposition of polysaccharides, mucopolysaccharides, glycoproteins, and sphingolipid caused by single defects in genes for specific lysosomal enzymes. There is considerable genetic heterogeneity and phenotypic variation, causing varied patterns of associated developmental abnormalities in the musculoskeletal, nervous, and other systems, which are evident early in life.

Molecular and Cellular Biology

Specific genetic defects leading to cardiac involvement include glycogen storage disease type II (Pompe's disease), a deficiency of alpha-1,4-glucosidase, which causes abnormal glycogen accumulation; mucopolysaccharidoses IH, IS, and II (Hurler's, Hunter's, and Scheie's syndromes), which are due to deficiencies of sulfatases and produce accumulation of proteoglycans and glycosaminoglycans; sphingolipidoses, with deficiency of alpha-galactosidase A (Fabry's disease), leading to accumulation of trihexosylglyceramine, and beta-glucocerebrosidase (Gaucher's disease), with accumulation of glucocerebroside.

Cardiac Involvement

Cardiomyopathy and valvular and coronary disease can result from abnormal accumulations of the specific substrates that are inadequately degraded in the lysosomal storage diseases.

THE FOLLOWING CRITERIA ARE REQUIRED FOR THE DIAGNOSIS OF HEART DISEASE DUE TO LYSOSOMAL STORAGE DISEASES.
Cardiac enlargement, with or without valvular insufficiency, or coronary artery disease with clinical and laboratory evi-

dence for absence of a specific enzyme or accumulation of its substrate.

MARFAN'S SYNDROME

The Disease

Marfan's syndrome is due to a congenital disorder of the microfibrillar component of connective tissue, which is inherited as an autosomal dominant. It is characterized by long extremities, a high-arched palate, pectus excavatum, scoliosis, lax joints and skin, and ectopia lentis.

Molecular and Cellular Biology

The underlying defect is in the synthesis of fibrillin, a large glycoprotein that is a major component of microfibrils, which constitute the ciliary zonules and provide the scaffolding for elastic tissue in the skin, periosteum and perichondrium, aorta, and heart valves. The defects result from point mutations in the fibrillin gene, which shares the genetic locus (15q21.1) for Marfan's syndrome.

Cardiac Involvement

The most common abnormalities are aneurysmal dilatation of the aortic root, aneurysms of the sinuses of Valsalva, and prolapse of the mitral and tricuspid valves. As dilatation of the aortic root progresses with age, there are increased hazards of aortic dissection with sudden death and of worsening aortic regurgitation. Because there is genetic polymorphism, cardiovascular abnormalities are not always accompanied by all components of the fully expressed syndrome.

THE FOLLOWING CRITERIA ARE REQUIRED FOR THE DIAGNOSIS OF HEART DISEASE DUE TO MARFAN'S SYNDROME.

Initial

Detection of one or more of the cardiovascular abnormalities known to occur with Marfan's syndrome and two or more other characteristics of the syndrome.

Definitive

Laboratory demonstration of altered fibrillin synthesis or the molecular genetic abnormality.

NEOPLASMS

The Disease

Primary tumors of the heart can be benign or malignant. Myxomas, fibromas, lipomas, and sarcomas are frequently discovered by echocardiography performed because of unexplained cardiac murmurs and symptoms suggesting endocarditis or heart failure. Secondary tumors may involve the pericardium, myocardium, and valves by contiguous spread from tumors in adjacent organs, by direct invasion of the venae cavae or pulmonary veins, by metastases from distant primary sites, or by involvement with diffusely disseminated lymphomas, sarcomas, and leukemias.

Molecular and Cellular Biology

Clones of autonomous and undifferentiated malignant cells may result from genetic mutations, activation of oncogenes or loss of suppressor oncogenes, and interaction with environmental factors. Metastases result when motile tumor cells attach to host cell membranes via secreted plasminogen activator and adherence glycoproteins, such as laminin and fibronectin, and invade via release of lysosomal hydrolases and collagenase.

Primary benign cardiac tumors are less frequent than primary malignant tumors or metastases to the heart but are clinically important because they can produce dramatic symptoms, are readily detectable by echocardiography and MRI, and are often curable by surgery.

Metastases to the heart are most frequent in the course of melanoma but are most commonly caused by cancer of the lung and breast. The pericardium is most frequently involved. Kaposi's sarcoma in patients with AIDS often metastasizes to the heart.

Nonbacterial thrombotic endocarditis can be associated with adenocarcinoma, lymphoma, and leukemia and can liberate microemboli; it is detectable by echocardiography and MRI.

Cardiac Involvement

Tumors of the pericardium can produce effusions that lead to cardiac tamponade. Myocardial tumors can cause arrhythmias, conduction disorders, and congestive heart failure. Tumors involving the great veins, endocardium, or valves can produce evidence of local obstruction, systemic or pulmonary embolism, and fever. Myxomas are most common in the left atrium, may produce no symptoms, or can mimic mitral stenosis, with murmurs and symptoms varying with body position and a typical "tumor plop." Occasionally, systemic manifestations can mimic subacute bacterial endocarditis. Myxomas are most often detected by echocardiography.

THE FOLLOWING CRITERIA ARE REQUIRED FOR THE DIAGNOSIS OF HEART DISEASE DUE TO NEOPLASM.

Initial
The clinical manifestations as described.

Definitive
1. **Demonstration of an intracardiac tumor by echocardiography, MRI, CT scan, or contrast ventriculography.**
2. **Evidence of neoplasm demonstrated by presence of tumor cells in pericardium, pericardial fluid, or myocardium.**

OBESITY

The Disease
Extreme generalized increase in body fat can lead to heart disease directly by producing increased circulating blood volume and cardiac output and indirectly by leading to hyperinsulinemia, hypertension, lipid abnormalities, and alveolar hypoventilation.

Molecular and Cellular Biology
Obesity that begins in early childhood is associated with both an increased number and an increased size of adipocytes; in adult-onset obesity, adipocytes are normal in number but increased in size. Since fat tissue is aerobic and vascular, requirements for blood flow are high; excess body fat increases resting demands for systemic flow, and the increase in body weight increases the muscular work of exercise. Secondary effects of obesity include hyperinsulinemia due to a decreased number of receptors and a postreceptor defect. Hyperinsulinemia is linked to hypertension, high triglycerides and low HDL in the serum, and altered thrombolytic activity, perhaps due to increases in plasminogen activator inhibitor of the endothelial type (PAI-I).

Cardiac Involvement
The heart may be affected in two ways. Increased body fat and blood volume lead to increased preload and afterload,

with resulting myocardial dilatation and hypertrophy, reduced diastolic compliance, and ventricular failure. In addition, there may be a reduction in alveolar respiration, with resulting disturbances in respiratory gas exchange, hypoxia, and pulmonary hypertension, causing the pickwickian syndrome.

THE FOLLOWING CRITERIA ARE REQUIRED FOR THE DIAGNOSIS OF HEART DISEASE DUE TO OBESITY.

Evidence of cardiac dilatation, hypertrophy, or failure in the presence of severe obesity and in the absence of other specific causes of heart disease.

PAGET'S DISEASE OF BONE (OSTEITIS DEFORMANS)

The Disease

Paget's disease of bone consists of excessive resorption of bone followed or accompanied by increased formation of new bone deposited in a disorganized pattern. The cause is unknown.

Molecular and Cellular Biology

Accelerated resorption of bone is mediated by large numbers of giant osteoclasts, leading to deposition of vascular connective tissue and followed by accelerated though disorganized formation of new bone. The augmented metabolism in the involved bones leads directly to increased regional blood flow to bone and indirectly to the overlying skin.

Cardiac Involvement

When over one-third of the bone mass is involved, an increase in cardiac output becomes evident. Since the disease predominates in older men in whom heart disease from other causes is prevalent, it is rarely the sole cause of symptoms.

THE FOLLOWING CRITERIA ARE REQUIRED FOR THE DIAGNOSIS OF HEART DISEASE DUE TO PAGET'S DISEASE OF BONE.

Ventricular dilatation or hypertrophy associated with increased cardiac output at rest in a patient with Paget's disease, in the absence of other cause for the cardiac manifestations.

PHEOCHROMOCYTOMA

The Disease

Pheochromocytomas are tumors of chromaffin cells that produce excessive amounts of the catecholamines norepinephrine and epinephrine. The release of the catecholamines can produce paroxysmal or fixed hypertension, often associated with headache, diaphoresis, orthostatic syncope, and a diabetic glucose tolerance curve. Occasionally, pheochromocytomas are inherited as an autosomal recessive trait, which produces the MEN type IIa and IIb syndromes, in which there are associated multiple endocrine neoplasia, such as medullary carcinoma of the thyroid, parathyroid adenomas, and hemangioblastoma of the cerebellum.

Molecular and Cellular Biology

The heart may be injured directly by the excessive catecholamines, with production of cardiomyopathy, or indirectly by systemic hypertension, which causes left ventricular hypertrophy and failure. The direct effects are mediated by the action of catecholamines on their sarcolemmal G-protein coupled receptors, thereby stimulating adenylate cyclase to convert adenosine triphosphate to cyclic adenosine monophosphate, which activates a protein kinase. The protein kinase phosphorylates calcium channels, and this enhances the entrance of calcium into the cell. Excessive and prolonged stimulation by catecholamines via these processes may lead to an accumulation of intracellular calcium and ultimately to cellular injury and decreased contractility.

Cardiac Involvement

Arrhythmias are common, and there can be deep inversions of precordial T waves and ECG evidence for left ventricular hypertrophy. Left ventricular dilatation and failure can occur.

THE FOLLOWING CRITERIA ARE REQUIRED FOR THE DIAGNOSIS OF HEART DISEASE DUE TO PHEOCHROMOCYTOMA.

Cardiac dilatation or failure in the presence of a functioning pheochromocytoma diagnosed by biochemical assays of catecholamine secretion, and demonstration of the tumor by CT scan, MRI, or other imaging technique.

POLYARTERITIS NODOSA

The Disease

Polyarteritis nodosa (PAN) is an acute necrotizing segmental arteritis of small- and medium-sized muscular arteries. It is most frequent in middle-aged men but can occur at any age and follow either a rapid or indolent course. Systemic effects include fever, anemia, rapid erythrocyte sedimentation rate (ESR), and elevated gamma globulin. The clinical manifestations vary with the pattern of organ involvement. There can be nodular and purpuric skin lesions, pulmonary infiltrates, bronchial asthma, retinitis, uveitis, abdominal pain, hepatomegaly mononeuritis multiplex, cranial nerve paralysis, and stroke. Renal involvement is frequent, with hematuria, proteinurea, and secondary hypertension.

Molecular and Cellular Biology

The cause is unknown but probably involves immune complexes that are deposited in blood vessels injured by mediators released from platelets and mast cells via the action of IgE. Many patients with PAN are infected with hepatitis B antigen, which forms such immune complexes with IgM. Complement is activated by the deposited complexes and attracts neutrophils, which engulf them and release proteolytic enzymes. Cell-mediated immune injury and delayed hypersensitivity may also be involved, and endothelial cells activated by cytokines may activate T-lymphocytes. All of these mechanisms may be involved in mediating vascular injury, which leads to thrombosis or formation of aneurysms.

Cardiac Involvement

By involving the coronary arteries, the disease may produce myocardial infarction, arrhythmias, conduction disturbances, hemorrhagic pericardial effusions, and congestive heart failure. The renal hypertension can produce left ventricular hypertrophy.

THE FOLLOWING CRITERIA ARE REQUIRED FOR THE DIAGNOSIS OF HEART DISEASE DUE TO POLYARTERITIS NODOSA.

The presence of one or more of the following: acute myocardial infarction, pericarditis, sudden hemorrhagic pericardial effusion, arrhythmias, conduction disturbances, or myocarditis, plus the demonstration of the characteristic lesion in a biopsy from any involved tissue.

PREGNANCY (PERIPARTUM CARDIOMYOPATHY)

The Disease

Dilated cardiomyopathy with congestive heart failure occurring for the first time immediately after delivery, immediately before delivery, or in the first 1 to 6 months postpartum is presumed to bear a relationship to the pregnant state, though the etiology remains unknown.

Molecular and Cellular Biology

The hemodynamic changes occurring with normal pregnancy are well delineated. They include a progressive increase in blood volume beginning in the first trimester, which is probably mediated by estrogen stimulation of the renin-angiotensin system and the effects of placental hormones on erythropoiesis, a gradual increase in cardiac output reaching 1.5 times normal by the third trimester, with a rise in both stroke volume and heart rate, and a fall in systemic resistance with widening of the pulse pressure, probably reflecting a combination of hormonal effects and placental flow. Physical examination and echocardiography show evidence of increased cardiac contractile force, mild dilatation of the right ventricle and sometimes the left, mild tricuspid and pulmonary regurgitation, and occasional pericardial effusion. If there is no preexisting heart disease and the pregnancy is not complicated by toxemia, the normal maternal heart will quickly revert to the pregravid state after delivery. When cardiac enlargement or dyspnea appears or worsens in the immediate prepartum or in the postpartum period, peripartum cardiomyopathy may be the cause.

Cardiac Involvement

In patients with peripartum cardiomyopathy, left ventricular failure develops quickly or insidiously, with echocardiographic evidence of dilatation of all chambers, but particularly of the left ventricle. About 50 percent of patients recover completely in the 6 months after pregnancy, but there is a high incidence of relapse with subsequent pregnancies. Other patients can progress to chronic congestive heart failure or death after the initial episode. The etiology is unknown, and the picture resembles other cases of dilated cardiomyopathy. However, biopsies from some patients show histologic evidence of myocarditis of uncertain etiologic significance.

THE FOLLOWING CRITERIA ARE REQUIRED FOR THE DIAGNOSIS OF HEART DISEASE DUE TO PREGNANCY (PERIPARTUM CARDIOMYOPATHY).

The occurrence of persistent left ventricular dilatation or the onset of left ventricular failure in the final month or first 6 months after pregnancy, in the absence of evidence for preexisting or acquired heart disease of other cause.

PROGRESSIVE MUSCULAR DYSTROPHY (DUCHENNE TYPE)

The Disease

This is the most common and most severe of the muscular dystrophies, and since it is inherited as an X-linked recessive, it occurs almost exclusively in males. Difficulty in ambulation usually begins between the ages of 1 and 6. Rising from the prone or seated position requires a striking and complex series of movements. The early pseudohypertrophy of the muscles below the knees, with later wasting of the upper limbs, differentiates this dystrophy clinically. Serum levels of creatine phosphokinase are elevated early in life.

Molecular and Cellular Biology

The disease is due to the absence or mutation of dystrophin, a 400-Kd protein, from the sarcolemmal membranes of skeletal and cardiac muscle. Dystrophin is a structural component that probably functions to help maintain membrane integrity during contraction. The phenotypic absence of dystrophin is due to the deletion or mutation of its large gene, which has 2000 kb, from its normal locus on the X chromosome at the Xp21 site. The abnormality of dystrophin explains the severe degenerative changes found in skeletal and cardiac muscle in patients with the disease. Mild mental impairment is frequent and probably reflects the absence of dystrophin from the brain, where it occurs normally.

Cardiac Involvement

Cardiomyopathy is frequent, but symptoms are obscured because of inactivity imposed by the severe skeletal muscle disease. ECG abnormalities are frequent, with deep Q waves in the limb and left precordial leads and tall R waves over the right precordium. Disturbances in intraventricular conduction are frequent, and there may be supraventricular tachycardias. Though ventricular failure can occur, most patients succumb from respiratory failure.

THE FOLLOWING CRITERIA ARE REQUIRED FOR THE DIAGNOSIS OF HEART DISEASE DUE TO MUSCULAR DYSTROPHY.

Initial

ECG abnormalities or evidence of left ventricular dilatation or dysfunction in the presence of clinical evidence of progressive muscular dystrophy.

Definitive

The cardiac manifestations as described plus the biochemical or molecular genetic evidence of the abnormality.

PROGRESSIVE SYSTEMIC SCLEROSIS (SCLERODERMA)

The Disease

In progressive systemic sclerosis, there is induration and fibrosis of the esophagus, kidneys, lungs, and myocardium, which resembles the process in the skin. Raynaud's phenomenon is common. Visceral involvement occasionally occurs in the absence of skin lesions.

Molecular and Cellular Biology

The disease results from loss of regulation of the synthesis and deposition by fibroblasts of collagen; there may also be immunologically mediated damage to vascular endothelial cells, which leads to occlusion of small vessels.

Cardiac Involvement

When the heart is involved directly in the disease process, there can be extensive myocardial fibrosis, which leads to decreased diastolic compliance, impaired impulse conduction, and arrhythmias. Renal involvement causes sytemic hypertension, and pulmonary fibrosis can produce pulmonary hypertension. These processes can secondarily affect the heart.

THE FOLLOWING CRITERIA ARE REQUIRED FOR THE DIAGNOSIS OF HEART DISEASE DUE TO PROGRESSIVE SYSTEMIC SCLEROSIS.

Disturbances in conduction or in ventricular diastolic function and evidence for progressive systemic sclerosis.

PULMONARY DISEASE (COR PULMONALE)

The Disease

Certain disorders of pulmonary function or structure can produce right ventricular hypertrophy, dilatation, or failure. Pulmonary artery hypertension, secondary to an increased pulmonary vascular resistance, is the underlying process that leads to acute or chronic right ventricular overload, dilatation, hypertrophy, and failure.

Pulmonary hypertension can result from disturbances in respiratory gas exchange, which lead to pulmonary vasoconstriction, polycythemia, and increased cardiac output. The principal diseases that produce pulmonary hypertension by these mechanisms include obstructive diseases of the lung, structural deformities of the chest wall, upper airway obstruction and sleep apnea, and neuromuscular diseases.

Pulmonary hypertension can also result from anatomic curtailment of the pulmonary vascular bed produced by acute massive embolization, recurrent multiple emboli, thrombosis, or occlusive vascular disease due to arteritis, sickle cell disease, or schistosomiasis. The capacity of the pulmonary vascular bed can also be reduced by diffuse fibrosing, granulomatous, or metastatic lesions.

Molecular and Cellular Biology

The mechanism by which hypoxia causes constriction of smooth muscle in the pulmonary resistance vessels is unknown, but its effect is increased by acidosis. Pulmonary vasoconstriction may depend on platelet and endothelial responses, which modulate the release of eicosanoids, nitric oxide, and endothelin. Prolonged vasoconstriction may lead to permanent structural changes in resistance vessels.

Obstruction of the pulmonary vascular bed by any pathologic process must be widespread to result in increased pulmonary resistance.

Hypoxia, acidosis, and other physiologic processes may act in concert with anatomic causes to produce pulmonary hypertension.

Cardiac Involvement

The presence of pulmonary arterial hypertension does not by itself warrant a diagnosis of pulmonary heart disease. Many conditions that are not primary disturbances of pulmonary structure or function can lead to secondary pulmonary hypertension; examples are congenital heart disease with left-to-right shunt, mitral stenosis or regurgitation, or an increase in left ventricular diastolic pressure due to failure or decreased diastolic compliance. Pulmonary disease as an etiologic diagnosis does not include such conditions, nor does it include pulmonary hypertension, either transient or fixed, caused by pulmonary disease but not accompanied by enlargement or failure of the right ventricle.

The disease process responsible should always be identified when a diagnosis is made of heart disease due to pulmonary disease; for example, pulmonary heart disease due to chronic obstructive pulmonary disease.

THE FOLLOWING CRITERIA ARE REQUIRED FOR THE DIAGNOSIS OF HEART DISEASE DUE TO PULMONARY DISEASE.

Initial

The occurrence of right ventricular dilatation, hypertrophy, or failure in the presence of a disease process that primarily involves the lungs, pulmonary vasculature, or respiratory gas exchange.

Definitive

The clinical manifestations as described plus significant pulmonary hypertension demonstrated by Doppler echocardiography or cardiac catheterization and the absence of left-sided heart disease.

RADIATION

The Disease

Acute or chronic inflammation and fibrosis of the heart due to therapeutic doses of ionizing radiation or rarely due to industrial accidents.

Molecular and Cellular Biology

Ionizing radiation typically injures the vascular endothelium through the generation of free radicals. This occurs in both the large coronary arteries and the microcirculation, resulting in endothelial cell death and capillary thrombosis and rupture. The resulting ischemia leads to myocardial fibrosis.

Cardiac Involvement

Occasionally patients will develop acute pericarditis following radiation therapy. More commonly there are chronic effects months or years after exposure. These may consist of symptoms due to failure of one or both ventricles because of fibrosis, or ischemic symptoms due to coronary artery involvement. Often, objective signs of ventricular failure are not severe and patients remain asymptomatic.

THE FOLLOWING CRITERIA ARE REQUIRED FOR THE DIAGNOSIS OF HEART DISEASE DUE TO IONIZING RADIATION.

Acute pericarditis or chronic ventricular failure following radiation exposure in the absence of other causes, or diffuse coronary artery disease following radiation exposure in the absence of typical risk factors for atherosclerosis.

REITER'S SYNDROME

The Disease

Reiter's syndrome consists of a triad of nonbacterial urethritis, arthritis, and conjunctivitis. In addition there may be fever, weight loss, dysentery, skin and mucous membrane lesions, adenopathy, splenomegaly, pericarditis, and aortic involvement.

Molecular and Cellular Biology

Chronic cardiac involvement most often occurs in patients with the histocompatibility antigen HLA-B27.

Cardiac Involvement

The most common manifestations are pericarditis and atrioventricular block, which occur with acute attacks. Less often, chronic manifestations may include aortic (and occasionally mitral) regurgitation. Aortic pathology involves focal medial necrosis. The aortic valve may be fibrotic and thickened with rolled cusp edges.

THE FOLLOWING CRITERIA ARE REQUIRED FOR THE DIAGNOSIS OF HEART DISEASE DUE TO REITER'S SYNDROME.

Pericarditis or conduction disturbances associated with an acute attack of Reiter's syndrome, or aortic or mitral regurgitation or conduction disturbances associated with chronic Reiter's syndrome in the absence of other causes.

RHEUMATIC FEVER/RHEUMATIC HEART DISEASE

The Disease

Rheumatic Fever

Rheumatic fever is a nonsuppurative complication of pharyngitis due to group A beta-hemolytic streptococcus. The major clinical manifestations, as originally noted in the Jones criteria, are carditis, arthritis, subcutaneous nodules, erythema marginatum, and chorea. In addition, minor manifestations include arthralgia, fever, elevated ESR, elevated C-reactive protein, and a prolonged P–R interval. While the disease follows streptococcal infection (with a latent period as short as a week), many patients do not remember having such an infection. A positive pharyngeal culture or abnormal antibody titers to streptolysin O, deoxyribonuclease, or hyaluronidase should be used in establishing that there was an antecedent streptococcal pharyngitis, although in some patients this is not possible. In general, two major Jones criteria or one major and two minor criteria, with evidence of streptococcal pharyngitis as noted above, are necessary for making the diagnosis. Exceptions to the Jones criteria for the diagnosis of acute rheumatic fever are as follows:

1. Chorea may be the only clinical manifestation of rheumatic fever.
2. Indolent carditis may be the only clinical manifestation in patients who seek medical attention months after the onset of the disease. Evidence of a preceding streptococcal infection may no longer be present.
3. In patients with a previous attack of rheumatic fever (who are at high risk for a recurrence), the diagnosis of valvulitis may be difficult unless the diagnosis of it involves a valve not previously affected. In these patients, only one major criterion, or several minor ones, may allow a presumptive diagnosis to be made.

Rheumatic Heart Disease

Rheumatic heart disease is a sequela of rheumatic fever, although as with the streptococcal infection, many patients do not remember having had rheumatic fever. Rheumatic heart disease may involve all of the cardiac valves, but tricuspid disease occurs in only about 10 percent and pulmonic disease is rare. The typical mitral valve involvement results in regurgitation, stenosis, or both. Aortic regurgitation or combined regurgitation and stenosis are common, although pure aortic stenosis is not.

Molecular and Cellular Biology

Rheumatogenic strains of group A streptococcus have multiple components that are either identical to or cross react with human cardiac tissue, such as capsular hyaluronate, membrane antigens, and cell wall polysaccharide. Although there is no definitive proof that these streptococcal antigens actually cause the cardiac damage, it is likely that immunologic reaction to these antigens does result in the manifestations of acute rheumatic fever. Furthermore, the M protein of these streptococci is a large molecule with moieties that are blastogens for human T cells. The pathologic changes of rheumatic fever are mostly nonspecific and involve fibrinoid degeneration of collagen. The specific Aschoff's body does not appear to correlate with the acute dilatation of severe myocarditis, but these bodies are found chronically in the hearts of patients with progressive rheumatic heart disease.

Cardiac Involvement

Rheumatic Fever

All layers of the heart may be involved. The pericardium typically is thickened with an inflammatory exudate, and pericardial effusion is common. Constrictive pericarditis is said not to occur. Myocarditis may result in ventricular dilatation, resulting in secondary valve ring dilatation and regurgitation. Congestive heart failure is not common (occurring in 5–10% of patients with carditis), but it may be severe. Since all layers of the heart are usually involved, evidence of myocarditis without accompanying valvulitis makes the diagnosis unlikely. Endocarditis (valvulitis) may result in mitral or aortic regurgitation. The characteristic murmurs are systolic (mitral regurgitation) or diastolic (aortic regurgitation, and the mid-diastolic Carey-Coombs murmur due to increased flow secondary to mitral regurgitation or due to an enlarged left ventricle and mitral valvulitis without regurgitation).

Rheumatic Heart Disease

Mitral valve deformities, with fusion of the commissures, thickening and eventual calcification of the leaflets, and thickening and shortening of the chordae, result in mitral stenosis with variable degrees of regurgitation. The predominant lesion may be regurgitation, although the leaflets are fused or deformed to some degree and not redundant as they appear in myxomatous mitral regurgitation. The aortic valve may be similarly affected, with thickening of the cusps and fusion of the commissures resulting in stenosis and regurgitation. The appearance and performance of the valves is best evaluated clinically by transthoracic or transesophageal echocardiography. Isolated aortic valve involvement (without mitral disease) is uncommon. Tricuspid valve deformity is less common (occurring in about 10%), and pulmonic valve disease is rare. Important sequelae include pulmonary congestion and eventually pulmonary hypertension and right heart failure in mitral stenosis and left ventricular failure in mitral regurgitation and aortic valve disease. Atrial fibrillation and embolic complications are responsible for much of the morbidity of chronic rheumatic heart disease. In addition, the patients are at risk for endocarditis (less commonly in pure mitral stenosis).

THE FOLLOWING CRITERIA ARE REQUIRED FOR THE DIAGNOSIS OF HEART DISEASE DUE TO ACUTE RHEUMATIC FEVER.

Endocarditis, myocarditis, or pericarditis during an attack of acute rheumatic fever diagnosed by the Jones criteria.

THE FOLLOWING CRITERIA ARE REQUIRED FOR THE DIAGNOSIS OF CHRONIC RHEUMATIC HEART DISEASE.

Valve deformity in a patient with a history of acute rheumatic fever. Mitral stenosis with typical commissural fusion, not due to a congenital lesion, even in the absence of a history of rheumatic fever.

RHEUMATOID ARTHRITIS

The Disease

Rheumatoid arthritis is characterized by a persistent inflammatory synovitis involving the peripheral joints, which is usually symmetric and which can lead to severe joint deformity. The disease is of unknown etiology and has various systemic manifestations, which may include cardiac involvement.

Molecular and Cellular Biology

Inflammatory infiltrates in rheumatoid arthritis contain a large proportion of T4 helper lymphocytes, in association with HLA-DR-positive macrophages. Various lymphokines elaborated by these cells have been found in synovial fluid, including gamma-interferon, interleukin-2, leukocyte and macrophage migration inhibition factors, and monocyte chemotactic factor. There is also B-cell involvement, with production of immunoglobulins such as rheumatoid factor. These findings have led to the conclusion that rheumatoid arthritis is immunologically mediated, although a specific inciting factor has not been identified.

Cardiac Involvement

Pericardial effusion is present in up to 50 percent of patients, although it is usually asymptomatic and rarely causes tamponade or chronic constrictive pericarditis. The glucose of the fluid is characteristically low (as it is in pleural fluid in these patients). In patients with a large number of subcutaneous nodules, inflammatory lesions may also be present in the myocardium or on the valves, but they rarely result in significant myocardial or valvular dysfunction, although aortic regurgitation can occur. Coronary arteritis, while often present pathologically in patients with diffuse rheumatoid arteritis, rarely causes myocardial infarction.

THE FOLLOWING CRITERIA ARE REQUIRED FOR THE DIAGNOSIS OF HEART DISEASE DUE TO RHEUMATOID ARTHRITIS.

Pericarditis, myocarditis, coronary arteritis, or aortic regurgitation in the presence of active rheumatoid arthritis, or constrictive pericarditis in the presence of chronic rheumatoid arthritis in the absence of more common etiologies.

SARCOIDOSIS

The Disease

Sarcoidosis is a granulomatous disease of unknown etiology that most often affects the lung. Additional organ involvement occurs in the skin, eyes, lymph nodes, heart, and rarely the brain. The acute form is accompanied by constitutional symptoms. A more chronic form usually presents with dyspnea. Many patients are asymptomatic when the disease is discovered on routine chest x-ray. About 10 percent have disease referable to organs other than the lungs. Pulmonary involvement may result in chronic respiratory failure due to interstitial lung disease. Laboratory abnormalities include hyperglobulinemia, eosinophilia, lymphopenia, hypercalcemia, and elevated levels of angiotensin-converting enzyme.

Molecular and Cellular Biology

Although the patients are often anergic and have depressed cellular immunity on examination of the blood, the sites of disease involvement are characterized by increased immune processes involving T helper cells. These lymphocytes and mononuclear phagocytes accumulate, with the development of noncaseating granulomas, which also involve epithelioid cells and giant cells. The characteristic cells may be identified in bronchoalveolar fluid obtained by lavage. The T helper cells release a variety of lymphokines, which attract monocytes and lead to the formation of granulomas. Thus the disease is characterized by an aberrant immune response, and the end result is organ fibrosis.

Cardiac Involvement

Although cardiac involvement is present in 20 to 30 percent of patients pathologically, clinical cardiac disease is present in only about 5 percent of those with sarcoidosis. The predominant manifestations are heart block, congestive heart failure, ventricular arrhythmias, and sudden death. Two-thirds of the patients who die of their heart disease do so suddenly, and this is especially true in younger patients. The cardiomyopathy may have a restrictive pattern or may present with ventricular dilatation resembling ischemic or idiopathic cardiomyopathy. Rare cardiac complications include pericardial effusion and ventricular aneurysm formation.

THE FOLLOWING CRITERIA ARE REQUIRED FOR THE DIAGNOSIS OF HEART DISEASE DUE TO SARCOIDOSIS.

ECG abnormalities (conduction disturbances, arrhythmias, or repolarization changes) or cardiomyopathy in the presence of systemic sarcoidosis.

SYSTEMIC ARTERIOVENOUS FISTULA

The Disease

Congenital arteriovenous fistulas most commonly involve the vessels of the lower extremities, although any vascular bed may be affected. Small fistulas do not cause symptoms, but large ones may deform an entire limb and may cause high-output congestive heart failure. Acquired fistulas may occur secondary to trauma or may be iatrogenic: intentionally created fistulas for use in hemodialysis or accidentally after femoral artery catheterization or any surgery near major vessels. Rarely, aortic aneurysms may erode into a neighboring vein, such as the inferior vena cava. Hereditary hemorrhagic telangiectasia (Osler-Weber-Rendu syndrome) may be associated with large hepatic or pulmonary fistulas and high-output cardiac failure. Pulmonary fistulas may be identified by x-ray. Kaposi's sarcoma may also lead to significant shunting.

Molecular and Cellular Biology

Congenital fistulas occur when there is an arrest of the normal vascular development in the fetus. They appear to be similar to normal fetal capillary networks.

Cardiac Involvement

If the fistulas are sufficiently large, there is a significant drop in systemic vascular resistance and an increase in blood volume. The stroke volume, heart rate, and cardiac output all rise. If a fistula can be temporarily occluded by pressure, physical findings may be temporarily altered. Left ventricular enlargement is common, and severe involvement will lead to high-output left ventricular failure. A continuous murmur is usually heard overlying the lesion, and left ventricular hypertrophy may be seen on the ECG or echocardiogram. Occasionally, endothelial infection in the fistula may mimic endocarditis.

THE FOLLOWING CRITERIA ARE REQUIRED FOR THE DIAGNOSIS OF HEART DISEASE DUE TO SYSTEMIC ARTERIOVENOUS FISTULA.

Left ventricular enlargement in the presence of a systemic arteriovenous fistula, in the absence of other causes of cardiomegaly, with reversal after closure of the fistula.

SYSTEMIC LUPUS ERYTHEMATOSUS

The Disease

Systemic lupus erythematosus is a multisystem disease of unknown etiology. Tissues are damaged because of the deposition of immune complexes or autoimmune antibodies. About 90 percent of the patients are women. Major organ involvement includes the musculoskeletal system (arthritis, myositis, ischemic bone necrosis), the skin (typical malar rash, oral ulceration, vasculitis, alopecia), the bone marrow (thrombocytopenia, anemia, leukopenia), the brain and peripheral nervous system (seizures, vasculitis, psychosis, peripheral neuropathy), the kidneys (glomerulonephritis, nephrotic syndrome, uremia), and the heart. In addition, patients often have splenomegaly and may also have lymphadenopathy, eye involvement, and vascular thrombosis due to circulating anticardiolipin antibodies ("lupus anticoagulant").

Molecular and Cellular Biology

Although the pathogenesis of lupus is unknown, there appears to be a genetic component, as there is an increased frequency of certain histocompatibility antigens (MB1/MT1 haplotype and HLA-DR2). In addition, some lupus patients have inherited deficiencies in complement, which may reduce the clearance of immune complexes. Viral and bacterial etiologies have been postulated, with the theory that microbial antigens may either act as nonspecific B-cell stimulators or elicit antibodies that cross react with human DNA. The preponderance of lupus in females may be explained in part by the fact that estrogen enhances antibody response, and patients with lupus have relatively prolonged estrogen stimulation due to an increased production of 16-alpha-hydroxyestrone. In addition, patients with lupus have a combination of B-cell hyperactivity and suppression of T helper and T suppressor lymphocytes. Thus, they are less able to suppress anti-DNA antibody synthesis. The abnormal antibodies produced in lupus include antibodies to DNA, RNA, RNA polymerase, ribonuclear proteins, histones, phospholipid, blood elements, and neurons.

Cardiac Involvement

Two-thirds of patients will develop pericarditis, which is often benign. Tamponade and constrictive pericarditis are unusual complications. Myocarditis occurs in about 10 percent of patients, and this can result in cardiomegaly, heart failure, and arrhythmias. Endocarditis has been traditionally described as "verrucous" (Libman-Sacks) lesions, which are seen on autopsy in about 10 percent. These were previously thought to be benign lesions with only rare hemodynamic consequences. However, more recent evaluation with echocardiography has revealed valvular thickening or vegetation-like lesions in about 30 percent and even more commonly (40%) in those lupus patients who have anticardiolipin antibodies. The size of these valvular masses varies, but very large masses may result in severe regurgitation and less often stenosis. Valve replacement has been necessary in some of these patients. In rare cases, mobile valvular thrombi have been seen on echocardiography, accompanied by cerebral and systemic embolization. An additional rare cardiac manifestation of lupus is myocardial infarction due to coronary vasculitis. There is also an incidence of accelerated atherosclerosis, possibly related to steroid use or hypertension.

ONE OF THE FOLLOWING CRITERIA IS REQUIRED FOR THE DIAGNOSIS OF HEART DISEASE DUE TO SYSTEMIC LUPUS ERYTHEMATOSUS.

1. **Pericarditis, cardiac enlargement, or heart failure in a patient with systemic lupus erythematosus and no other causes of such heart disease.**
2. **Libman-Sacks endocarditis or valvular thrombi seen on echocardiography in patients with systemic lupus erythematosus.**

TOXIC AGENT

The Disease

A variety of chemicals and drugs may cause cardiac damage. This may be manifest as an acute reaction, with inflammation and necrosis, or as a chronic cardiomyopathy. In some instances, both courses may occur (as with anthracyclines or ethanol).

Molecular and Cellular Biology

The mechanisms of cardiac damage vary with the offending agent. In the case of the anthracyclines, the exact mechanism is unknown. However, the drugs bind to DNA, inhibiting DNA and RNA polymerases. They may cause lipid peroxidation and may bind to cardiolipins and actin. They also inhibit adenosine triphosphate production, interfere with the sodium-potassium pump in the sarcolemma, and interfere with mitochondrial oxidative phosphorylation by inhibiting coenzyme Q. Myocardial necrosis may result from excess accumulation of calcium in the myocardium. The damage to myocardial cells in culture is similar to that which occurs to tumor cells in culture.

In contrast, cocaine may produce cardiotoxicity by causing coronary vasoconstriction and hypersensitivity reactions. The accompanying increased oxygen demands (increased heart rate and blood pressure) and impaired coronary flow may cause ischemia and infarction.

A common form of cardiac toxicity results from the electrophysiologic effects of commonly used antiarrhythmics, with prolongation of action potential duration and repolarization and, in some instances, the production of arrhythmias.

Cardiac Involvement

The type of cardiac involvement depends on the damaging agent. Patients with chronic anthracycline toxicity have dilated cardiomyopathy, which is dose dependent. The acute toxicity is manifested by arrhythmias and occasionally myocarditis or pericarditis. Cocaine toxicity is manifested by myocardial ischemia and occasionally infarction. This may be especially prominent in patients with underlying coronary artery disease. Patients may also have malignant arrhythmias and sudden death, probably related to excessive sympathomimetic stimulation and vasoconstriction.

THE FOLLOWING CRITERIA ARE REQUIRED FOR THE DIAGNOSIS OF HEART DISEASE DUE TO A TOXIC AGENT.

Evidence that exposure to a drug or exogenous chemical has produced or increased a significant disorder of cardiac function or structure.

TRANSPLANTATION

The Disease

Donors and recipients of transplanted hearts are matched for body size and blood ABO groups. If the allografts are well selected and well preserved, they generally function well hemodynamically. Pulmonary hypertension in the recipient can cause problems, since the donor right ventricle may be unprepared for abrupt confrontation with an increased afterload. Donor hearts are attached to the posterior portions of the native right atrium and left atrium and to the pulmonary artery and aorta, so atrial parasystole may be seen. Since the hearts are denervated, the Frank-Starling response is initially paramount in modulating cardiac output. Sympathetic stimulation is mediated via circulating catecholamines. Ischemia does not elicit angina.

Rejection of the allograft by the recipient's immune system is the major therapeutic problem. Infection and secondary tumors can occur as a result of immunosuppressive therapy.

Molecular and Cellular Biology

The rejection reaction begins when major histocompatibility components (classes I and II) are ingested by macrophages, which process the antigens and present them to helper and cytotoxic T-lymphocytes. These in turn secrete interleukin-2, which leads to proliferation of cytotoxic T-lymphocytes, to antibody production, and ultimately to cardiac myolysis and graft rejection. Arteriosclerosis of the allograft coronary arteries is a frequent complication and may be immunologically mediated, perhaps with involvement of endothelial and platelet-derived growth factors.

Cardiac Involvement

Early graft rejection may cause no symptoms, and the diagnosis depends on detection of the graded histologic changes in serial endomyocardial biopsies. With later rejection, there may be fever, arrhythmias, and ventricular failure. Echocardiography is useful in detecting and following wall movement abnormalities in the course of rejection. Graft arteriosclerosis may be evident on angiography but may be best delineated by intracoronary ultrasonography. It is a major cause of late graft failure.

THE FOLLOWING CRITERIA ARE REQUIRED FOR THE DIAGNOSIS OF HEART DISEASE DUE TO TRANSPLANTATION.

The clinical or laboratory manifestations noted in a patient with a transplanted heart.

TRAUMA

The Disease

Injury to the heart or great vessels may result from penetrating or blunt chest trauma. Once thought of as an esoteric form of heart disease, traumatic heart disease is now recognized as a common cause of death, especially in the young. Car accidents are the most commonly encountered causes of blunt trauma, although it may also result from blows to the chest received in fights, falls, or sporting events. In recent years, seat belt and air bag injuries have been added to the more common steering wheel injuries, during which the heart is compressed between the sternum and spine. Penetrating chest injuries are usually due to use of firearms or knives. Iatrogenic cardiac trauma may occur due to cardiopulmonary resuscitation or catheters used for diagnosis, angioplasty, valvuloplasty, and ablation. In addition, instrumentation of the esophagus (for stricture dilation) may rarely result in pericardial perforation. Foreign bodies may also reach the pericardial sac through the esophagus or bronchi.

Cardiac and Great Vessel Involvement

The primary acute manifestations of trauma to the heart and great vessels are exsanguination, pericardial tamponade, and aortic disruption. Lesions that may present with subacute and chronic manifestations include valvular disruption, left-to-right shunts, ventricular and aortic aneurysm or pseudoaneurysm formation, myocardial injury due to contusion or to coronary artery injury, coronary fistulas, ventricular septal defect, and pericarditis (which can lead to constriction).

Rupture of the heart may be accompanied by obvious gross chest wall trauma, but it may also occur without such signs.

Valvular disruption may result from leaflet tears or rupture of chordae or papillary muscles. These may occur due to blunt trauma as well as penetrating wounds. With blunt trauma, the aortic valve is most often involved, followed by the mitral and tricuspid.

Blunt chest trauma may result in intimal disruption of the aorta. Most often, this occurs at the isthmus, but in about 10 percent of patients this may occur just above the aortic valve or at other locations. Only 10 to 20 percent of patients with aortic disruption reach the hospital, but these patients may be successfully treated if the diagnosis is suspected and recognized. Transesophageal echocardiography is valuable in the diagnosis of aortic tears and intimal disruption.

Myocardial contusion may mimic infarction, both in its ECG and clinical manifestations. These may include repolarization changes as well as the development of Q waves. Clinically, patients may have arrhythmias, cardiac failure, and late aneurysm formation. Direct coronary artery injury may also cause infarction, especially in patients with preexisting coronary atherosclerosis. Late sequelae may include coronary aneurysm and fistula formation.

THE FOLLOWING CRITERIA ARE REQUIRED FOR THE DIAGNOSIS OF HEART DISEASE DUE TO TRAUMA.

Initial

The occurrence of chest trauma and one or more of the following: arrhythmias, conduction disturbance, myocardial contusion or infarction, pericarditis, hemopericardium, pneumopericardium, valvular regurgitation, aortic disruption, ventricular septal defect, ventricular aneurysm or pseudoaneurysm, coronary aneurysm or fistula, or aortic aneurysm or pseudoaneurysm formation.

Definitive

Confirmation of the clinical finding by echocardiography, angiography, or other imaging technique.

UNKNOWN ETIOLOGY

The cause of a patient's heart disease should be stated as "Unknown" in those patients who present with either definite structural changes in the heart or abnormal cardiac function for which no specific etiology can be determined.

UREMIA

The Disease

Although the kidney may recover completely from acute disease, sustained or severe disease results in progressive loss of nephrons and chronic renal failure. Uremia, which has multisystem consequences, results. The syndrome has many metabolic and endocrinologic manifestations. These include disorders of fluid and electrolyte balance, hematologic abnormalities, secondary hyperparathyroidism, renal osteodystrophy and osteomalacia, serum lipid abnormalities, hyperglycemia, hyperuricemia, infertility, skin rashes, gastrointestinal disorders, neuromuscular disorders, lung disease, and cardiovascular disease.

Molecular and Cellular Biology

As renal damage progresses, there is compensatory hypertrophy of surviving nephrons, but these are eventually damaged by the burden of increased glomerular pressure and flow. Cellular function is aberrant throughout the body in uremia. Cellular sodium and potassium ATPase activity is decreased, and energy-dependent ion fluxes across cell membranes are impaired. Since active ion pumping accounts for a significant proportion of energy production, some patients become hypothermic. The generalized decrease in active ion transport also results in increased intracellular sodium and decreased intracellular potassium. The increased intracellular sodium results in an increase in intracellular fluid volume superimposed on an increased extracellular volume due to a decrease in glomerular filtration. Despite decreases in intracellular potassium (which may be aggravated by inadequate potassium intake, diarrhea, vomiting, and diuretics), serum potassium is often high because of the accompanying metabolic acidosis. This hyperkalemia may have direct cardiac consequences. Hyperglycemia may result from a decreased cellular response to insulin as well as decreased glucose utilization by peripheral tissues. Long-term abnormalities in lipids may have cardiovascular consequences. Uremic patients have hypertriglyceridemia due to decreased lipoprotein lipase and hepatic triglyceride lipase activity and possibly to increased production by the liver. In addition, synthesis of high-density lipoprotein is often decreased.

Cardiac Involvement

Cardiac disease is the most common cause of death in patients on dialysis. Hypertension is present in most uremic patients. Its absence may be due to excessive fluid losses with diarrhea or vomiting. Hypertension is due to fluid overload, high renin levels, sympathetic overactivity, or a combination of these factors. Uremic patients with hypertension often have a high cardiac output and low systemic vascular resistance due to anemia. With erythropoietin administration, there is an increase in hematocrit and viscosity, which results in an increase in vascular resistance, and the blood pressure may rise.

The increased afterload in hypertensive uremic patients may cause left ventricular failure with congestive symptoms. Alternatively, fluid retention can cause circulatory congestion, which may be successfully treated with dialysis. Heart failure is the most common cause of cardiac death in dialysis patients, followed by myocardial infarction, and rarely pericarditis.

Uremic patients may have accelerated coronary (and other) atherosclerosis, which is multifactorial in etiology. Coronary artery bypass surgery may be successfully carried out in uremic patients, although with an increase in morbidity. Occasionally, angina may occur in uremic patients in the absence of coronary atherosclerosis, possibly due to a combination of anemia, hypertension, left ventricular hypertrophy, and decreased vasodilator reserve.

Pericarditis is common in uremic patients, and one-third to one-half have pericardial effusion on echocardiography. The effusions reflect an inflammatory process, which may also affect the pleura. Although large hemorrhagic effusions with tamponade may occur, tamponade is an uncommon cause of death in uremia.

There is some evidence that left ventricular hypertrophy and dysfunction may occur in uremia in the absence of other factors such as hypertension and coronary disease, although anemia, fluid overload, and hypercalcemia with its resultant myocardial calcifications may be causes. Surgically created arteriovenous fistulas can contribute to high-output failure.

THE FOLLOWING CRITERIA ARE REQUIRED FOR THE DIAGNOSIS OF HEART DISEASE DUE TO UREMIA.

Pericardial effusion, cardiomyopathy, congestive heart failure, or myocardial calcification occurring in the course of chronic uremia in the absence of other underlying cause for the specific manifestation.

The Anatomic Cardiac Diagnosis

Nomenclature

Diseases of the Aorta
  Aneurysm of the Aorta
  Aortic Dissection
  Aortitis
    Aortic Arch Syndrome (Pulseless Disease,
      Takayasu's Disease)
    Giant Cell Aortitis
    Spondylitic Aortitis
    Syphilitic Aortitis
  Atherosclerosis of the Aorta
  Cystic Medial Degeneration
    Idiopathic
    Marfan's Syndrome
  Dilatation of the Aorta
  Embolism to the Aorta
  Rupture of the Aorta
  Thrombosis of the Aorta
Diseases of the Pulmonary Vasculature
  Aneurysm of the Pulmonary Artery
  Arteriosclerosis
    Atherosclerosis
    Medial Hypertrophy
    Intimal Fibrosis
  Arteritis
  Arteriolitis
  Dilatation of the Pulmonary Artery
  Embolism to a Pulmonary Artery
  Thrombosis of a Pulmonary Artery
  Sclerosis of Pulmonary Veins
Diseases of the Coronary Arteries
  Arteritis
    Infective
    Polyarteritis Nodosa
  Atherosclerosis
  Embolism to a Coronary Artery
  Stenosis of a Coronary Orifice
Diseases of the Endocardium and Valves
  Calcification of the Mitral Annulus
  Endocardial Fibroelastosis

Endocardial Fibrosis (Endomyocardial Fibrosis)
Endocarditis
    Infective Endocarditis
    Lupus Valvulitis (Atypical Verrucous
       Endocarditis)
    Nonbacterial Thrombotic Endocarditis
       (Marantic Endocarditis, Terminal
       Endocarditis)
    Rheumatic Valvulitis and Endocarditis
    Rheumatoid Valvulitis
Fibromyxomatous Degeneration of a Valve
   (Mucoid Degeneration)
Intracardiac Thrombosis (Endocardial
   Thrombosis)
Neoplasm of the Endocardium
    Myxoma
    Papillary Fibroma (Papilloma)
Rupture of Chordae Tendineae
Valvular Deformity (With or Without Stenosis
   or Regurgitation)
    Aortic Valve Deformity Causing Stenosis
    Aortic Valve Deformity Causing
       Regurgitation
    Mitral Valve Deformity Causing Stenosis
    Mitral Valve Deformity Causing
       Regurgitation
    Tricuspid Valve Deformity Causing Stenosis
    Tricuspid Valve Deformity Causing
       Regurgitation
    Pulmonic Valve Deformity Causing Stenosis
    Pulmonic Valve Deformity Causing
       Regurgitation
    Valvular Vegetations
Diseases of the Myocardium
  Cardiomyopathy
    Adipose Infiltration of the Myocardium
    Amyloidosis
    Friedreich's Ataxia
    Hemochromatosis
    Hypothyroidism
    Lysosomal Storage Diseases
       Glycogen Storage Disease
       Mucopolysaccharidoses
    Nodular Glycogen Infiltration
       (Rhabdomyoma)

Progressive Muscular Dystrophy
Enlargement of the Heart
  Left Ventricular Enlargement
    Left Ventricular Hypertrophy
    Hypertrophic Cardiomyopathy
  Right Ventricular Enlargement
  Left Atrial Enlargement
  Right Atrial Enlargement
Myocardial Fibrosis
Myocardial Infarction
Myocarditis
  Hypersensitivity
  Infective Myocarditis
  Idiopathic Myocarditis
  Lupus Myocarditis
  Progressive Systemic Sclerosis (Scleroderma)
  Rheumatic Myocarditis
  Rheumatoid Myocarditis
  Sarcoidosis
Neoplasm
Rupture of the Myocardium: Free Wall,
  Interventricular Septum, or a Papillary
  Muscle
Ventricular Aneurysm
Diseases of the Pericardium
  Cysts
  Fibrosis or Calcification
  Hemopericardium
  Neoplasm
  Pericardial Effusion (Hydropericardium)
  Pericarditis
  Pneumopericardium
  Congenital Absence of the Left Pericardium
Anomalies of Cardiac Position
  Dextrocardia
    Dextrocardia with Situs Inversus
    Dextrocardia with Situs Solitus
  Levocardia with Situs Inversus
Anomalies of the Aorta and Aortic Arch System
  Coarctation of the Aorta
  Right Aortic Arch
  Vascular Ring
Anomalies of the Pulmonary Arteries
  Pulmonary Arteriovenous Fistula
  Pulmonary Vascular Sling

Diseases of the Aorta

ANEURYSM OF THE AORTA

The term *aneurysm* is applied only to a saccular or sharply demarcated fusiform dilatation of the aorta. In the thoracic aorta, syphilis was formerly the commonest cause of aneurysms. However, atherosclerosis is now the usual etiologic factor in this location and in the vast majority of abdominal aortic aneurysms. Congenital and traumatic aneurysms are rare. Marfan's syndrome may be associated with aneurysmal dilatation of the supravalvular aorta.

Atherosclerotic aneurysm is a consequence of medial injury and attenuation associated with extensive intimal plaque formation. The loss of muscle and elastic tissue, coupled with increasing lateral stress as distention proceeds, results in fusiform or globular dilatation. It is most frequently found in the abdominal aorta between the origin of the renal arteries and the bifurcation. Atherosclerotic aneurysms may be multiple. They commonly contain lamellated thrombus, which may embolize distally. Complications include leakage of blood, frank rupture, and erosion of vertebrae. Disruption of the aneurysmal wall with massive retroperitoneal or intraperitoneal hemorrhage is a frequent cause of death. The tear is found in the widest, and consequently the thinnest, portion of the area of dilatation; it rarely occurs at the ends or margins.

Syphilitic aneurysm results from aortitis predominantly involving the adventitia, the outer media, and vasa vasorum. The inflammation and obliteration of the vasa vasorum cause destruction and loss of the musculoelastic media with subsequent stretching and dilatation of the residual fibrous and scarred wall. Lamellated thrombus frequently lines and partially fills the aneurysmal sac. Complications include compression of adjacent structures such as the bronchus and recurrent laryngeal nerve and rupture and erosion of resistant neighboring structures such as the sternum and vertebrae.

Aortic aneurysms may exist without producing symptoms and are frequently discovered on routine physical examination of the abdomen or chest x-ray. Echocardiography is most useful in diagnosis. A complete evaluation may require computed tomography (CT) scan, magnetic resonance imaging (MRI), or transesophageal echocardiographic examination. Thoracic aneurysms may produce pain, cough, hoarseness, dysphagia, a tracheal tug, inequality of the pulse and blood pressure in the arms, and localized or diffuse pulsation when there is impingement on the chest wall. There may be concomitant aortic regurgitation. Abdominal aneurysms are most commonly discovered as pulsating masses, which produce pain as they enlarge or press on adjacent vertebrae and nerves, or are discovered serendipitously in abdominal x-ray or echocardiographic examination. If rupture occurs, severe pain, signs of peritoneal irritation, or shock may ensue. Pain may be a sign of incipient rupture. Aneurysms equal to or greater than 5 cm in diameter have a greater frequency of rupture.

THE FOLLOWING CRITERION IS REQUIRED FOR THE DIAGNOSIS OF ANEURYSM OF THE AORTA.

A saccular or sharply demarcated fusiform dilatation of the aorta demonstrated by x-ray, echocardiogram, CT, MRI, or angiography.

AORTIC DISSECTION

Dissection of the aorta is caused by a forceful penetration of blood between the layers of the vessel, characteristically separating the outer third from the inner two-thirds of the media. In more than 90 percent of patients, an intimal tear is the precipitating event. However, the initial injury may be caused by hemorrhage from the vasa vasorum into an area of preexisting cystic medial degeneration where subsequent expansion leads to rupture through the aortic intima. The intimal tear provides an opening for extension of the lesion, with the systemic blood pressure as a driving force. The intimal tear is located most frequently in the proximal 3 cm of the aorta. It is usually transverse or circumferential and measures from 1 to 4 cm in length. The second most common site is close to the insertion of the ligamentum arteriosum.

Dissection may progress for short distances proximally, and induce aortic regurgitation or coronary occlusion, or distally, and continue throughout the entire length of the aorta. Rupture through adventitia may produce massive hemorrhage into the pericardial sac, pleural space, peritoneal cavity, mediastinum, or retroperitoneal area. Infrequently, the hematoma reenters the main aortic lumen to form a so-called double-barreled aorta. This artificially created channel may remain functional and become endothelialized, or it may be closed by thrombus formation and fibrosis. In most instances in which the dissection continues throughout the entire length of the aorta, small branches such as the intercostals may be severed; large branches, such as the renal, mesenteric, and iliac vessels, may be restricted by a continuation of the pathologic process within their walls.

Aortic dissection occurs predominantly in men in the middle or older age groups, particularly in the presence of systemic hypertension. Persons with Marfan's syndrome or aortic coarctation are particularly prone to this process.

The cardinal symptom of aortic dissection is the sudden onset of severe, continuous tearing or crushing pain in the chest that radiates to the back and is generally unaccompanied by electrocardiographic (ECG) evidence of myocardial infarction. The other manifestations of aortic dissection depend largely on involvement of aortic branches. Thus signs and symptoms of myocardial, cerebral, renal, mesenteric, or iliac arterial insufficiency can appear.

Physical findings include agitation, the murmur of aortic regurgitation, asymmetric diminution of arterial pulses, and systolic bruits over the areas where the aortic lumen is narrowed. Systemic blood pressure is usually well maintained at the onset.

A chest x-ray may show widening of the aorta. Transesophageal and transthoracic echocardiography demonstrate aortic widening, double echoes from the aortic wall, and an intimal flap within the lumen of the aorta. These lesions may also be demonstrated by CT scan, MRI, or aortography.

THE FOLLOWING CRITERIA ARE REQUIRED FOR THE DIAGNOSIS OF AORTIC DISSECTION.

Initial

The characteristic pain associated with one or more of the following: aortic regurgitation, widening of the thoracic aorta, or asymmetric decreases in arterial pulse volume.

Definitive

Evidence on aortography or any of the noninvasive methods referred to above of an intimal flap and separation of the aorta into true and false lumens.

AORTITIS

Aortic Arch Syndrome (Pulseless Disease, Takayasu's Disease)

Aortic arch syndrome is primarily a disease of young women and is seen most often in Asians. The lesions involve the aortic arch and the origins of the great vessels from the arch, including the coronary ostia. There is adventitial sclerosis, scarring of the media with disruption of the musculoelastic coats, and marked obliterative intimal fibrous thickening. Lymphocytes and plasma cells infiltrate the wall. Although rare giant cells are seen, this is not a usual feature. Thrombosis may be superimposed.

Clinically, the aortic arch syndrome is characterized by loss of pulses in the arms and a variety of manifestations of ischemia in those areas supplied by the major branches of the aortic arch. Similar findings may also be produced by syphilis, atherosclerosis, and giant cell aortitis, although these entities usually cause aneurysmal dilatation rather than obliteration.

THE FOLLOWING CRITERIA ARE REQUIRED FOR THE DIAGNOSIS OF AORTIC ARCH SYNDROME.

Angiographic demonstration of narrowing of the lumen of the aorta or narrowing or obliteration of the brachiocephalic vessels arising from it, in the absence of other known cause in a patient under the age of 40.

Giant Cell Aortitis

Giant cell aortitis is an inflammatory lesion of the aorta that occurs in older age groups. It can occur as an isolated phenomenon but most commonly is part of a syndrome involving medium-sized arteries, particularly the temporal artery. Involvement of the carotid system may result in blindness and central nervous system disturbances. All major branches of the aorta can be involved. The media, particularly its inner portion, is disrupted by an infiltration of lymphocytes, with accompanying macrophages and plasma cells. Fragmentation of the internal elastic membrane or the elastic lamellae of the aorta evokes a foreign body giant cell reaction. The overlying intimal fibrosis in smaller muscular arteries such as the temporal artery can produce striking luminal narrowing. Biopsy of the temporal artery may demonstrate these characteristic lesions. Giant cell aortitis is associated with polymyalgia rheumatica in approximately 40 percent of patients.

THE FOLLOWING CRITERIA ARE REQUIRED FOR THE DIAGNOSIS OF GIANT CELL AORTITIS.

Reduction in the lumen of the aorta demonstrated by angiography or other methods, usually associated with obliteration or narrowing of its major branches, plus histologic evidence of giant cell arteritis.

Spondylitic Aortitis

Ankylosing spondylitis may be accompanied by aortic regurgitation. This is the result of aortic medial scarring with dilatation of the ring comparable to that seen in syphilis. Adventitial sclerosis, obliterating intimal thickening of the vasa vasorum, and aortic intimal fibrosis, as well as scarring of the media, characterize this lesion. Thickening of the aortic cusps, with rolling of the edges, accompanies commissural separation and may be related to valvular inflammation. As in syphilis, however, most cases of valvular insufficiency are secondary to ring dilatation. A similar lesion is seen in Reiter's syndrome.

THE FOLLOWING CRITERION IS REQUIRED FOR THE DIAGNOSIS OF SPONDYLITIC AORTITIS.

The association of aortic regurgitation with ankylosing spondylitis.

Syphilitic Aortitis

In syphilitic aortitis, involvement is most frequent in the ascending portion and arch of the aorta, less common in the thoracic part, and rare in the abdominal segment. The vessel wall is thickened and inelastic, and the lumen may be dilated. The intima contains well-defined, pearly-white, hyaline, smooth-surfaced elevations of variable size. Longitudinal wrinkling of the intima is fairly characteristic. Atheromatous deposits in the area of involvement are exaggerated and may complicate and obscure its appearance. The intimal plaques may encroach on the orifice of any arterial branch, including the ostium of either or both coronary arteries. This encroachment frequently causes stenosis or almost complete obliteration of the orifices.

There is an increase of connective tissue in the adventitia, thickening and endothelial proliferation in the vasa vasorum, and perivascular infiltration of lymphocytes and plasma cells. The media is penetrated in flame-shaped fashion by thin-walled vascular channels and collections of lymphocytes and plasma cells. These lesions accompany areas of scarring where the elastic lamellae are ruptured and the smooth muscle cells replaced by collagen. Occasionally, the larger cell aggregates form miliary gummata with central areas of necrosis. Rarely, a few multinucleated giant cells may appear. The intima is irregularly thickened by proliferation of connective tissue.

In one-third to one-half of all patients with syphilitic aortitis, the aortic valve is affected. As a result of inflammatory change in the underlying aortic wall and dilatation of the ring, the commissures are separated, leading to aortic regurgitation. The lateral parts of the aortic cusps may coalesce with the intima of the aorta, leading to further separation of the commissures. In advanced forms of the disease, the margins of the cusps show thickening and rolling toward the ventricular aspect, which may be either mechanical or inflammatory in origin. Further cicatrization may reduce the cusps to cordlike structures and increase the degree of regurgitation.

In addition to fibrous proliferation, the affected leaflets and the aorta show endothelial proliferation in the vasa vasorum and infiltration by lymphocytes and plasma cells.

Syphilitic aortitis usually becomes clinically manifest only when there are complications such as aortic dilatation, aneurysm, aortic regurgitation, or coronary ostial stenosis. Aortitis may cause systolic murmurs, heard at the base of the heart; a ringing quality to the aortic component of the second sound; and radiologic evidence of dilatation, exaggerated pulsation, or calcification of the ascending aorta.

A diagnosis of syphilitic aortitis requires serologic demonstration of prior infection by *Treponema pallidum*, especially since widening of the aortic arch is frequent with systemic hypertension and in patients over 40 years of age.

THE FOLLOWING CRITERIA ARE REQUIRED FOR THE DIAGNOSIS OF SYPHILITIC AORTITIS.

Initial

Widening or aneurysm of the ascending aorta, aortic regurgitation, or coronary ostial stenosis.

Definitive

Serologic evidence of syphilis.

ATHEROSCLEROSIS OF THE AORTA

Atherosclerosis of the aorta is characterized initially by intimal change. Endothelial injury or activation results in the specific binding of inflammatory cells to the endothelium and the release of cytokines and other mediators of inflammation. Intra- and extracellular lipid accumulates in this layer, associated with an increase in subendothelial connective tissue rich in mucopolysaccharide ground substance. As it ages, the center undergoes degeneration, with liberation of lipoprotein and crystalline cholesterol, which form a central grumous mass. Reactive proliferation of fibrous tissue and varying degrees of inflammatory response, consisting of lymphocytes and mononuclear cells, accompany the lesion throughout its evolution. The lipid-rich plaque frequently undergoes calcification, giving the area of involvement of the aorta a brittle character.

As the plaque expands, the underlying musculoelastic media becomes compressed, attenuated, and scarred. The internal elastic lamella may be frayed and fragmented, and the components of the plaque may penetrate and further destroy the media.

The degree of involvement of the aorta by atherosclerosis is least in the ascending portion and increases in severity from the arch to the abdominal segment. It is most marked just proximal to the bifurcation. Elsewhere in the vessel, pronounced lesions occur about the orifices of the branches and at points of fixation to surrounding structures. In children and young adults, the disease has an affinity for that segment of the aorta just distal to the aortic valve and for the posterior wall of the descending thoracic aorta, particularly about the orifices of intercostal arteries.

The degenerating plaque may rupture into the lumen. This complication is common but usually causes no detectable difficulty unless extruded components of the plaque and an associated thrombus embolize to a vessel of importance. However, thrombosis and aneurysm also may result from atherosclerosis.

Atherosclerosis of the aorta produces clinical symptoms based on the severity of the structural complications such as aneurysm, embolization (especially from pedunculated, mobile atherosclerotic material), thrombosis, or impingement on the orifice of arteries, with reduction in regional blood flow. A systolic ejection murmur at the base of the heart resulting from aortic dilatation may be present. The aorta is elongated, tortuous, and widened, as demonstrated by chest x-ray, echocardiography, CT scan, MRI, or aortography. The descending aorta becomes readily visible and often curves to the left. Calcific plaques may frequently be seen in the aortic knob and in the abdominal aorta. Transesophageal echocardiography is an especially sensitive and specific technique for demonstrating sessile and mobile atheromata in the ascending aorta, arch, and proximal descending aorta.

ONE OF THE FOLLOWING CRITERIA IS REQUIRED FOR THE DIAGNOSIS OF ATHEROSCLEROSIS OF THE AORTA.

1. **Demonstration of calcification or irregularity of outline by radiography, MRI, CT, or echocardiography.**
2. **Echocardiographic demonstration of atherosclerotic plaque.**
3. **Evidence of occlusion of major aortic branches in the absence of any other demonstrable cause.**

CYSTIC MEDIAL DEGENERATION

Idiopathic

The changes of idiopathic cystic medial degeneration involve the aorta with moderate frequency and are a frequent concomitant of aging.

Slitlike spaces between the lamellae of the media of the aorta are filled with a homogeneous, basophilic, mucoid material. An increase in and coalescence of these spaces produce cysts or cavities due to degeneration of muscle and elastic tissue. The abnormal mucoid substance is metachromatic and stains as acid mucopolysaccharide; its origin is unknown, but it may be a consequence of degeneration induced by intimal hyperplasia and medial hypertrophy of the vasa vasorum. Marked dilatation of the ascending aorta and dissecting hematoma are the most significant complications of this disorder. The dilatation of the ascending aorta often assumes a characteristic triangular shape.

ONE OF THE FOLLOWING CRITERIA IS REQUIRED FOR THE DIAGNOSIS OF IDIOPATHIC CYSTIC MEDIAL DEGENERATION OF THE AORTA.

1. **Aortic dissection occurring in the absence of any other cause.**
2. **Marked dilatation of the ascending aorta in the absence of syphilis, Marfan's syndrome, Ehlers-Danlos syndrome, or any other known cause.**

Marfan's Syndrome

In Marfan's syndrome, a hereditary disease, the degeneration in the aorta is similar to that seen in the idiopathic form, but it is a consequence of mutations in the gene that codes for a microfibrillar component of elastic tissue known as fibrillin. (See page 22.) Dilatation of the aorta and aneurysm of a sinus of Valsalva are consequences of the medial cystic degeneration; secondary aortic regurgitation may result. As in the idiopathic form of cystic medial degeneration, the most frequent complication is aortic dissection.

THE FOLLOWING CRITERIA ARE REQUIRED FOR THE DIAGNOSIS OF CYSTIC MEDIAL DEGENERATION DUE TO MARFAN'S SYNDROME.

Evidence of Marfan's syndrome and any one of the following: dilatation of the aorta, aneurysm of a sinus of Valsalva, or aortic dissection.

DILATATION OF THE AORTA

The thoracic aorta can become dilated as a consequence of hemodynamic factors such as systemic hypertension, aortic valvular disease, or increased aortic blood flow. Dilatation of the thoracic and abdominal aorta may result from structural alterations due to atherosclerosis, syphilis, Marfan's syndrome, or idiopathic cystic medial degeneration.

Dilatation of the ascending aorta may produce systolic murmurs at the base of the heart, which may radiate into the neck. If the aortic ring is widened (annuloaortic ectasia), the murmur of aortic regurgitation may be present.

THE FOLLOWING CRITERION IS REQUIRED FOR THE DIAGNOSIS OF DILATATION OF THE AORTA.

Demonstration of an increase in the transverse diameter of the aorta by chest x-ray, echocardiography, MRI, CT, or aortography.

EMBOLISM TO THE AORTA

Emboli to the aorta may originate from thrombi in the left atrium, left atrial appendage, or left ventricle. Thrombi developing over an ulcerated atherosclerotic plaque can also give rise to more distal emboli. Emboli usually lodge at the bifurcation of the aorta and can occlude the iliac arteries. The sudden onset of pain, numbness, weakness, or paresthesias in the lower extremities, accompanied by coldness, pallor, mottled cyanosis, and absent pulsations in the same areas, is clinical evidence of an embolus lodged at the aortic bifurcation. However, sudden massive thrombosis of the terminal aorta can give rise to the same clinical picture. Aortography may delineate the site of obstruction.

THE FOLLOWING CRITERIA ARE REQUIRED FOR THE DIAGNOSIS OF EMBOLISM TO THE AORTA.

The sudden onset of the symptoms and signs of acute obstruction of the lower aorta and demonstration of a site of obstruction or a filling defect by aortography or a noninvasive method. It may be impossible to distinguish this condition from in situ thrombosis of the distal aorta.

RUPTURE OF THE AORTA

Rupture of the aorta may result from trauma or may be associated with aortic dissection or aneurysm formation. Coarctation of the aorta more rarely leads to rupture. Complete rupture may be rapidly fatal, but with slow bleeding into the esophagus, pericardial sac, pleural spaces, mediastinum, or abdomen, death may be postponed for hours or days. Evidence of blood loss and shock are the major clinical manifestations.

**THE FOLLOWING CRITERIA ARE REQUIRED FOR THE
DIAGNOSIS OF RUPTURE OF THE AORTA.**

**Following trauma or in the presence of aortic aneurysm,
dissection, or coarctation, demonstration of extravasation of
blood from the aorta into one of the areas noted above.**

THROMBOSIS OF THE AORTA

Thrombosis of the aorta most commonly results from
atherosclerosis. Gradual occlusion of the lumen of the
terminal aorta can result in the development of collateral
circulation to the lower extremities, so that their blood
supply is fairly well maintained and they remain warm
and their color normal. However, symptoms may include
impotence and intermittent claudication, with pain appearing in the hips, thighs, and gluteal areas (Leriche
syndrome).

Clinically, rapid occlusion of the lower portion of the
aorta by thrombosis may be indistinguishable from occlusion due to embolism.

**THE FOLLOWING CRITERIA ARE REQUIRED FOR THE
DIAGNOSIS OF THROMBOSIS OF THE AORTA.**

**The gradual onset of the symptoms and signs of obstruction
of the lower aorta and the demonstration of a site of obstruction by aortography or a noninvasive test. It may be impossible to distinguish this condition from aortic embolism.**

Diseases of the Pulmonary
Vasculature

ANEURYSM OF THE PULMONARY ARTERY

True aneurysms of the pulmonary artery should be distinguished from the general dilatation that may complicate chronic pulmonary hypertension. While degenerative and inflammatory vascular diseases that commonly
involve the aorta are seen rarely in the pulmonary artery,
syphilis, infective endocarditis, and trauma are encountered in association with pulmonary arterial aneurysms.
An increased incidence of aneurysm of the pulmonary
trunk or its branches and of pulmonary dissection is also
found in the presence of severe pulmonary hypertension,
particularly when associated with congenital anomalies
of the heart and great vessels. Patent ductus arteriosus,
large ventricular or atrial septal defects, mitral obstruc-

tion, and recurrent pulmonary thromboembolism are therefore common predisposing conditions. Aneurysms of the main trunk are usually present when the pulmonary valve is congenitally absent or incompetent. Pulmonary arterial aneurysms may rupture either into the pericardial sac, resulting in tamponade, or into the lung, following which massive hemoptysis occurs.

THE FOLLOWING CRITERION IS REQUIRED FOR THE DIAGNOSIS OF ANEURYSM OF THE PULMONARY ARTERY.

Demonstration by echocardiography, angiography, MRI, or CT of aneurysm of the pulmonary artery.

ARTERIOSCLEROSIS

Sustained pulmonary arterial hypertension, regardless of the cause, may give rise to one or more of the following arteriosclerotic lesions: atherosclerosis, medial hypertrophy, or intimal fibrosis. These pathologic changes are encountered in the presence of left-to-right intracardiac shunts with large pulmonary blood flow; pulmonary parenchymal disease such as the pneumoconioses; pulmonary thromboemboli; idiopathic or primary pulmonary hypertension, alveolar hypoxia due to chronic bronchitis, hypoventilation, or exposure to high altitude; and protracted pulmonary venous hypertension such as that encountered in mitral obstruction or protracted or recurrent left ventricular failure. In mitral obstruction and left ventricular failure, the distribution of lesions is greatest in the dependent portions of the lung.

Although these arteriosclerotic lesions represent a response to increased intravascular pressure, they may themselves contribute to the levels of pressure encountered.

Atherosclerosis

Atherosclerosis of the major pulmonary arteries increases in incidence and extent with advancing years and is almost universally present, although in minor form, after the age of 40. The severity of this process appears to be independent of systemic atherosclerosis. Marked deposition of lipids and fibrous intimal plaques in the major pulmonary arteries are rare in the absence of chronic pulmonary hypertension, but in its presence, these changes become considerably more severe and widespread, especially at points of vessel division, and appear at an earlier age. Even in marked pulmonary hypertension, these lesions do not rival the corresponding disease in the aorta. They rarely ulcerate, thrombose, or lead to medial hypertrophy. They rarely produce clinical manifestations and are not detected prior to death.

Medial Hypertrophy

The earliest characteristic finding in pulmonary hypertension, regardless of cause, is muscular hyperplasia in the media of muscular arteries and arterioles. The vessels come to resemble the thick-walled pulmonary arteries and arterioles of the fetal lung. It has been suggested that smooth muscle hyperplasia is stimulated by chronic spasm in response to persistent pressure elevation, but the process may be related to endothelial injury, as in the arterial lesion. The exact nature of the stimulus causing the cells to multiply is unknown. There is evidence that this lesion is reversible if pulmonary arterial pressure falls.

THE FOLLOWING CRITERION IS REQUIRED FOR THE DIAGNOSIS OF MEDIAL HYPERTROPHY OF THE PULMONARY ARTERIES AND ARTERIOLES.

Demonstration of the characteristic histopathologic lesion on lung biopsy.

Intimal Fibrosis

Intimal fibrosis with occasional formation of longitudinal smooth muscle bundles is a more advanced response to pulmonary hypertension than is medial hypertrophy. It also occurs as the result of organization of thromboemboli. Consequently, the origin of pulmonary hypertension in some patients has been attributed to repeated episodes of thromboembolism because the dominant pulmonary arterial structural reaction is intimal fibrosis. The intimal sclerosis seen with chronically excessive pulmonary blood flow at low pressure, as in atrial septal defect or anomalous pulmonary venous connection, may also be due to the organization of small mural thrombi. Segmental intimal sclerosis in major pulmonary arteries has been described after intrauterine rubella infection, possibly in response to damage of the elastica in the media. Intimal fibrosis is believed to be reversible with subsidence of pulmonary hypertension.

THE FOLLOWING CRITERION IS REQUIRED FOR THE DIAGNOSIS OF INTIMAL FIBROSIS OF THE PULMONARY ARTERIES AND ARTERIOLES.

Demonstration of the characteristic histopathologic lesion on lung biopsy.

ARTERITIS

Inflammatory lesions of the pulmonary arteries occur as part of generalized collagen-vascular disease, including rheumatic fever, rheumatoid arthritis, dermatomyositis, polyarteritis nodosa, and Wegener's and sarcoid granulomatosis. There are differences in the intensity of necrosis, inflammation, and thrombosis in the various diseases, but the reactions are identical to those in systemic arteries in each disease.

Hypersensitivity angiitis, which also may be generalized, has a predilection for pulmonary arteries. There may be a necrotizing panarteritis, with many eosinophilic leukocytes in the exudate, rendering the reaction indistinguishable from polyarteritis nodosa. A granulomatous arteritis with eosinophilic infiltrate is characteristically found in pulmonary schistosomiasis. The ova released by adult worms in the liver, distal colon, or urinary bladder enter the inferior vena cava, usually by portal-to-systemic venous shunts, and are carried to the lungs, where their spines apparently contribute to entrapment in muscular pulmonary arteries with a luminal diameter of 100 to 1000 μ. Here, a T-cell-mediated immune response leads to granuloma formation that differs strikingly from the usual bland thrombosis accompanying other forms of emboli.

These lesions may result in increased resistance to blood flow and pulmonary hypertension.

ONE OF THE FOLLOWING CRITERIA IS REQUIRED FOR THE DIAGNOSIS OF PULMONARY ARTERITIS.

1. Demonstration of the characteristic histopathologic finding on lung biopsy.
2. Pulmonary hypertension and extrapulmonary histopathologic demonstration of a systemic disease known to produce pulmonary arteritis.

ARTERIOLITIS

Necrotizing arteriolitis is the characteristic pathologic finding in the presence of severe pulmonary hypertension from any cause. It is always superimposed on arteriolosclerosis. It consists of focal fibrinoid necrosis of the media, with an acute inflammatory response in all layers of the vessel wall. Details of cells and fibers are lost in the homogeneous eosinophilic transformation of the media. A similar reaction may occur in the muscular pulmonary arteries. Thrombi form in these areas, and the necrotic vessels may rupture. Healing of such lesions is unusual because they occur in the terminal stage of disease. There is evidence that the complex plexiform and angiomatoid lesions seen in association with this arteriolitis develop when pseudoaneurysms occur in ruptured, damaged vessels. At this stage, the disease is known as plexogenic pulmonary arteriopathy.

Arteriolitis is encountered in the presence of pulmonary hypertension so severe that the levels of pressure approach, or occasionally exceed, their counterparts in the systemic arterial circulation. These lesions in turn contribute to the level of pulmonary arterial pressure encountered. The usual disorders associated with this process are certain cases of mitral obstruction, multiple pulmonary thromboemboli, primary (idiopathic) pulmonary hypertension, and congenital lesions of the heart and great vessels associated with large pulmonary blood flow. In congenital heart disease, the direction of intracardiac shunt is from right to left at this stage. The same lesions have been associated with cirrhosis of the liver and acquired immunodeficiency disease (AIDS).

Arteriolitis does not appear to be reversible, and the level of pulmonary arterial pressure does not fall in response to either surgical correction of the underlying lesion or pulmonary vasodilating agents.

THE FOLLOWING CRITERION IS REQUIRED FOR THE DIAGNOSIS OF ARTERIOLITIS.

Demonstration of the characteristic histopathologic findings on lung biopsy.

DILATATION OF THE PULMONARY ARTERY

The main pulmonary artery and its major branches may be congenitally dilated or become dilated following an increase in pulmonary arterial pressure or flow. Dilatation distal to areas of stenosis is often present. In some instances, the cause of dilatation is unknown.

Dilatation of the pulmonary artery may produce systolic murmurs at the upper left sternal border.

**THE FOLLOWING CRITERION IS REQUIRED
FOR THE DIAGNOSIS OF DILATATION OF THE
PULMONARY ARTERY.**

**Demonstration of an increase in the transverse diameter of
the pulmonary artery by chest x-ray, echocardiogram, CT,
MRI, or angiography.**

EMBOLISM TO A PULMONARY ARTERY

The pulmonary circulation filters materials exceeding 10
to 15 μ in diameter. Emboli consisting of bland or infected
thrombi, bone marrow, tumor cells, amniotic fluid, fat,
parasites, injected foreign materials, and air may lodge
in the pulmonary arterioles or arteries, depending on
their size. Deep venous thrombosis is the cause of over 90
percent of pulmonary embolism. Circulatory stasis; hy-
percoagulable states, in particular those due to deficiency of antithrombin III, protein C, and protein S; carcinoma; inflammatory diseases of the pelvic organs and
lower extremities; mural thrombosis; tumors; and infective endocarditis of the right heart are frequent causes.
The clinical picture in pulmonary arterial embolism is
variable, ranging from syncope, vascular collapse, and
sudden death following massive occlusion to the insidious
development of severe pulmonary hypertension and refractory right ventricular failure following repeated show-
ers of small emboli.

The sudden onset of unexplained dyspnea or tachypnea
is the most frequent symptom of pulmonary emboli, while
pleuritic chest pain, hemoptysis, pleural effusion, and
pleural friction rub are present only when infarction
has occurred. The ECG is generally normal. With large
embolism, it can show right bundle branch block; right
deviation of the electrical axis; tall, peaked P waves
in leads II, III, and aVF; a deep S in lead I; and a
Q3–T3 pattern. Most of these findings are transitory.
Atrial arrhythmias and precordial T-wave inversion may
occur.

Chest x-rays may be normal or show evidence of local
infarction, local reduced vascular filling, central pulmonary arterial distention, or right ventricular enlargement. The arterial PO_2 may be low, but this is an incon-
stant finding. Elevation of pulmonary arterial pressure
may be detected by right heart catheterization or Doppler
echocardiography. Echocardiography may also show right
heart dilatation.

ONE OF THE FOLLOWING CRITERIA IS REQUIRED FOR THE DIAGNOSIS OF EMBOLISM TO A PULMONARY ARTERY.

Initial

Unexplained dyspnea or tachypnea in the presence of clinical, x-ray, or ECG evidence of pulmonary embolism.

Definitive

1. **The presence of typical filling defects on pulmonary angiography.**
2. **A radionuclide lung scan showing ventilation-perfusion mismatch in a pattern suggesting embolization with high positive predictive accuracy.**

THROMBOSIS OF A PULMONARY ARTERY

Primary thrombosis in the pulmonary arteries is rare and may indicate defects in the intrinsic clotting mechanism or a tendency of the red blood cells to agglutinate (as occurs in sickle cell anemia or polycythemia). It can also result from chest trauma or from impingement and narrowing of vessels associated with tumors. Thrombi are found frequently in cases of cyanotic congenital heart disease, such as tetralogy of Fallot, because pulmonary blood flow is reduced, and the polycythemic response to hypoxemia leads to increased blood viscosity. Because the conditions under which thrombosis is likely to occur also predispose to embolism, and since the clinical features of both processes may be indistinguishable, it is often difficult, if not impossible, to ascertain on clinical grounds whether intravascular thrombi are local or embolic in origin.

THERE ARE NO RELIABLE CLINICAL CRITERIA TO DIFFERENTIATE BETWEEN PULMONARY EMBOLISM AND THROMBOSIS IN SITU OF A PULMONARY ARTERY.

SCLEROSIS OF PULMONARY VEINS

Obliterative sclerosis of small intrapulmonary veins can occur without evidence of antecedent inflammation or other pulmonary parenchymal lesions. The walls of the veins are the site of fibrosis, and the lumina are severely narrowed or occluded. Secondary changes in the lung are indistinguishable either from those due to extrinsic compression of pulmonary veins by scarring or tumor or from those due to mitral obstruction.

The clinical syndrome is a nonspecific one of progressive pulmonary congestion in the absence of other abnormalities known to be capable of producing pulmonary venous hypertension. Diagnosis prior to death is difficult and unusual.

THE FOLLOWING CRITERION IS REQUIRED FOR THE DIAGNOSIS OF SCLEROSIS OF PULMONARY VEINS.
Lung biopsy that demonstrates characteristic lesions of the intrapulmonary veins.

Diseases of the Coronary Arteries

ARTERITIS

Infective

Infective arteritis results most commonly from septic emboli in infective endocarditis and more rarely by direct extension from contiguous suppurative processes such as tuberculous pericarditis. The inflammation can spread to all coats of the artery and lead to myocardial infarction, mycotic aneurysms, or myocardial abscesses. The diagnosis is rarely made before death, since the primary disease usually dominates the clinical picture.

NO RELIABLE CRITERIA EXIST FOR THE DIAGNOSIS OF INFECTIVE ARTERITIS.

Polyarteritis Nodosa

The outstanding features of arteritis due to polyarteritis nodosa are inflammation of all layers of the coronary arteries, with conspicuous medial and adventitial involvement and perivascular infiltration. Necrosis of the wall may result in the formation of aneurysms or rupture of a vessel. Thrombosis or obliteration of the lumen by scar formation can result in small areas of myocardial infarction. Ventricular enlargement and failure may be secondary to coronary arteritis or hypertension, which is a frequent manifestation of vascular involvement elsewhere, especially in the kidney. Arteritis secondary to lupus erythematosus may be identical to that seen in polyarteritis nodosa. Kawasaki disease in infants and young children may also cause coronary artery lesions that are indistinguishable from polyarteritis nodosa, and it may lead to coronary aneurysms or myocardial infarction.

THE CRITERIA REQUIRED FOR THE DIAGNOSIS OF POLYARTERITIS NODOSA ARE ON PAGE 27.

ATHEROSCLEROSIS

Atherosclerosis of the coronary arteries is a progressive disorder of the vascular wall that results in the narrowing of the lumen by intimal plaques and loss of normal vasomotor control. The initiating event is injury to the endothelium that opens it to abnormal communication with both the cells of blood on the luminal side and the smooth muscle cells of the media on the abluminal side. Blood monocytes are induced to adhere to the endothelium, invade the potential subendothelial space within the intima, reside there, proliferate, and ingest lipid, whereby they become foam cells. The interaction of "activated" endothelial cells with these monocyte-derived macrophages, T-lymphocytes, and platelets invokes an inflammatory response that attracts medial smooth muscle cells to migrate through the internal elastic lamina and induces them to proliferate in the intima. The cells may be converted from the contractile to the synthetic phenotype and induced to secrete abnormally large amounts of matrix macromolecules. The cytokines and growth factors produced by all of the cells listed act in paracrine and autocrine fashion to sustain the development of the lesion. If the injurious stimuli are removed, the lesions may regress almost completely.

The factors that can injure the endothelium to induce atherosclerosis are many. Cholesterol, in particular the form included in oxidized low-density lipoprotein (LDL), is estimated to account for 50 percent of atherosclerosis. Other prominent damaging molecules and agents include hypertension, the products of cigarette smoke including tobacco glycoproteins, hyperglycemia both directly and through the formation of sugar-protein adducts called advanced glycation end products, and possibly infection with the herpes and cytomegalovirus agents in susceptible individuals.

The earliest lesions may be seen at birth or in childhood, are called "fatty streaks," and consist of bloated foam cells residing just under the endothelium. In the progression of this lesion, two simultaneous processes are opposed: the intimal lesions expand, tending to narrow the lumen, and the artery wall dilates, tending to maintain the lumen. The predominance of the former leads to progressive obliteration of the vessel lumen and the various syndromes of myocardial ischemia. While the earliest lesion may consist of little more than foam cells, the mature lesion of adulthood is far more complex. This stage is referred to as a "fibrous plaque" and in addition to macrophages includes variable quantities of smooth muscle cells (both of which may be filled with cholesterol and cholesteryl esters) and T-lymphocytes, all embedded in a dense extracellular matrix of proteoglycans, collagen, and elastic fibers with extracellular lipid including cholesterol crystals deposited in a lipid core. Mural platelet thrombi cover various portions of the lesion at various times. While the fatty streak is yellow, flat, and nonprotruding, the fibrous plaque is white and protrudes into the lumen. Fraying, fragmentation, and rupture of the internal elastic lamina may occur, and the media underlying the intimal mass may thin due to atrophy and fibrous replacement. Because of the enhanced oxygen needs of the thickened wall, or because of the overabundance of angiogenic factors such as basic fibroblast growth factor (bFGF), the adventitial cuff external to sites of atherosclerosis may contain a rich and abnormally fragile capillary plexus of vasa vasorum.

Coronary angiography, coronary fiberoptic angioscopy, and intravascular echocardiography in vivo and serial sectioning post mortem have revealed the topography and dimensions of the lesions and allowed their correlation with the ischemic syndromes. The advanced disease is characterized by diffuse involvement along the entire course of the epicardial arteries. The majority of lesions are eccentric, irregularly protruding into the lumen as lumps arising from a diseased, thickened intima. When the process obliterates approximately 75 percent of the cross-sectional area, coronary vasodilatory flow reserve is exhausted and any increase in myocardial demand or further reduction in arterial supply will result in myocardial ischemia. Lesions of this size with relatively intact and smooth surfaces result in the "stable" ischemic syndromes: exertional angina and silent myocardial ischemia. When large or small lesions fissure or ulcerate, they develop varying amounts of intramural thrombus, which may extend into the remaining lumen, potentially resulting in totally occlusive thrombosis. Thus, disrupted plaques of varying mass result in the "unstable" ischemic syndromes: unstable angina and more frequent silent ischemia, myocardial infarction, and sudden death. The sequelae of plaque disruption and occlusive thrombosis are dependent in part on whether a collateral circulation has developed, the extent of protection being approximately related to the extent of blood flow distal to the site of disruption. Calcification is common.

ONE OF THE FOLLOWING CRITERIA IS REQUIRED FOR THE DIAGNOSIS OF ATHEROSCLEROSIS OF THE CORONARY ARTERIES.

Initial

Classic anginal syndrome in the absence of other known cause.

Definitive

1. **Demonstration by coronary angiography, angioscopy, intravascular echocardiogram, CT scan, or MRI of obstructive coronary disease.**
2. **Anginal syndrome in the presence of evidence of reversible myocardial ischemia by a noninvasive method.**

EMBOLISM TO A CORONARY ARTERY

Embolism to a coronary artery occurs most commonly in the course of infective endocarditis. Emboli can also originate from thrombi on prosthetic valves or components of these valves, from mural thrombi on the left side of the heart, or from valve fragments released from mitral or aortic valves during an intervention. Coronary artery catheterization, angioplasty, atherectomy, and thrombolysis may result in embolism.

Emboli can produce myocardial infarction or myocardial abscesses. The anterior descending branch of the left coronary is the vessel involved most frequently.

THE FOLLOWING CRITERIA ARE REQUIRED FOR THE DIAGNOSIS OF EMBOLISM TO A CORONARY ARTERY.

Myocardial infarction in the presence of infective endocarditis, intravascular or intra-aortic procedure, or evidence by imaging techniques of other ventricular source, aortic or mitral prosthesis, or homograft.

STENOSIS OF A CORONARY ORIFICE

Stenosis of a coronary orifice is now most often the result of atherosclerosis, whereas previously syphilitic aortitis was the most common cause. Trauma during cardiac surgery and a dissecting hematoma of the aorta can also result in compression of the coronary arteries at their origin.

Anginal syndrome, myocardial fibrosis, and myocardial infarction can result from these lesions. These manifestations of coronary insufficiency are most frequently due to coronary atherosclerosis or aortic valvular lesions; hence the diagnosis of coronary ostial stenosis requires arteriographic demonstration.

THE FOLLOWING CRITERION IS REQUIRED FOR THE DIAGNOSIS OF STENOSIS OF A CORONARY ORIFICE.

Angiographic evidence of coronary ostial stenosis.

Diseases of the Endocardium and Valves

CALCIFICATION OF THE MITRAL ANNULUS

The zone of attachment of the mitral valve, and occasionally that of the aortic valve, marks the site of a fibrocalcific deposit that is frequent in older persons. Mitral annular calcification is frequently associated with this. The deposits of calcium are variable in extent and mainly involve the junctional myocardium immediately below the valve annulus. These lesions usually do not produce obstruction or regurgitation and are not related to antecedent endocarditis. The valves are usually not involved, or only slightly so at their base, and valvular function usually remains undisturbed. However, the calcification occasionally may extend into the mitral leaflets and produce mitral regurgitation. In rare instances the calcific deposits may affect the conduction system; they may ulcerate, producing emboli, or serve as a nidus for endocarditis.

The characteristic finding is that of annular calcification detected by echocardiography, x-ray, or other imaging technique.

THE FOLLOWING CRITERION IS REQUIRED FOR THE DIAGNOSIS OF CALCIFICATION OF THE MITRAL ANNULUS.

Echocardiographic or other evidence of calcium between the left atrium and left ventricle.

ENDOCARDIAL FIBROELASTOSIS

Endocardial fibroelastosis is characterized by diffuse thickening of the endocardium, primarily of the left ventricle, giving it a milky-white appearance and relatively smooth lining. In addition to left ventricular involvement, the left atrium is frequently affected; although the endocardium of the right ventricle may show some thickening, it is always less prominent than on the left. There is a characteristic hyperplasia of fibroelastic tissue in and beneath the endocardium, with extension of fibrous bands into the myocardium.

The etiology and pathogenesis of endocardial fibroelastosis as an isolated phenomenon are unknown. Mumps virus infection in utero has been implicated. It may be present at birth and cause death from left ventricular failure in infancy. The occurrence of patchy areas of endocardial thickening in association with congenital malformations, notably those involving left-sided valves (aortic stenosis or atresia, mitral stenosis), and coarctation of the aorta is considered a "secondary" reaction to hemodynamic stress and injury.

The clinical picture of endocardial fibroelastosis is frequently that of an infant who fails to thrive and manifests signs of progressive left ventricular failure. Heart murmurs are inconspicuous, although an apical systolic murmur may occasionally reflect mitral regurgitation. The chest x-ray usually shows marked cardiac enlargement, and the ECG primarily reflects left ventricular enlargement.

The diagnosis is made with certainty only at necropsy or with endocardial biopsy. However, endocardial fibroelastosis may be considered to be present if in such clinical situations the following are excluded: active myocarditis, glycogen storage disease, and cardiovascular malformations, notably anomalous origin of the left coronary artery from the pulmonary artery. Endocardial fibroelastosis may rarely occur or persist in young adults and cause a restrictive cardiomyopathy. In older individuals, localized fibroelastosis may be secondary to myocardial infarction.

THE FOLLOWING CRITERION IS REQUIRED FOR THE DIAGNOSIS OF ENDOCARDIAL FIBROELASTOSIS.

Histopathologic evidence of endocardial fibroelastosis on endomyocardial biopsy.

ENDOCARDIAL FIBROSIS (ENDOMYOCARDIAL FIBROSIS)

This lesion is characterized by extensive endocardial and subendocardial fibrosis. The opaque, milky-white endocardium differs from that of endocardial fibroelastosis in that there is no increase in elastic tissue. The sclerosing process frequently extends to the inner myocardium. It is most common in Africa but has also been described in other parts of the world. The fibrosis tends to involve the inflow surface of the left ventricle, particularly toward the apex. It may extend upward to involve the posterior mitral valve, causing mitral regurgitation.

While focal degrees of endocardial thickening may be seen in other patients with hypertrophy of the heart of unknown cause, it is never so extensive as that found with endocardial fibrosis. The same pathologic findings are noted at the end-stage of the hypereosinophilic syndrome.

Patients with endocardial fibrosis may have an enlarged heart and evidence of ventricular failure. The diagnosis is rarely made prior to death.

THE FOLLOWING CRITERION IS REQUIRED FOR THE DIAGNOSIS OF ENDOCARDIAL FIBROSIS (ENDOMYOCARDIAL FIBROSIS).

Histopathologic evidence of endocardial fibrosis on endo-myocardial biopsy.

ENDOCARDITIS

Infective Endocarditis

A wide variety of bacteria may cause endocarditis. The majority of cases are caused by *Streptococcus viridans* and are seen in patients with valves previously damaged by rheumatic fever or deformed by congenital defects. Infection can also occur on prosthetic valves and with congenital anomalies such as patent ductus arteriosus and ventricular septal defect. Other bacteria known to cause infection include staphylococcus, pneumococcus, beta-hemolytic streptococcus, *Haemophilus influenzae*, meningococcus, and salmonella. These often cause infection of previously normal valves, especially in debilitated patients. Fungi can also be the cause of infection, particularly in intravenous drug addicts, and the responsible organism is usually *Candida albicans*.

The valves are the site of a destructive process with superimposed vegetations. The vegetations are located principally on the contact surfaces of the valves but may extend to contiguous mural endocardial surfaces, chordae tendineae, and papillary muscles. The left side of the heart is preponderantly involved, although right-sided endocarditis is common in drug addicts.

The vegetations consist of masses of fibrin with enmeshed red cells. Bacteria grow on the surface and are entrapped within the friable fibrin mass. The underlying valve or mural endocardium is ulcerated, necrotic, and variably invaded by polymorphonuclear leukocytes and may be the site of frank abscess formation. An acute inflammatory reaction may be seen throughout the involved valve. As the infection is prolonged, either because of the nature of the infecting organism or because of antibiotic therapy, the lesion may contain large numbers of mononuclear cells. Evidences of repair are seen in the proliferation of connective tissue in the valve and in the growth of granulation tissue into the vegetation itself. With control of the infection, the vegetations undergo fibrosis, hyalinization, and often calcification, forming irregular nodular masses and deforming the valve.

Serious consequences of the active stages include destruction of a portion of the valve leaflet, perforation or aneurysm of a leaflet, rupture of the chordae tendineae, annular or myocardial abscess, and embolization. If the patient survives to the healed stage, such defects may be the cause of continuing hemodynamic disability.

The clinical picture is characterized by fever, anemia, splenomegaly, new or changing murmurs, and embolic phenomena involving the skin, mucous membrane, brain, spleen, kidneys, and extremities. Right-sided endocarditis is frequently associated with septic emboli to the lungs; this can occur in narcotic addicts. Shaking chills, sweating, clubbing, and arthralgias are common. Osler's nodes, Janeway lesions, and splinter hemorrhages, although well-known as associated findings, are not often seen today. With severe valvular damage, signs and symptoms of valvular regurgitation may become prominent, and ventricular failure may develop abruptly. In many patients, valvular vegetations may be demonstrable by echocardiography, especially transesophageal echocardiography.

THE CRITERIA REQUIRED FOR THE DIAGNOSIS OF INFECTIVE ENDOCARDITIS AND VALVULAR VEGETATIONS ARE ON PAGES 19 AND 90.

Lupus Valvulitis (Atypical Verrucous Endocarditis)

Valvulitis can occur in association with systemic lupus erythematosus. The lesions may vary in size from small verrucae to large vegetations and consist of granular fibrinous masses in which red and white blood cells are enmeshed. When present, hematoxylin bodies provide a distinctive feature of the lesion. Infiltration with macrophages and lymphocytes is present at the bases of the fibrinous masses, and occasionally there are plasma cells and evidence of organization. The masses are usually located on the ventricular aspect of the valves and extend in some cases onto the neighboring mural endocardium. The mitral and tricuspid valves are most often involved. Perforation of the valve and rupture of the chordae tendineae have not been described with the lesion.

These lesions rarely produce valvular obstruction or regurgitation and hence are not recognized clinically. However, superimposition of infective endocarditis is not unusual and may produce significant deformity of the valves.

THE CRITERIA REQUIRED FOR THE DIAGNOSIS OF LUPUS VALVULITIS ARE ON PAGE 41.

Nonbacterial Thrombotic Endocarditis (Marantic Endocarditis, Terminal Endocarditis)

Nonbacterial thrombotic endocarditis is seen most frequently in patients with chronic wasting diseases such as malignant tumors with metastases or severe malnutrition. The origin of the lesion is not clear. The lesion consists of firm, gray, yellow, or pink flat or raised nodules along the line of closure of the mitral valve and occasionally of the aortic valve. The lesions are larger than rheumatic verrucae and occasionally may be seen as large polypoid or pedunculated vegetations. The underlying valves may show some degenerative change. The mural endocardium and the chordae tendineae are usually not involved. The vegetations consist largely of agglutinated platelets and an admixture of red blood cells and fibrin, often with some evidence of organization at the periphery. Polymorphonuclear leukocytes are rarely found in these lesions, and bacteria are not present. However, these vegetations may become infected with bacteria, leading to valvular endocarditis. Embolic phenomena, particularly cerebral, occasionally occur with this type of endocarditis. These lesions may occasionally be demonstrated by echocardiography. The lesion is rarely recognized prior to death.

THE FOLLOWING CRITERIA ARE REQUIRED FOR THE DIAGNOSIS OF NONBACTERIAL THROMBOTIC ENDOCARDITIS.

Sterile valvular vegetations demonstrable by echocardiography or embolic phenomena in patients with malignant or other chronic wasting diseases.

Rheumatic Valvulitis and Endocarditis

During the acute phase of rheumatic heart disease, tiny, wartlike nodules (verrucae), 1 to 3 mm in size, occur along the line of closure of the valvular leaflets. These are firm and occur singly, in clusters, or in a continuous chain. Being strongly adherent, they do not easily become emboli. The mitral valve is most frequently affected, followed closely in frequency by the aortic valve. The tricuspid valve is involved less often and less severely, and the pulmonic valve is affected only rarely. Verrucae may be present along the chordae tendineae, which become swollen and fused. The affected leaflets are edematous and often adhere to each other.

The vegetations consist of small platelet and fibrin thrombi deposited on damaged proliferated endocardial cells. The underlying valvular tissue is edematous and contains a cellular infiltrate. The verrucae undergo organization, with an ingrowth of connective tissue cells, and the surface becomes covered by a smooth layer of endothelium. Within the leaflet and in the valve ring there is also a concomitant diffuse inflammatory process characterized by edema, an ingrowth of capillaries, the presence of polymorphonuclear cells, and occasionally Aschoff's bodies. Subsidence of this interstitial valvulitis is followed by an increase in connective tissue and an ingrowth of new blood vessels.

The acute insult to the valves, with or without recurrent attacks of rheumatic carditis, leads to progressive scarring and deformity. The leaflets become fused, retracted, thickened, vascularized, and calcified. The edges of the aortic valve cusps become thickened and rolled; the fusion of the cusps may be so extensive that the valve assumes a bicuspid appearance. The chordae tendineae also become fused, thickened, and shortened, thus adding to the mechanical deformity of the valve. At this stage, the valves contain masses of hyaline fibrous tissue, numerous thick-walled blood vessels, irregular collections of calcium, and foci of lymphocytes and monocytes. These structural alterations in the leaflet lead to stenosis of the orifice and incompetence of the valve and to valvular obstruction or regurgitation, or both.

Some thickening and vascularization of the mitral valve, slight fusion and thickening of the chordae tendineae, and slight fusion of the commissures of the cusps of the aortic valve are not infrequent incidental necropsy findings in older patients. Whether they are all due to rheumatic inflammation or whether other disease processes are implicated is not clear.

The endocardium of the left atrium just above the posterior leaflet of the mitral valve is often the site of a zone of fibrinoid necrosis with associated Aschoff's cells. Aschoff's bodies are frequently observed in the endocardium of atrial appendages and ventricular endocardium.

THE CRITERIA REQUIRED FOR THE DIAGNOSIS OF RHEUMATIC VALVULITIS ARE ON PAGE 36.

Rheumatoid Valvulitis

The unusual but specific form of rheumatoid involvement of valves is the presence of granulomas. These have central areas of fibrinoid necrosis surrounded by palisaded rows of macrophages and are identical to the subcutaneous rheumatoid nodule. They are usually accompanied by similar granulomatous involvement of pericardium and pleura.

The valvular lesions rarely produce valvular obstruction or regurgitation and hence are not recognized clinically.

THE CRITERIA REQUIRED FOR THE DIAGNOSIS OF RHEUMATOID VALVULITIS ARE ON PAGE 37.

FIBROMYXOMATOUS DEGENERATION OF A VALVE (MUCOID DEGENERATION)

Fibromyxomatous degeneration of the mitral and aortic valves may lead to regurgitation. The central skeleton of fibrous tissue is transformed into a loose accumulation of connective-tissue ground substance, and the outer layers of the leaflets are secondarily thickened by increases in collagen and elastic fibers. Involvement of the annulus may lead to dilatation of the orifice. Both leaflets of the mitral valve may be thickened and enlarged and balloon into the left atrium. Usually, the posterior leaflet is more seriously affected; the anterior leaflet is sometimes spared entirely. The histologic appearance is similar to that in patients with Marfan's syndrome, but other stigmata of that syndrome may be absent. The diseased valves may be the seat of superimposed infective or nonbacterial thrombotic endocarditis. The attenuated or elongated chordae tendineae contribute to valvular malfunction. They may rupture, with abrupt appearance of severe mitral regurgitation. Fibromyxomatous degeneration is the most common cause of the mitral valve prolapse syndrome.

THE FOLLOWING CRITERION IS REQUIRED FOR THE DIAGNOSIS OF FIBROMYXOMATOUS DEGENERATION OF A VALVE.

Histologic evidence of fibromyxomatous change at operation or evidence for congenital or familial mitral valve prolapse.

INTRACARDIAC THROMBOSIS (ENDOCARDIAL THROMBOSIS)

Intracardiac thrombosis may result from inflammation, injury, necrosis and fibrosis, and slowing and abnormal eddying of the bloodstream. Thrombi may form on the endocardium of any of the cardiac chambers and are especially frequent in the atrial appendages. They may be the source of systemic or pulmonary emboli.

Thrombi are often found in the atrial appendages, most often associated with atrial dilatation, atrial fibrillation, and ventricular failure. They are best detected by transesophageal echocardiography and are often preceded or accompanied by distinctive, swirling, intra-atrial echoes ("smoke"). Ball, or globoid, thrombi occasionally lie free in the atrial chambers or may be attached to the atrioventricular orifices. They are most often found in association with obstruction of the mitral or tricuspid valves.

In the ventricles, the majority of mural thrombi form as complications of myocardial infarction, particularly with ventricular failure. Although they are found predominantly in the left ventricle, they may involve both sides of the interventricular septum. In ventricular aneurysms incidental to myocardial infarction, mural thrombosis is common. The large thrombi are attached at their bases and are friable and laminated and may be organized. Thrombosis of the ventricles is also seen in heart disease due to alcoholism or dilated cardiomyopathy.

Mural thrombi may be the source of systemic or pulmonary emboli. Intracardiac thrombi may be demonstrated by contrast angiography, transthoracic and especially transesophageal echocardiography, CT, and MRI.

ONE OF THE FOLLOWING CRITERIA IS REQUIRED FOR THE DIAGNOSIS OF INTRACARDIAC THROMBOSIS.

Initial

Evidence of systemic embolization in the presence of myocardial infarction, atrial fibrillation, intermittent valvular obstruction, or dilated cardiomyopathy.

Definitive

Evidence of an intracardiac mass using echocardiography (especially transesophageal echocardiography), CT, MRI, or contrast angiography. Differentiation of tumor from thrombus may require multiple imaging techniques.

NEOPLASM OF THE ENDOCARDIUM

Myxoma

Myxomas of the endocardium are almost invariably benign and are usually single. Their precise cellular origin is unknown. They occur most frequently in the atria, predominantly on the left, and their location determines their hemodynamic effects. Left atrial myxomas, particularly if they are pedunculated, can produce intermittent obstruction of the mitral orifice. Obstruction of venous flow into the left atrium may also cause pulmonary hypertension. Sudden movement of the tumor mass with atrial systole can cause an audible early diastolic sound. Myxomas in the right atrium can produce intermittent obstruction of the tricuspid orifice. Similarly, myxomas arising in the ventricles can produce intermittent obstruction to outflow from the right or left ventricle. Such intermittent obstruction can cause the sudden onset of severe hemodynamic abnormalities in patients who have no antecedent history of heart disease, and the signs and symptoms may be unique in their alterations with changes in body position.

Right-sided myxomas can produce emboli to the pulmonary arteries and left-sided myxomas, emboli to the peripheral arteries. In addition, the presence of the tumor mass itself can cause fever, weight loss, alterations in serum globulins, and an anemia that is sometimes hemolytic.

Myxomas are most frequently detected by echocardiography. Other imaging techniques such as CT, MRI, and contrast angiography may also be used.

Papillary Fibroma (Papilloma)

Papillary fibromas of the heart valves are rare lesions that can produce murmurs and intermittent or fixed obstruction of the valve orifices. The findings, as with myxomas, depend on the anatomic location, size, and shape of the masses, which may arise from thrombus material rather than from valvular tissues. Although previously classified as neoplasms, they are now considered to be non-neoplastic and secondary to organization of thrombi on the surface of a valve or the mural endocardium.

ONE OF THE FOLLOWING CRITERIA IS REQUIRED FOR THE DIAGNOSIS OF NEOPLASM OF THE ENDOCARDIUM.

1. **Demonstration by echocardiography, CT, MRI, or contrast angiography of an intracavitary tumor mass.**
2. **Histologic demonstration of myxomatous tissue in an embolus removed from a peripheral artery.**
3. **Demonstration of tumor tissue removed from the endocardium.**

RUPTURE OF CHORDAE TENDINEAE

Rupture of chordae tendineae is most often spontaneous. It may also occur as a result of nonpenetrating crushing injury, infective endocarditis, rheumatic valvulitis, or fibromyxomatous degeneration.

The physiologic consequence of rupture of the chordeae tendineae depends on the number and type of chordae that are torn. When there is significant impairment of valve support during systole, valvular regurgitation results, which may lead to rapid development of pulmonary or systemic congestion. With rupture of a single cord, the only finding may be a systolic murmur or the characteristic echocardiographic abnormality.

While the sudden appearance of mitral or tricuspid regurgitation following trauma or occurring during the course of infective endocarditis or rheumatic valvulitis suggests rupture of the chordae tendineae, tear or perforation of a valve or detachment of a papillary muscle may be associated with the same findings.

THE FOLLOWING CRITERION IS REQUIRED FOR THE DIAGNOSIS OF RUPTURE OF CHORDAE TENDINEAE.

Demonstration of ruptured chordea tendineae by echocardiography or at operation.

VALVULAR DEFORMITY (WITH OR WITHOUT STENOSIS OR REGURGITATION)

This section describes anatomic deformities of the heart valves that can be identified clinically and pathologically. These deformities may or may not result in physiologic abnormalities. Additional descriptions of the physiologic consequences of these deformities on blood flow across the valves and on physical signs are given later in this section (in connection with congenital diseases of the cardiac valves) and in Section 3.

Valvular deformities can range from mild fibrosis and thickening to severe abnormalities of valve structure that cause severe valvular dysfunction (stenosis and insufficiency). Deformities can be congenital or can result from degenerative disease, infectious endocarditis, rheumatic fever, syphilis, or trauma, can be chemically caused as in carcinoid heart disease, or can arise as a primary abnormality in a previously normal valve. Progression of the abnormality in a valve primarily damaged by inflammation or congenital abnormality may be secondary to chronic hemodynamic trauma caused by blood turbulence or jet impact.

Inflammation of a valve in single or recurring episodes leads to healing with proliferation of granulation tissue, which matures to produce dense, collagenized scar tissue. Thick-walled small arteries extend into the valve substance from the base of the valve. Such neovascularization is particularly prominent in rheumatic heart disease. The dense fibrous tissue in a scarred valve interrupts and replaces the normal collagen and elastic tissue skeleton of the valve. Inflammation with subsequent scarring leads to fusion of the commissures of the atrioventricular valves. Chordae tendineae are shortened, thickened, and fused. Scarring with or without calcification produces a relatively rigid, unyielding valve, with consequent disturbances in valve function producing stenosis and regurgitation. Frank perforation of a valve may occur during infective endocarditis. Similarly, a defect at the free edge and lie of closure of a valve in the form of irregular scalloping or extensive erosion may be seen after infection and may result in abnormalities of valve closure.

Echocardiographic studies are the most effective means for the early detection and evaluation of valvular deformities. Angiography with contrast medium can also demonstrate valvular deformities and the associated stenosis or insufficiency. When valvular deformity is included in the Anatomic Cardiac Diagnosis, the type of deformity should be specified (e.g., calcified, immobile mitral leaflets; ruptured chordae tendineae with flail leaflet; myxomatous degeneration). The terms *stenosis* and *regurgitation* denote functional consequences of the anatomic abnormality and should be used in the Physiologic Cardiac Diagnosis.

Aortic Valve Deformity Causing Stenosis

In older persons without a history of rheumatic fever, the aortic cusps may become sclerotic and calcified, resulting in rigidity and deformity. Among patients under the age of 70, the commonest predisposing cause is a congenitally bicuspid or monocuspid valve; these are subjected to abnormal hemodynamic stresses of their structure. In patients over 70, aortic stenosis most frequently develops in normally tricuspid valves, which can become severely deformed by fibrosis and calcification. Rheumatic fever is now a less common cause of aortic stenosis.

Deformities of the aortic valve may be heralded by systolic murmurs at the cardiac base and by echocardiographic evidence for mild thickening of the valve cusps, sometimes with calcification, before there is evidence for significant limitation in motion of the leaflets or evidence for stenosis or regurgitation as detected by Doppler echocardiographic studies or by cardiac catheterization and use of contrast agents. Repeated examinations over the years may demonstrate slow progression of the valve deformity, with increased thickening and calcification of the cusps and restriction of valve opening. Doppler studies demonstrate an increased flow velocity across the valve indicating a transvalvular pressure gradient. Valve area may be calculated from the "law of continuity," using in the calculation measured flow velocities in the aortic root and left ventricular output tract and the measured area of the left ventricular outflow tract. Prolapse and flail movement of valve cusps are also best demonstrated by echocardiography. Angiography with contrast medium can show a valve that bulges convexly into the aorta during systole, forming a dome, with decreased mobility and an eccentric orifice. A narrow jet of contrast medium may be seen to enter the aorta during systole. (See also pages 157–159 and 221.)

Prosthetic tissue valves in the aortic position may become fibrotic and calcified with time, leading to rigid cusps, a narrowed opening during systole, and aortic stenosis.

THE FOLLOWING CRITERIA ARE REQUIRED FOR THE DIAGNOSIS OF AORTIC VALVE DEFORMITY WITH OR WITHOUT AORTIC STENOSIS.

Initial

The characteristic systolic murmur.

Definitive

1. **Evidence for thickening, calcification, or other deformity of the valve cusps, or impaired cusp excursion during the cardiac cycle as detected by echocardiography, angiocardiography, or other imaging techniques, or**
2. **Evidence by echocardiography or other imaging techniques for valve deformity causing a decrease in the valve orifice during systole, with or without evidence for valve obstruction (stenosis) by Doppler echocardiography or hemodynamic measurement.**

Aortic Valve Deformity Causing Regurgitation

Aortic valve deformity causing aortic regurgitation most commonly results from myxomatous degeneration of the valve. In older individuals, the same degenerative process described as a cause of aortic stenosis may be accompanied by aortic regurgitation due to failure of the thickened immobile cusps to coapt effectively during diastole. Mild degrees of aortic regurgitation may be detected in a large proportion of elderly individuals by sensitive Doppler flow methods, suggesting that some fibrosis and retraction of aortic valve cusps may be a frequent concomitant of aging. (See also pages 155 and 223.)

Rheumatic fever is a less common cause of aortic deformity leading to aortic regurgitation, as is rheumatoid arthritis with involvement of the valve leaflets or spondylitis deformans, which can cause widening of the aortic root. Among patients with Marfan's syndrome, there may be marked prolapse of one or more aortic leaflets; widening of the aortic ring, often with aneurysms of the aortic root, may lead to failure of the leaflets to coapt in diastole. Either process can lead to aortic regurgitation. Similar widening of the aortic root may be caused by long-standing arterial hypertension, but an association with aortic regurgitation is less frequent. Prosthetic tissue valves in the aortic position can become deformed by fibrosis and shrinkage, causing aortic regurgitation.

THE FOLLOWING CRITERIA ARE REQUIRED FOR THE DIAGNOSIS OF AORTIC VALVE DEFORMITY CAUSING REGURGITATION.

Initial

The characteristic diastolic murmur.

Definitive

Echocardiographic evidence for valve thickening, calcification, or shrinkage leading to a demonstrable failure of the leaflets to coapt fully in diastole, with evidence for regurgitation by Doppler flow studies or contrast angiography.

Mitral Valve Deformity Causing Stenosis

Rheumatic fever remains the principal cause of mitral valve deformity leading to stenosis. Echocardiography can show early thickening, calcification, and diminished excursion of the valve leaflets, often accompanied by thickening and shortening of chordae tendineae. As these deformations progress, the effective orifice of the valve during diastole decreases. M-mode echocardiography shows anterior movement of the posterior leaflet during diastole and slow diastolic closure of the valve (diminished E to F slope). On two-dimensional study there is fusion of the commissures, anterior bowing of the anterior leaflet during diastole, and a diminished valve area. Doppler examination shows increased velocity of flow across the mitral valve during diastole and a pressure gradient. The mitral valve orifice area may be expressed as a function of decay of the pressure gradient across the valve (prolonged pressure half-time). Transesophageal echocardiography may be necessary for precise evaluation of deformities of the mitral leaflets and the valve infrastructure. As deformation proceeds, the evidence for mitral stenosis increases, as reflected in auscultatory, Doppler echocardiographic, and hemodynamic studies. Contrast ventriculography can show dome-shaped, anterior bulging of the mitral valve into the ventricle during diastole, with a jet of diastolic flow that is diminished in size. Prosthetic tissue valves in the mitral position may become stenotic as a result of fibrosis and calcification. (See also pages 162 and 224.)

THE FOLLOWING CRITERIA ARE REQUIRED FOR THE DIAGNOSIS OF MITRAL VALVE DEFORMITY WITH OR WITHOUT STENOSIS.

Initial

The characteristic diastolic murmur.

Definitive

1. **Echocardiographic evidence for thickening, deformity, and calcification of the mitral leaflets with any reduction in their ability to separate at their commissures during diastole, but no hemodynamic evidence for valvular stenosis, or**
2. **Echocardiographic evidence of deformity of the mitral valve leaflets and infrastructure sufficient to limit opening of the mitral orifice during diastole, with significant mitral stenosis evident by Doppler echocardiographic or hemodynamic measurement.**

Mitral Valve Deformity Causing Regurgitation

Mitral deformity that can result in mitral regurgitation is most commonly due to myxomatous degeneration, which may also cause mitral valve prolapse. Valve deformity due to rheumatic fever produces a combination of mitral stenosis and regurgitation when scarred or shrunken leaflets are unable to open and close normally because of rigidity or associated abnormalities of chordae tendineae. Mild degrees of mitral valve deformity consisting of thickening and calcification are common in individuals who show no other clinical abnormalities or may be associated with systolic regurgitant murmurs and minimal degrees of regurgitation detected by Doppler echocardiographic studies.

Rupture of chordae tendineae can occur without obvious cause or can be related to myxomatous changes and mitral valve prolapse, infectious endocarditis, or trauma. Valve tissue may become untethered and can demonstrate flail movement. Infective endocarditis may produce destruction or perforation of mitral leaflets and can lead to significant regurgitation. Prosthetic tissue valves in the mitral position may undergo deterioration, which leads to mitral regurgitation. (See also pages 160 and 226.)

THE FOLLOWING CRITERIA ARE REQUIRED FOR THE DIAGNOSIS OF MITRAL VALVE DEFORMITY CAUSING REGURGITATION.

Initial

The characteristic systolic murmur.

Definitive
1. **Evidence by echocardiography or other imaging technique for mitral valve prolapse or the other deformities listed above, or**
2. **Evidence for mitral regurgitation by Doppler flow studies or contrast ventriculography.**

Tricuspid Valve Deformity Causing Stenosis

Deformity of the tricuspid valve causing stenosis is most commonly due to rheumatic fever; mitral stenosis is also present in most patients. Tricuspid stenosis can also be associated with carcinoid tumors, but these more often cause tricuspid regurgitation. The valve commissures are fused, and the leaflets are thickened. The dome-shaped valve leaflets can be seen protruding into the right ventricle during systole on echocardiography or contrast ventriculography. (See also pages 169 and 229.)

THE FOLLOWING CRITERIA ARE REQUIRED FOR THE DIAGNOSIS OF TRICUSPID VALVE DEFORMITY WITH OR WITHOUT STENOSIS.

Initial
The characteristic diastolic murmur.

Definitive
1. **The valve deformities noted above, demonstrated by echocardiography or other imaging techniques, or**
2. **Evidence for a pressure gradient across the tricuspid valve during diastole demonstrated by Doppler flow studies or cardiac catheterization.**

Tricuspid Valve Deformity Causing Regurgitation

Deformity of the tricuspid valve leading to regurgitation can be caused by myxomatous degeneration with associated prolapse of the leaflets, rheumatic fever with thickening and deformity of the leaflets and accompanying tricuspid stenosis, carcinoid syndrome, cardiac tumors, and infective endocarditis. Trauma can cause prolapse of one or more leaflets. However, tricuspid regurgitation most commonly results from dilatation of the tricuspid annulus associated with right ventricular enlargement, pulmonary hypertension, and congestive heart failure, with no intrinsic deformity of the valve leaflets. (See also page 229.)

THE FOLLOWING CRITERIA ARE REQUIRED FOR THE DIAGNOSIS OF TRICUSPID VALVE DEFORMITY WITH OR WITHOUT REGURGITATION.

Initial

The characteristic systolic murmur.

Definitive

1. Demonstration of the valve deformities described above by echocardiography or other imaging techniques, or
2. Demonstration of tricuspid regurgitation by Doppler flow studies or contrast ventriculography.

Pulmonic Valve Deformity Causing Stenosis

Valve deformity producing pulmonic stenosis is most commonly congenital, and the thickened valve cusps are dome-shaped as they bulge into the pulmonary artery during systole. Post-stenotic dilatation of the pulmonary artery and subvalvular muscular hypertrophy are often associated. Rheumatic fever is rarely a cause. Echocardiography or contrast ventriculography can demonstrate the typical deformities. (See also pages 165 and 227.)

THE FOLLOWING CRITERIA ARE REQUIRED FOR THE DIAGNOSIS OF PULMONIC VALVE DEFORMITY WITH OR WITHOUT STENOSIS.

Initial

The characteristic systolic murmur.

Definitive

1. Demonstration by echocardiography or contrast ventriculography of the valvular deformity, or
2. Evidence for a systolic pressure gradient across the valve by Doppler flow studies or cardiac catheterization.

Pulmonic Valve Deformity Causing Regurgitation

Deformity of the pulmonic valve leading to regurgitation is most often congenital and rarely is due to infectious endocarditis. Pulmonary regurgitation is a frequent finding on routine Doppler flow studies and is most commonly due to myxomatous changes in the valve leaflet or to dilatation of the valve ring. Pulmonic regurgitation may be associated with pulmonary hypertension or pulmonary artery aneurysms, without intrinsic abnormalities of the leaflets. (See also page 228.)

THE FOLLOWING CRITERIA ARE REQUIRED FOR THE DIAGNOSIS OF PULMONIC VALVE DEFORMITY WITH OR WITHOUT REGURGITATION.

Initial

The characteristic diastolic murmur.

Definitive

1. **Any of the abnormalities of the pulmonary valve described above.**
2. **Evidence for pulmonary regurgitation by Doppler flow studies or regurgitation into the right ventricle of contrast material injected into the pulmonary artery.**

Valvular Vegetations

Valvular vegetations due to infective endocarditis can occur on any valve and are best identified clinically by echocardiography. They consist of a mixture of cellular debris, living and dead bacteria, fibrin, platelets, and blood cells. Transthoracic echocardiography provides better sensitivity and definition; it can detect lesions as small as 1 mm. The technique permits serial observations of vegetations for their size, contour, degree of movement during the cardiac cycle (which can interfere with valve movement), and changes in dimension due to shrinkage during treatment or to fragmentation and embolization.

THE FOLLOWING CRITERIA ARE REQUIRED FOR THE DIAGNOSIS OF VALVE DEFORMITY DUE TO A VEGETATION.

Initial

Clinical evidence of infective endocarditis.

Definitive

Identification by echocardiography or other imaging technique of a mass attached to a valve in the presence of clinical evidence for infective endocarditis and in the absence of evidence for other cause, such as tumor, thrombus, or flail movement of a valve segment.

Diseases of the Myocardium

CARDIOMYOPATHY

Adipose Infiltration of the Myocardium

Adipose infiltration of the myocardium is seen particularly in obese persons with excess epicardial fat. The right ventricle is predominantly involved. Adipose tissue extends into the myocardium, infiltrating between fibers, which may undergo atrophy and extensive replacement when the infiltration is extremely severe. The role of such adipose infiltration in the production of clinical heart disease due to obesity is not clearly established. Rarely adipose tissue may infiltrate the right ventricle extensively, causing dyskinesis and cardiac arrhythmias (arrhythmogenic right ventricular dysplasia). Focal deposit of fat in the interatrial septum can often be identified by echocardiography.

THE FOLLOWING CRITERIA ARE REQUIRED FOR THE DIAGNOSIS OF ADIPOSE INFILTRATION OF THE MYOCARDIUM.
1. **Histologic evidence of fatty infiltration of myocardium.**
2. **Echocardiographic evidence of deposition of masses in the interatrial septum consistent with fatty deposits.**

Amyloidosis

In the isolated or senile form, in that associated with a plasma cell dyscrasia, and the familial form, amyloid (a fibrillar protein of several biochemical types) is deposited in the interstitium of the myocardium and conduction system. The myofibers are surrounded, compressed, rendered atrophic, and eventually replaced by amyloid. Neighboring muscle fibers may be hypertrophied, but the weight of the heart is often not increased. Multiple small subendocardial nodules may be present in the atria.

In the systemic or secondary form, amyloid is predominantly deposited in the small arteries and arterioles, although it may also be deposited in the interstices of the myocardium.

Extensive involvement can occasionally lead to cardiac enlargement and to disordered ventricular filling with congestive phenomena. The echocardiogram displays an increase in wall thickness and asymmetric thickening of the interventricular septum. The ventricular myocardium has a speckled appearance, and there is increased echogenecity. Enlarged atria and pericardial effusion may be present. Ventricular restriction and reduced ventricular compliance are demonstrable on Doppler study. The ECG may show left axis deviation, prolongation of the P–R interval, or complete atrioventricular block. Atrial fibrillation is a common finding. The voltage of the

QRS complexes and T waves often is reduced, and there may be poor progression of R waves in the precordial leads.

THE CRITERIA REQUIRED FOR THE DIAGNOSIS OF AMYLOIDOSIS ARE ON PAGE 5.

Friedreich's Ataxia

Myocardial degeneration without pericardial or valvular disease has frequently been found in Friedreich's ataxia. There is cardiac enlargement, with focal destruction of myofibers, replacement fibrosis, and hypertrophy of intact fibers. Focal interstitial myocarditis characterized by infiltration by lymphocytes and occasionally by polymorphonuclear leukocytes may be observed. Small coronary arteries are often involved and may be occluded. The conduction system may be involved in this process.

THE CRITERIA REQUIRED FOR THE DIAGNOSIS OF FRIEDREICH'S ATAXIA ARE ON PAGE 12.

Hemochromatosis

Involvement of the myocardium is common in hemochromatosis and consists of the accumulation of hemosiderin within the myofibers and interstitium. This begins as perinuclear deposition and spreads to involve much of the fiber. It is associated with degenerative changes within the fiber, fragmentation, and focal scarring.

Cardiac enlargement and conduction disturbances commonly occur. Disturbances in ventricular filling may be terminal.

THE CRITERIA REQUIRED FOR THE DIAGNOSIS OF HEMOCHROMATOSIS ARE ON PAGE 13.

Hypothyroidism

In myxedema, the properties of collagen and mucoproteins are probably altered, and soluble complexes are converted into unstable gels. These are deposited in the interstitium of the heart and in the pericardium. Consequently, an increase in basophilic and metachromatic material can be demonstrated between muscle fibers and in the pericardium, particularly in untreated patients. The deposits in the pericardium are probably the cause of the frequently observed pericardial effusion. The functional significance of the myocardial deposits is unknown. Myocytes also accumulate glycoproteins.

THE CRITERIA REQUIRED FOR THE DIAGNOSIS OF HYPOTHYROIDISM ARE ON PAGE 17.

Lysosomal Storage Diseases

Glycogen Storage Disease

Abnormal glycogen deposition in the myocardium due to alpha-1, 4-glucosidase deficiency (Pompe's disease) results in marked cardiac enlargement, particularly of the left ventricle and ventricular septum. The myofibers are infiltrated and swollen with glycogen and contain few myofibrils. Left ventricular failure may result from this lesion. In some instances, subaortic obstruction is produced by encroachment of the thickened interventricular system on the left ventricular outflow tract.

Huge deposits of glycogen can also be found in the tongue, skeletal muscle, and other organs.

THE CRITERIA REQUIRED FOR THE DIAGNOSIS OF GLYCOGEN STORAGE DISEASE ARE ON PAGES 21–22.

Mucopolysaccharidoses

This group of genetic disorders is characterized by inborn errors of metabolism that result in the deposition of excess quantities of mucopolysaccharides in connective tissue. Fibroblasts are swollen and vacuolated, and there is an increase in intercellular ground substance. In the heart, there is nodular thickening of the valves and shortening and thickening of the chordae tendineae. Regurgitation or obstruction of the mitral or aortic valves may result, as may pulmonic regurgitation. Deposition of mucopolysaccharide in the intima of coronary vessels, with reactive intimal fibrous proliferation, may produce striking narrowing. Enlargement of the heart is usually attributable to valvular defects, but direct involvement of myocardial connective tissue may play a role.

THE CRITERIA REQUIRED FOR THE DIAGNOSIS OF MUCOPOLYSACCHARIDOSES ARE ON PAGES 21–22.

Nodular Glycogen Infiltration (Rhabdomyoma)

This form of cardiac glycogen deposition is most often observed in association with tuberous sclerosis. The nodular lesions usually occur in the ventricular septum but may be present in the wall of any of the chambers or the atrial septum. They compress surounding normal myofibers and are made up of a lacy network of cell membranes encompassing large vacuolar spaces that contain gly-cogen. The masses so formed may seriously encroach on the lumina of the chambers.

Symptoms in infancy may result from left ventricular failure or arrhythmias. In older children and adults with tuberous sclerosis (manifested by mental retardation, intracranial calcification, or adenoma sebaceum), cardio-megaly may be the only evidence of glycogen deposition in the heart.

THE FOLLOWING CRITERIA ARE REQUIRED FOR THE DIAGNOSIS OF CARDIOMYOPATHY DUE TO NODULAR GLYCOGEN INFILTRATION (RHABDOMYOMA).

Demonstration by echocardiography or other imaging tech-niques of local mural or septal tumor masses in patients with tuberous sclerosis.

Progressive Muscular Dystrophy

The heart in progressive muscular dystrophy may show fine or gross areas of fibrosis. Residual atrophic myofi-bers are encompassed by the fibrous tissue. Other muscle fibers are hypertrophied.

THE CRITERIA REQUIRED FOR THE DIAGNOSIS OF PROGRESSIVE MUSCULAR DYSTROPHY ARE ON PAGE 30.

ENLARGEMENT OF THE HEART

Enlargement of the heart results from hypertrophy of the myocardium or dilatation of the cardiac chambers or a combination of these changes. One chamber or all four may be involved, depending on the nature of the underly-ing disease and its degree of progression.

Left Ventricular Enlargement

Left Ventricular Hypertrophy

Hypertrophy of the left ventricle is an adaptive response to increased pressure or volume work or to loss of contrac-tile units. Since myocardial cells are terminally differen-tiated, they cannot increase in number, but they can increase in diameter and length. Their intracellular com-ponents such as mitochondria and sarcomeres can in-crease in size and number, and the nuclei can become polyploid. Other cells, particularly interstitial fibroblasts, can increase in number and may synthesize more col-lagen I and III, leading to fibrosis.

Sarcomeres may proliferate in parallel in response to pressure overload, leading to concentric hypertrophy, or in series in response to volume overload, leading to longitudinal hypertrophy. The initial stimulus to ventricular hypertrophy is probably mechanical, reflecting increased wall stress and stretching. It is not clear how this stimulus is linked to subsequent increases in protein synthesis via activation of tissue growth factors and of nuclear proto-oncogenes such as *c-myc* and *c-fos*, which activate genes regulating the synthesis of a variety of growth factors and of contractile proteins such as myosin heavy chains. The process may lead to shifts of myosin heavy-chain isoforms to the beta form and to changes in membrane Na-K-ATPase, alterations that can modify the contractile properties of the hypertrophied cells.

As hypertrophy progresses, changes in ventricular architecture occur. There is thickening of the free wall, interventricular septum, papillary muscles, and trabeculae carneae, which may reduce the lumen of the chamber. When hypertrophy occurs without dilatation, it is termed concentric. When dilatation accompanies hypertrophy, it produces eccentric hypertrophy, with gradual enlargement of the ventricle; the trabeculae carneae and papillary muscles are flattened and less prominent than in concentric hypertrophy. Thickening of the wall is beneficial by reducing tangential stress in accordance with Laplace's law, but marked hypertrophy may decrease diastolic compliance and elevate end-diastolic pressure.

The adaptive response of the hypertrophied heart may ultimately be limited by an inability of the coronary vascular supply to increase proportionately and by increased formation of fibrous tissue; ventricular performance then deteriorates unless afterload and preload are reduced. "Physiologic" hypertrophy may occur in the hearts of highly trained athletes, but thickness of the free wall measured echocardiographically rarely exceeds 13 mm, just above normal limits.

Hypertrophic Cardiomyopathy

Hypertrophy of the left ventricle can sometimes occur in the absence of recognizable cause, with varying degrees of muscle necrosis and patchy fibrosis, destruction and disorganization of myocytes and muscle bundles. Hypertrophy may be generalized or regional and in its most dramatic form can produce obstruction of the left ventricular outflow tract. It usually appears early in life and in about 50 percent of patients is familial, inherited as an autosomal dominant. In some kindreds, the disease is linked to missense mutations of a gene on chromosome 14q1 which regulates the structure of the beta-myosin heavy chain. The disease exhibits genetic heterogeneity, and varying mutations of beta-myosin have been identified; it is not yet clear how they affect muscle structure in hypertrophic cardiomyopathy.

The obstructive form of hypertrophic cardiomyopathy is associated with marked, asymmetric hypertrophy of the interventricular septum, which can abut the anterior leaflet of the mitral valve as it moves forward during systole, causing obstruction to outflow of blood from the ventricle. This type of dynamic obstruction produces a systolic murmur at the base, which is increased during the Valsalva maneuver, after ventricular premature beats, or other processes that foster apposition of the asymmetric septum and the anterior mitral leaflet during systole by decreasing ventricular size or increasing inotropy. Echocardiography is the most sensitive technique for demonstrating asymmetric septal hypertrophy and systolic anterior motion of the anterior mitral leaflet. As with the murmur, it may be necessary to use provocative maneuvers to elicit obstruction if it is not present at rest. Doppler interrogation of the left ventricular outflow tract in systole will characteristically reveal an increased flow velocity peaking in late systole, corresponding to a late systolic gradient. Mitral regurgitation is frequently an associated finding.

Echocardiography can demonstrate generalized systolic obliteration of the cavity in hypertrophic cardiomyopathy, as it sometimes will in pronounced hypertrophy resulting from severe aortic stenosis or arterial hypertension. Nonobstructive cardiomyopathy is recognized echocardiographically as abnormal thickening of any wall of the left ventricle; one clinically distinct form is limited to the ventricular apex.

Clinical Findings

Generally, hypertrophy does not cause symptoms except those related to decreased diastolic compliance. Hypertrophic cardiomyopathy of the obstructive type may be asymptomatic or can produce angina, light-headedness, syncope, hypotension, acute left ventricular failure, and even sudden death. Enlargement of the left ventricle usually causes the point of maximal impulse to be displaced to the left and downward on physical examination. The apical thrust tends to be prolonged and vigorous, and a fourth heart sound is commonly present.

Mild to moderate hypertrophy may not alter the ECG. However, marked hypertrophy of the left ventricle does cause changes in the ECG, which are due primarily to the increase in muscle mass and strength of the cardiac dipole, the more horizontal position of the heart within the thorax, and patchy myocardial fibrosis, which may cause conduction delay in the anterosuperior division of the left bundle branch. These factors alter the position of the mean frontal plane QRS axis, the voltage of the QRS complex, and the morphology of the ventricular repolarization complex. The hypertrophied left ventricle becomes more horizontal in the thorax, causing a leftward and superior shift of the QRS axis forming angles of $+29$ to -30 degrees. When conduction delay occurs in the anterosuperior division of the left bundle branch, the QRS axis becomes even more superior, forming angles of -40 to -90 degrees. In some subjects with left ventricular hypertrophy, the QRS axis remains in a more vertical position ($+30$ to $+90$ degrees).

An increase in voltage of the QRS complex is the most specific ECG criterion for left ventricular hypertrophy (specificity averaging 80–90% when compared to autopsy or echocardiographic measurement of left ventricular mass). However, the sensitivity of voltage criteria for left ventricular hypertrophy is poor (averaging <40%). Several sets of voltage criteria for left ventricular hypertrophy have been proposed. In general, high voltage is said to be present (at normal standardization 1 mV = 10 mm) if the arithmetic sum of the R-wave amplitude in lead I and the S-wave amplitude in lead III equals or exceeds 25 mm (2.5 mV); the maximum amplitude of the R or S waves in any limb lead equals or exceeds 20 mm (2.0 mV); the amplitude of the R wave in lead aVL equals or exceeds 13 mm (1.3 mV); the arithmetic sum of the S-wave amplitude in V_1 and the R-wave amplitude in V_5 or V_6 equals or exceeds 35 mm (3.5 mV); or the amplitude of the R wave in V_5 or V_6 equals or exceeds 30 mm (3.0 mV).

Two distinctive ECG abnormalities may characterize hypertrophic cardiomyopathy: (1) large Q waves in precordial leads in the presence of asymmetric septal hypertrophy and (2) large deeply inverted left precordial T waves in the apical form of hypertrophic cardiomyopathy.

While voltage criteria for left ventricular hypertrophy are useful, several factors (in addition to the basic error of the method) limit their reliability. These include inaccurate and variable position of the precordial electrodes, obesity, unusual shape of the thorax, and extensive pleural or pericardial effusion. In addition, in normal young adults aged 25 to 35 years, precordial QRS voltages often exceed values for the mature adult, further reducing the specificity of voltage criteria for left ventricular hypertrophy.

In children, the voltage of the QRS complex tends to be higher than in adults. Hence voltage criteria for left ventricular hypertrophy in children are different. Left ventricular hypertrophy can be suspected when the sum of R in lead I and S in III is more than 30 mm; the sum of R in V_5 and S in V_2 is greater than 60 mm; and the R/S ratio in V_1 is less than the maximum normal for the age: under 1 year, 0.8; 1 to 5 years, 0.2; and 6 to 14 years, 0.1 or less. The intrinsicoid deflection in V_6 may exceed 0.04 second, but this is a late manifestation of left hypertrophy, as are depressions of S–T segments and inversions of T waves in the left ventricular leads (I, aVL, V_4–V_6).

Left ventricular hypertrophy is most reliably demonstrated by echocardiography, which can accurately define left ventricular dimensions, volume, and mass and wall thickness. Left ventricular dilatation is determined from echocardiographic measurements of diastolic dimensions and is defined in the adult as an internal dimension of 5.3 cm or greater. The upper limit of left ventricular end-diastolic volume in the normal adult is 90 ml/m². Echocardiographic estimates of mass are derived from measurements of left ventricular internal dimension, thickness of the interventricular septum, and thickness of the posterior wall. The range in the normal adult is 100 to 250 gm with indexed values of 125 gm/m² or less in men and 110 gm/m² or less in women. Left ventricular wall thickness greater than 1.2 cm also defines left ventricular hypertrophy.

ONE OF THE FOLLOWING CRITERIA IS REQUIRED FOR THE DIAGNOSIS OF ENLARGEMENT OF THE LEFT VENTRICLE.

Initial

1. A displacement of the point of maximum impulse downward and to the left on physical examination (unless there

is accompanying right ventricular enlargement, in which case this sign becomes less specific).
2. High voltage of the QRS complex plus S–T segment depression and T-wave inversion in precordial leads V_5 and V_6 with or without similar ST–T changes in leads I and aVL. Possible left ventricular hypertrophy is recognized when high voltage is present without the repolarization abnormality.
3. In infants, left axis deviation with an rS complex in the right precordial leads and increased voltage of the R wave in the left precordial leads.

Definitive

1. Echocardiographic demonstration of dilatation or hypertrophy of the left ventricle.
2. Demonstration of left ventricular dilatation or hypertrophy by CT, MRI, or contrast ventriculography.

Right Ventricular Enlargement

Hypertrophy of the right ventricle results in thickening and increased prominence of the trabeculae carneae. Hypertrophy of the right ventricular infundibulum, the crista supraventricularis, and the papillary muscles also occurs. Pure hypertrophy of the right ventricle is usually caused by chronic pressure overloads. Considerable hypertrophy may be present without overall enlargement of the heart apparent on chest x-ray.

Marked hypertrophy may lead to a decrease in compliance of the right ventricular wall and elevation of the end-diastolic pressure in the right ventricle. Muscle hypertrophy, particularly of the right ventricular outflow tract or infundibulum, may be so marked as to cause an obstruction to right ventricular ejection.

Dilatation of the right ventricle tends to broaden and flatten the trabeculae carneae. A dilated right ventricle may secondarily displace the left ventricle toward the left and lift the cardiac apex off the diaphragm, as is typical of tetralogy of Fallot.

Dilatation is usually due to right ventricular failure or volume overload, as in left-to-right shunts at the atrial level or regurgitation across the tricuspid or pulmonary valves. Hypertrophy typically accompanies chronic dilatation. Dilatation without hypertrophy can result from the sudden appearance of pulmonary hypertension following massive pulmonary embolism.

Enlargement of the right ventricle can cause an epigastric pulsation. Considerable hypertrophy can result in a pronounced systolic pulsation along the left border of the sternum.

Marked hypertrophy of the right ventricle can lead to changes in the ECG that are in part related to a change in position of the heart in the thorax and in part to an increase in muscle mass. The mean electrical axis of the QRS may be shifted rightward. The axis is usually at +100 to +120 degrees but occasionally is as far to the right as +180 degrees. The QRS duration remains normal. If large R waves occur in the right precordial leads, especially if in V_1 the R is preceded by a Q wave, the pattern is suggestive of right ventricular hypertrophy. Additional ECG data suggestive of right ventricular hypertrophy are R/S ratio in V_1 greater than 1.0, R/S ratio in V_5 or V_6 less than 1.0, R-wave amplitude in V_1 5 mm or more, and R or R' amplitude in V_1 greater than 8 mm if QRS configuration is RSR'. In more advanced stages, there are depression of the S–T segments and negative T waves in leads II, III, aVF, and the right precordial leads V_1–V_3.

The changes in the mean electrical axis that suggest an ECG diagnosis of right ventricular hypertrophy in adults are not applicable to infants. Infants normally may have considerable right axis deviation at birth and shortly thereafter. However, in infants, if a Q wave precedes the large r in V_1 or V_{3R}, the pattern is diagnostic of right ventricular hypertrophy unless ventricular inversion with congenitally corrected transposition of the great arteries or papillary muscle infarction is present. With hypertrophy, the R/S ratio in V_1 or V_{3R} may exceed 6.0 up to 3 months of age, 4.0 up to 6 months, 2.0 up to 5 years, and 1.0 up to 15 years, while the R/S ratio in V_6 is 1.0 or less. With hypertrophy, the amplitude of R in V_1 or V_{3R} may exceed 20 mm in infants under 1 year or 16 mm in children over this age. Right hypertrophy is likely if there is an RSR' in V_1, with a normal QRS duration, and the height of one of the two R waves exceeds 8 mm, especially if the R/S ratio is larger than 1.0. The direction of T waves in right ventricular leads (V_{3R}, V_1–V_2) is upright in the first 24 hours of life, but after a few days, and certainly after 3 weeks of age, T waves in the right precordium are normally negative and remain so up to 1 year of age. Thus between age 3 weeks and 1 year, a positive T wave may appear in right V leads due to right ventricular hypertrophy; this is usually seen only when the QRS criteria for hypertrophy previously described are also present. Depression of the S–T segment in leads II, III, and aVF is seen with advanced right hypertrophy.

The chest x-ray may show changes induced by hypertrophy and dilatation. In the posteroanterior projection, the apex of the heart can be rounded and elevated. Frontal, lateral, and the right oblique projections can show bulging of the left upper and ventral (anterior) cardiac borders due to increased prominence and dilatation of the right ventricular outflow tract and main pulmonary artery.

Echocardiography is the most useful technique for detection and measurement of right ventricular dilatation and hypertrophy. Right ventricular hypertrophy is defined as wall thickness more than 5 mm.

ONE OF THE FOLLOWING CRITERIA IS REQUIRED FOR THE DIAGNOSIS OF RIGHT VENTRICULAR ENLARGEMENT.

Initial

1. **Pronounced systolic pulsation or heave along the left border of the sternum or under the xiphoid process in the epigastrium.**
2. **Right deviation of the electrical axis coupled either with depression of S–T segments and inversion of T waves in leads II, III, aVF, and V_1–V_3 or a single, tall peak or R in V_1.**
3. **In the frontal projection of the chest x-ray, unusual prominence of the central pulmonary arteries (indicating that pulmonary hypertension is present) and rounding and elevation of the apex of the heart. Enlargement of the main pulmonary artery and right atrium, accompanied by enlargement of the ventricular region of the heart.**
4. **In the lateral x-ray projection, encroachment of the heart on the retrosternal clear space, as well as dorsal displacement of the posterior margin of the intrathoracic inferior vena cava.**

Definitive

Echocardiographic evidence of dilatation or hypertrophy of the right ventricle.

Left Atrial Enlargement

Hypertrophy of the left atrium produces a thickened muscular atrial wall and prominent pectinate muscles in the base of the atrial appendage. Hypertrophy of the left atrium is usually the result of chronically increased left atrial pressure, as in left ventricular failure and mitral valve dysfunction.

Left atrial dilatation of variable degree usually accompanies left atrial hypertrophy. Dilatation is sometimes extreme, especially in chronic mitral regurgitation. Dilatation is often seen in both chronic pressure and chronic volume overloads (as in mitral regurgitation and, less strikingly, in large left-to-right shunts through ventricular septal defects or a patent ductus arteriosus). Atrial dilatation often occurs in the presence of chronic atrial fibrillation and tends to perpetuate the arrhythmia.

The ECG criteria for atrial enlargement are not very accurate and are less sensitive and specific than echocardiographic criteria. However, certain features may assist in the diagnosis. In left atrial enlargement, there is often an intra-atrial block, as shown by an increased duration of the P wave (exceeding 0.07 second in infants under 1 year old; 0.08 second from 1–12 years; 0.09 second from 12–16 years, and above 0.11 second in adults). The mean electrical axis of the P wave is shifted to the left (usually falling between $+30$ and -30 degrees). In V_1, the P wave may be biphasic, with the second and negative component 0.04 second in duration or longer and 1 mm (0.1 mV) or more in depth. There may or may not be notching of the P wave.

The size of the left atrium can be estimated on chest x-ray. However, the method does not permit accurate or quantitative measurements. Qualitatively left atrial enlargement may be recognized as a double density on the right heart border and an increase in cardiac opacity in this region. The left or right main bronchi are elevated by an enlarged left atrium.

Echocardiography is the method of choice for determining left atrial size. Left atrial dimension is measured at end–systole at the maximum dimension from the leading edge of the posterior wall of the aorta to the dominant line representing the posterior wall of the left atrium. In the normal adult, left atrial enlargement is present when left atrial size exceeds 4.0 cm or 2.2 cm/m^2.

ONE OF THE FOLLOWING CRITERIA IS REQUIRED FOR THE DIAGNOSIS OF LEFT ATRIAL ENLARGEMENT.

Initial

1. **A wide P wave, with a leftward P axis at or near 0 degrees and a prominent deep negative component to a diphasic P wave in V_1.**

2. **An abnormal frontal cardiac configuration on the chest x-ray due to one, and preferably several, of the following features: widening of the subcarinal angle; abnormal elevation of the right or left main bronchi, or both; a prominent second contour along the mid right heart border; straightening or convexity along the left heart border in the region of the left atrial appendage.**

Definitive

Demonstration of dilatation of the left atrium by echocardiography or other imaging techniques.

Right Atrial Enlargement

Hypertrophy of the right atrium, which results in a thickened muscular wall and prominent pectinate muscles, is usually due to chronically increased right atrial pressure, as in right ventricular failure, tricuspid valvular disease of acquired or congenital origin, or chronic atrial fibrillation.

Dilatation of the right atrium is usually accompanied by hypertrophy, but this is variable in degree. Dilatation tends to be most marked in the presence of chronic tricuspid regurgitation, especially when caused by congenital heart disease. Both dilatation and hypertrophy may result from large left-to-right shunts due to atrial septal defects or anomalous pulmonary venous connection to the right side of the heart.

Right atrial enlargement is best detected and measured by echocardiography.

ONE OF THE FOLLOWING CRITERIA IS REQUIRED FOR THE DIAGNOSIS OF RIGHT ATRIAL ENLARGEMENT.

Initial

A P wave that is less than 0.12 second in duration associated with large (>2.5 mm), sometimes peaked P waves in leads II, III, and aVF and a large upright initial component of a biphasic deflection in V_1.

Definitive

Demonstration of right atrial dilatation or hypertrophy by echocardiography or other imaging techniques.

MYOCARDIAL FIBROSIS

Replacement of the myocardium by fibrous tissue can occur in a wide variety of disorders and can be local or diffuse, minute or massive, and subendocardial, transmural, or subepicardial. Fibrosis is most often seen in patients with impaired coronary arterial flow and consequent myocardial necrosis. However, when recurrent ischemia occurs, as in angina pectoris, patchy myocardial fibrosis often develops even in the absence of necrosis. It may also be encountered in patients with healed myocarditis of rheumatic or other origin. Fibrosis is also found in patients with congestive or hypertrophic cardiomyopathy in the absence of coronary or inflammatory disease and can accompany severe hypertrophy and dilatation due to chronic valvular disease.

Ventricular fibrosis may lead to ventricular failure, cardiac dilatation, or asynergy. If it involves the conduction system, various forms of conduction abnormalities may result. Fibrosis of a papillary muscle, following transmural or subendocardial infarction, may cause mitral regurgitation.

Although myocardial fibrosis is a common accompaniment of many cardiac disorders, there are no signs or symptoms particular to it, and hence it is rarely recognized clinically, unless it results from a myocardial infarction or myocarditis due to progressive systemic sclerosis. It may be identified clinically with endomyocardial biopsy.

THE FOLLOWING CRITERIA ARE REQUIRED FOR THE DIAGNOSIS OF MYOCARDIAL FIBROSIS.

1. Evidence of any chronic disease capable of inducing myocardial fibrosis.
2. Demonstration of fibrosis in myocardial biopsy.

MYOCARDIAL INFARCTION

Infarction of the myocardium results from cessation of coronary blood flow due in the vast majority of cases to an occlusive thrombus that has formed at the site of rupture of an atherosclerotic plaque. It can also result from anomalous origin of the left coronary artery from the pulmonary artery and a variety of other causes.

Depending on the site of occlusion and the extent of collateral blood supply, the area of ischemic necrosis or infarction of the heart may vary from focal and minute to diffuse and massive. The extent of irreversible myocardial death is time dependent and generally proceeds as a wave front from the center to the periphery of the ischemic area. Infarcts do not ordinarily involve the myocardial wall uniformly throughout their extent. The same infarct may be transmural in one area and subendocardial or intramural in another. When the infarct involves the pericardium, it may be followed by fibrinous pericarditis; when it involves the endocardium, it may be followed by mural thrombosis. Generally, the process does not involve all of the muscle fibers within a circumscribed area, nor is the involvement uniform in age. Hence there is commonly a mixture of healthy and dead or dying muscle, infiltrated with leukocytes. Shrinkage following removal of necrotic muscle begins between the first and second week, when young granulation tissue appears. In the next few weeks this is replaced by fibrous tissue. The lesion becomes a scar within 2 or 3 months.

Obstruction of the anterior descending branch of the left coronary artery causes infarction of the apical portion of the anterior wall of the left ventricle and the contiguous portion of the interventricular septum. Obstruction of the right coronary artery causes infarction of the diaphragmatic or inferior wall of the left ventricle and the contiguous interventricular septum. Obstruction of the left circumflex artery causes infarction of the lateral or posterobasal walls of the left ventricle. Obstruction of the left main coronary artery causes extensive and often fatal infarction of the left ventricle. Very rarely, there may be isolated infarction of the right ventricle or of one of the atria. In conjunction with infarction of the inferior wall of the left ventricle, a substantial minority (5–30%) will show right ventricular infarction, and about 15 percent will show infarction of the atria, the right more often than the left. Obstruction of the right main coronary artery or of the left circumflex artery before the origin of the sinus node artery may produce pathologic changes in the sinoatrial and atrioventricular nodes, the His bundle, and the bundle branches; if the obstruction is distal to the origin of the sinus node artery, the sinoatrial node may be spared. Obstruction of coronary arteries may be associated with severe degeneration, necrosis, and fibrosis of any of the specialized structures resulting in atrioventricular, bundle branch, or fascicular blocks.

The typical patient with myocardial infarction presents with severe retrosternal chest pain or discomfort of a pressing or squeezing character not relieved by rest or nitroglycerin. The pain may also be felt in the neck, jaw, left shoulder or arm, or occasionally in the midback. Sweating, fainting, nausea, weakness, and occasionally vomiting, along with a subjective sense of doom, accompany the other symptoms. The attack may be preceded by a period of days or weeks marked by anginal episodes that progressively increase in duration and severity. In some patients, pain and other symptoms may be slight, may even be absent, or may not fit the characteristics described.

The physiologic consequences of an infarct depend on its location and mass and include ventricular failure, cardiogenic shock, and ventricular and supraventricular tachyarrhythmias as well as other disorders of impulse formation and transmission.

Clinical Findings

The patient may appear acutely ill and agitated, frequently is sweating, and often has pallor, cyanosis, and hypotension. The heart may be of normal size in the absence of antecedent disease. Heart sounds are often soft. A fourth heart sound is frequently present, and there may be paradoxical splitting of the second sound. A pericardial friction rub, a third heart sound, pulsus alternans, evidence of pulmonary congestion, and a wide variety of arrhythmias may be present. In some patients, only minimal signs, if any, of physiologic derangement may be noted.

Subsequent to the attack the patient may have a fever, leukocytosis, increased erythrocyte sedimentation rate, and a significant rise in the serum levels of several intracellular enzymes. Measurements of the MB isoenzyme of creatine kinase and the isoenzymes 1 and 2 of lactic dehydrogenase are most widely used. The serum concentrations of the enzymes increase to varying degrees, in proportion to the size of the infarct. The increase in creatine kinase is considered the most sensitive and specific laboratory test for acute myocardial infarction. The rise is detected in 2 to 3 hours, peaks at 24 hours, and declines to normal in 3 to 4 days. Lactic dehydrogenase (primarily isoenzyme 1) rises to its peak 3 to 6 days after the onset of acute myocardial infarction and returns to normal 1 to 2 weeks later. However, occasionally there is no elevation of temperature, white cell count, or enzymes, especially if the area of necrosis is small.

Characteristic ECG changes accompany most, although not all, infarctions. Three types of changes are seen:

alterations of the QRS complex, elevation of S–T segments, and serial T-wave changes; in the diagnosis of myocardial infarction, the most reliable of these are abnormalities of the QRS. The long-standing ECG subdivision of acute myocardial infarction into two main types or locations—transmural and subendocardial, based on the presence or absence of abnormal Q waves—has not been supported by anatomic evidence and is no longer considered valid. The descriptive phrases *Q-wave infarction* and *non-Q-wave infarction* have replaced *transmural* and *subendocardial*.

Changes in the QRS complex consist of either a Q wave that is larger than normal and usually wider than 0.03 second in duration in those leads that face the area of infarction or a loss of amplitude of R or disappearance of the R wave in one or more of the precordial V leads.

Elevation of the S–T segment will be found during the acute phase of the infarction in those leads facing the area of necrosis. This S–T elevation is usually accompanied by a reciprocal depression in the leads opposite those facing the infarction. For example, in anterior myocardial infarction the S–T is elevated in lead I and depressed in lead III, whereas in inferior myocardial infarction the S–T is elevated in standard leads II and III and depressed in standard lead I.

Serial T-wave changes occur over a period of several days. The T wave at first may be biphasic but later becomes inverted in the leads facing the area of myocardial infarction. With healing, negative T waves may revert to normal or may persist indefinitely.

Estimation of the sites of myocardial infarction can be determined from the ECG findings. Since the V leads are actually anterior precordial leads, they will reflect the various forms of anterior myocardial infarction. Depending on the site of these anterior infarcts, standard leads I and II as well as lead aVL will also be involved. Inferior myocardial infarctions are located for the most part on the diaphragmatic surface of the left ventricle. Lead aVF faces this area. Thus in inferior myocardial infarction, leads II, III, and aVF will contain the diagnostic evidence.

In anteroseptal myocardial infarctions, the changes will be found in leads V_1, V_2, and V_3 and without abnormality in the standard or aV leads. Anterior or apical myocardial infarction will show its effects in V_2, V_3, or

V_4, whereas anterolateral myocardial infarction will produce changes in V_4–V_6 as well as leads I and II. When the entire anterior wall is involved in the necrotic process, all six V leads will be affected. When infarction is located high on the lateral wall near the base, the effect will be noted in lead aVL only. The precordial V leads taken in the fourth intercostal space (the usual site) will not be abnormal. When a deep Q and elevated S–T segment or serial T-wave changes appear in aVL, one can confirm this diagnosis by finding these same abnormalities in the V leads taken two interspaces above the usual position, that is, in the second intercostal space. Inferior (diaphragmatic) myocardial infarction affects leads II, III, and aVF. If the inferior myocardial infarction extends laterally, as occasionally occurs, abnormalities will be noted not only in leads II, III, and aVF but also in V_5 and V_6.

True posterior (posterobasal or dorsal paravertebral, not diaphragmatic) infarcts are associated with an increase in size and duration (30 msec or longer) of R in V_1 and a large upright T wave in this lead. They are usually accompanied by an inferior or a lateral infarct.

Anatomically, subendocardial infarctions may completely encircle the interior of the left ventricle with a ringlike type of necrosis, or they may be focal. They are less frequently associated with total coronary occlusions and may result from acute increases in myocardial oxygen demand, early thrombolysis (spontaneous or induced), or coronary spasm. The ECG evidence consists of depression of the S–T segments in all leads except aVR. The S–T segment is elevated in the latter because it faces the interior of the left ventricle and hence the injured surface. Abnormal Q waves may or may not be present. The depression of the S–T segments remains fixed for several days, rather than disappearing in minutes or hours, as is the case with the transitory S–T segment abnormalities of coronary insufficiency.

Although the papillary muscles of the left ventricle may be infarcted along with subendocardial infarction, papillary muscles may be scarred or infarcted separately. Hence infarction of the posteromedial papillary muscle is associated with the depression of the S–T segment in V_1–V_4, and infarction of the anterolateral papillary muscle with these changes in V_4–V_6.

The ECG abnormalities of acute myocardial infarction generally evolve in a fairly characteristic way as a function of time after onset of the disease. Thus, the ECG may be used as a guide to the age of the infarct. In the large majority of patients, the onset of acute myocardial infarction is associated with deviations in position of the S–T segment. Sometimes the initial ECG manifestation is deeply inverted or large upright (depending on location of the infarct) T waves in the precordial leads. This repolarization abnormality is usually followed by S–T deviations in a few hours. Occasionally, the initial ECG abnormality may not occur for several days and rarely not for 2 or 3 weeks after the clinical onset of infarction. Completely normal serial ECGs are very rare in acute myocardial infarction. The S–T segment becomes isoelectric in 1 to 3 weeks in the majority of patients. Persistence of S–T elevations beyond this interval suggests the presence of akinetic or dyskinetic scar or aneurysm. Change in the polarity of T waves usually follows the S–T segment displacement by a few hours but sometimes is simultaneous with it. Serial changes in the amplitude of T waves continue for 6 to 8 weeks. Ultimately the T waves may return to normal or remain abnormal for prolonged periods of time or permanently. The abnormal Q wave is usually manifested several hours after the onset of infarction but may occur quickly, sometimes in association with the initial S–T segment displacement. It usually remains a permanent ECG abnormality, but in a significant number of patients (20–30%) after a year or longer, the Q wave disappears or becomes physiologic in duration or amplitude. The sequential pattern of ECG abnormalities that occurs in acute myocardial infarction may reflect the serial pathologic and pathophysiologic events: ischemia, injury, inflammation, necrosis, healing, fibrosis, and collagenosis.

The complications of myocardial infarction include arrhythmias, shock, ventricular failure, atrioventricular and intraventricular conduction disturbances, rupture of the myocardium or a papillary muscle, hemopericardium, myocardial fibrosis, ventricular asynergy, ventricular aneurysm, and mural thrombosis. Severe left ventricular failure and cardiogenic shock are generally associated with infarction of more than 30 to 35 percent of the left ventricle.

Echocardiography is useful in supporting the diagnosis of myocardial infarction by demonstrating segmental wall motion abnormalities. The infarcted area fails to thicken during systole and presents as a thin echodense segment. Localized areas of hypokinesis, akinesis, or dyskinesis may be present. Complications of myocardial infarction such as ventricular aneurysm, pseudoaneurysm, pericardial effusion, papillary muscle rupture, flail mitral leaflet, and mural thrombi can also be demonstrated by echocardiography. Doppler study may identify mitral regurgitation and flow across a ruptured interventricular septum. Echocardiography is of special value for demonstration of mural thrombi in the atrium or ventricle.

ONE OF THE FOLLOWING CRITERIA IS REQUIRED FOR THE DIAGNOSIS OF RECENT (ACUTE) MYOCARDIAL INFARCTION.

1. The following abnormalities in the ECG even in the absence of symptoms or abnormalities in serum enzymes: large Q waves associated with changes in the S–T segments and T waves in specific and appropriate leads that indicate the location of the infarct; serial S–T segment and T-wave changes that are specifically located but that occur without abnormal Q waves may also be used for the diagnosis but are less reliable.

2. The following abnormalities of the ECG coupled with specific enzyme alterations: serial T-wave changes, without elevation of S–T segments or abnormal Q waves in appropriate leads, indicating specific locations of the infarct. The T-wave changes must be localized and not widespread.

3. Compatible history and characteristic enzyme changes without ECG abnormalities provided that wall motion abnormalities are identified by imaging techniques.

ONE OF THE FOLLOWING CRITERIA IS REQUIRED FOR THE DIAGNOSIS OF PREVIOUS (OLD) MYOCARDIAL INFARCTION IN THE ABSENCE OF A DOCUMENTED PREVIOUS MYOCARDIAL INFARCTION.

1. Abnormal Q waves in appropriate ECG leads, indicating specific locations of the infarct, or abnormally small R waves in two or more adjacent V leads.

2. Arteriographic evidence of coronary occlusion or narrowing and corresponding ventricular asynergy or ventricular wall abnormality not due to ischemia alone.

MYOCARDITIS

Hypersensitivity

Myocarditis associated with hypersensitivity reactions, with or without accompanying vascular lesions, can occur in association with sensitivity reactions to drugs or heterologous serum. Eosinophils may predominate, or the reaction may consist principally of histiocytes and neutrophils. The principal clinical manifestations are the appearance of cardiac enlargement, ventricular failure, arrhythmias, and nonspecific changes in the final ventricular deflections (S–T and T). Echocardiography displays ventricular dilatation and reduced indices of systolic function.

THE FOLLOWING CRITERIA ARE REQUIRED FOR THE DIAGNOSIS OF MYOCARDITIS ASSOCIATED WITH HYPERSENSITIVITY REACTIONS.

Initial

Evidence of hypersensitivity reactions or systemic eosinophilia unrelated to any other obvious cause and one or more of the principal clinical manifestations previously described.

Definitive

Histopathologic evidence of hypersensitivity on endomyocardial biopsy.

Infective Myocarditis

Myocarditis can occur in association with infectious diseases of bacterial, fungal, rickettsial, viral, or parasitic origin. The lesions may consist of focal abscesses in which specific organisms may be present, or they may consist of focal or diffuse interstitial infiltration of histiocytes, lymphocytes, or polymorphonuclear leukocytes between the muscle fibers and in the perivascular connective tissue. Varying degrees of myocardial injury from fatty change to frank necrosis of the muscle cells can result.

In certain diseases, such as those produced by diphtheria toxin, *Trypanosoma cruzi* (Chagas' disease), and *Toxoplasma* (toxoplasmosis), the primary damage is to the myofiber itself, resulting in necrosis of muscle, with a secondary inflammatory response. Rarely, in the course of hematogenous disseminated tuberculosis or secondary or tertiary syphilis, focal granulomatous myocardial lesions occur. *Plasmodium*, usually *falciparum* and rarely *vivax*, can in severe cases produce capillary thrombi, with ischemic changes in the muscle. Healing occurs by fibrous replacement of areas of necrosis.

The clinical manifestations are protean and range from transitory nonspecific ECG changes to rapid or sudden death. Cardiac dilatation, ventricular failure, shock, conduction disturbances, sinus tachycardia or bradycardia, and atrial or ventricular arrhythmias can be encountered. The ECG may show abnormal S–T and T waves and the echocardiogram reduced systolic function. Serum levels of intracellular enzymes may become increased. Constitutional and specific manifestations of the basic infection (fever, leukocytosis, increased erythrocyte sedimentation rate, and positive blood cultures) are usually present.

THE FOLLOWING CRITERIA ARE REQUIRED FOR THE DIAGNOSIS OF INFECTIVE MYOCARDITIS.

Initial

The presence of an infection, as demonstrated by appropriate clinical and laboratory findings, and evidence of one or more of the following: appearance of cardiac enlargement, ventricular failure, shock, conduction defect, arrhythmias, or transient abnormal changes in the S–T segments or T waves.

Definitive

Demonstration of infective myocarditis by endomyocardial biopsy.

Idiopathic Myocarditis

Idiopathic myocarditis, of unknown cause but probably secondary to a viral infection, occurs primarily in adults. There is cardiac enlargement and diffuse myocardial inflammation. Disseminated areas of necrosis of myofibers with histiocytic reaction and areas of replacement fibrosis may be present. Wide bands of lymphocytes, histiocytes, plasma cells, and occasionally numbers of eosinophils may separate and replace muscle fibers. Endomyocardial biopsy may establish the diagnosis.

In some instances of isolated myocarditis, the reaction is characterized by the presence of large numbers of giant cells. Some appear to be of muscular origin; others are of the Langhans type. They may make up part of a diffuse reaction or may be arranged in discrete granulomas in association with lymphocytes and mononuclear cells arrayed about areas of necrosis of variable size. No organisms are demonstrable. The terms *nonspecific granulomatous myocarditis* and *giant cell myocarditis* are also employed to designate this form of disease.

The clinical course is marked by the appearance of considerable cardiac enlargement and ventricular failure, with rapid progression to death. The diagnosis is rarely made prior to death.

THE FOLLOWING CRITERIA ARE REQUIRED FOR THE DIAGNOSIS OF IDIOPATHIC MYOCARDITIS.

Clinical and biopsy evidence of myocarditis in the absence of a demonstrable cause.

Lupus Myocarditis

The myocarditis of systemic lupus erythematosus is a focal interstitial lesion. The cellular infiltrate consists of polymorphonuclear leukocytes and macrophages, as well as plasma cells and lymphocytes. Deposition of fibrin in association with infiltrates may produce a lesion with superficial resemblance to Aschoff's bodies, but true rheumatic granulomas are not seen. Areas of myocardial necrosis have been described but, when present, seem to be secondary to vasculitis with obliteration. The arteritis is necrotizing in type, with fibrinoid mural changes and associated leukocytic infiltration. Thrombosis may be superimposed on these lesions.

THE CRITERIA REQUIRED FOR THE DIAGNOSIS OF LUPUS MYOCARDITIS ARE ON PAGE 41.

Progressive Systemic Sclerosis (Scleroderma)

Myocardial involvement in progressive systemic sclerosis may take the form of interstitial fibrosis with encroachment on and replacement of myofibers. There is often associated intimal fibrosis of small arteries, but this lesion is not constant, nor is it so located as to explain the myocardial scarring.

Interstitial fibrosis may be extensive enough to produce ventricular failure through loss of myofibers or disturbances in ventricular filling. The fibrosis may also involve the conduction system. More commonly, progressive systemic sclerosis produces pulmonary heart disease by extensive interstitial fibrosis of the lungs, with obliterative disease of the pulmonary vasculature.

THE CRITERIA REQUIRED FOR THE DIAGNOSIS OF PROGRESSIVE SYSTEMIC SCLEROSIS (SCLERODERMA) ARE ON PAGE 30.

Rheumatic Myocarditis

The anatomic hallmark of rheumatic heart disease is Aschoff's nodule. This is a focal, granulomatous lesion occurring in close proximity to blood vessels and consisting of a central core of swollen fibrinoid material surrounded by large, often multinucleated basophilic cells with large vacuolated nuclei having a prominent nucleolus (Aschoff's cells), a sprinkling of smaller mononuclear cells, and occasionally a few polymorphonuclear leukocytes. Evolutionary changes occur with the passage of time. The nodule is gradually replaced by connective tissue and after several months becomes a fibrous scar.

Aschoff's nodules are usually most abundant in the myocardium of the left ventricle and interventricular septum and less common in the right ventricle. They also occur in the atrial myocardium and left atrial appendage. Lesions morphologically resembling Aschoff's nodules have been observed at other sites, such as the valves, pericardium, pleura, around the joints, and in the adventitia of the major blood vessels.

In addition to the pathognomonic Aschoff's nodule, active rheumatic myocarditis is characterized by edema of the interstitial connective tissue and a variable cellular exudate consisting of lymphocytes, polymorphonuclear leukocytes, Anitschkow's myocytes, and sometimes plasma cells and eosinophils. The cardiac muscle fibers may occasionally show degenerative changes or frank necrosis. As the acute stage of the process subsides, the edema and cellular infiltrate disappear, leaving behind small focal interstitial and myocardial scars.

Active rheumatic myocarditis is manifested clinically by an increase in heart size and by the appearance of ventricular failure, conduction disturbances, or atrial arrhythmias.

THE FOLLOWING CRITERIA ARE REQUIRED FOR THE DIAGNOSIS OF RHEUMATIC MYOCARDITIS.

A change in heart size or clinical appearance of ventricular failure or echocardiographic evidence of impaired ventricular function in association with infection with beta-hemolytic streptococcus of group A or one of the other major or minor criteria of rheumatic fever (see page 36).

Rheumatoid Myocarditis

Rheumatoid granulomas consisting of central areas of fibrinoid necrosis surrounded by palisaded rows of macrophages can occasionally be seen in the myocardium of patients with widespread joint involvement. The lesions rarely produce clinical evidence of cardiac involvement. The latter can be suspected if ventricular failure appears in a patient with active rheumatoid arthritis.

THE CRITERIA REQUIRED FOR THE DIAGNOSIS OF RHEUMATOID MYOCARDITIS ARE ON PAGE 37.

Sarcoidosis

Involvement of the myocardium in sarcoidosis may occasionally occur in the course of the generalized disease. There is replacement of myofibers by discrete and conglomerate epithelioid tubercles, which are noncaseous. These lesions are characteristically made up of closely aggregated epithelioid cells with multinucleated giant cells. Replacement of myofibers is irregular, and the conduction system may be involved. Enlargement of the heart is observed in instances where replacement is extensive. Hypertrophy of residual fibers is present. Rarely there may be extensive replacement of myocardium, simulating myocardial infarction. This may result from diffuse granulomatosis or granulomatous vasculitis of coronary arteries leading to ischemia.

Sarcoid heart disease is to be distinguished from that form of granulomatous disease that involves only the heart. This latter disease, characterized by a more diffuse type of reaction, with less of a tendency to form discrete well-defined granulomas, is best classified as isolated myocarditis, granulomatous type.

THE CRITERIA REQUIRED FOR THE DIAGNOSIS OF SARCOIDOSIS ARE ON PAGE 38.

NEOPLASM

Primary intramural tumors of the heart are rare. They may be benign or malignant and may arise from any of the tissues that make up the cardiac wall. Tumors may originate in adipose tissue (lipoma and liposarcoma), fibrous tissue (fibroma and fibrosarcoma), vessels (lymphangioma, hemangioma, and angiosarcoma), and striated muscle (rhabdomyosarcoma). The tumors displace and replace muscle fibers and may involve the conducting system, impinge on the cardiac chambers, occlude valve orifices, and produce protruding surface masses.

Metastatic tumor in the myocardium is fairly common. Carcinoma of the lung is the most frequent source of such involvement, probably because of its high incidence and its intrathoracic location. However, all malignant tumors can involve the myocardium, including malignant lymphoma. Although multiple nodules may replace cardiac muscle, they are rarely extensive enough to affect myocardial function. Primary cardiac lymphoma may occur independently, although it is associated more often with AIDS.

Myocardial tumors may cause cardiac arrhythmias or disturbances in conduction. They may also interfere with valve function or, more rarely, result in ventricular failure. X-rays may show nonspecific cardiac enlargement. Occasionally, the heart shape may be so deformed as to suggest a mass. Echocardiography can identify intracavitary tumors, extension of tumor from one of the great veins to the ventricular cavity, and paracardiac tumors. The intra-atrial myxoma, frequently a mobile mass, moves into the atrioventricular valve orifice during diastole and is usually attached by a stalk to the interatrial septum.

THE CRITERIA REQUIRED FOR THE DIAGNOSIS OF NEOPLASM ARE ON PAGE 24.

RUPTURE OF THE MYOCARDIUM: FREE WALL, INTERVENTRICULAR SEPTUM, OR A PAPILLARY MUSCLE

Rupture or perforation of the myocardium may result from trauma or myocardial infarction. There is usually an abrupt appearance of one or more of the following: left ventricular failure, pulmonary congestion, hemopericardium, pericardial tamponade, ventricular septal defect, shock, and electromechanical dissociation. Rupture of a capillary muscle may produce mitral regurgitation.

Free wall rupture due to infarction, which may occur as early as 1 to 2 days after onset of infarction, usually occurs between the fourth and seventh postinfarct days and is unusual after 2 weeks. Perforation of the interventricular septum may follow anteroseptal or posteroseptal myocardial infarction in the first 2 weeks of illness and is suggested by the sudden appearance of the harsh pansystolic murmur of ventricular septal defect, often accompanied by a thrill, at the left lower stenal border. Rupture of a papillary muscle due to infarction may also occur in the first 2 weeks of illness and usually produces mitral regurgitation of a severe degree and the rapid appearance of pulmonary edema. It is usually associated with the appearance of a loud apical systolic murmur.

Perforation of the heart by a cardiac catheter may not be attended by an abnormality of cardiac function until the catheter is withdrawn and bleeding occurs into the pericardial sac. It can be suspected when blood cannot be withdrawn through the catheter. Pacemaker wires may also perforate the heart.

ONE OF THE FOLLOWING CRITERIA IS REQUIRED FOR THE DIAGNOSIS OF RUPTURE OF THE MYOCARDIUM.

Free Wall

Echocardiographic or clinical evidence of hemopericardium or pseudoaneurysm in the appropriate clinical setting.

Interventricular Septum

Demonstration by echocardiogram or other imaging techniques of perforation of the interventricular septum with a left-to-right shunt at the ventricular level.

Papillary Muscle

Abrupt onset of severe mitral regurgitation, flail leaflet, or both demonstrated by echocardiography or other imaging techniques.

VENTRICULAR ANEURYSM

Myocardial infarction is the most common cause of aneurysm. Trauma is a less common etiology. The usual locations are apical, posterior, and, much more rarely, septal. Often a thrombus adheres to the wall of the ventricle and may partially or completely fill the pouch. In many instances, however, the lining is white, smooth or corrugated, and glistening. Pericardial adhesions often form over it. Rupture of a cardiac aneurysm is rare. The wall of the aneurysm consists of dense scar, with occasional groups or bands of muscle fibers and thickened endocardium, and it may be calcified.

The physiologic consequence of aneurysm of the heart is asynergy. If the asynergic area is small, asynergy may be insignificant, but if large, it can produce intractable ventricular failure, cardiac arrhythmias, or mural thrombi with or without systemic emboli. Mitral regurgitation is a frequent concomitant.

A double apical impulse may be felt. An aneurysm can sometimes be noted on an ordinary chest film as a bulge along the ventricular border but more frequently is iden-

tified on fluoroscopy by the typical paradoxical or reduced motion of the ventricular wall. The most reliable
noninvasive method for the diagnosis of ventricular aneurysm is echocardiography. Contrast ventriculography
can also be diagnostic. Persistent elevation of the S–T
segments in ECG leads with abnormal Q waves also
suggests aneurysm.

**THE FOLLOWING CRITERION IS REQUIRED FOR THE
DIAGNOSIS OF AN ANEURYSM OF THE HEART.**

**Demonstration of a localized bulge of the left ventricle, with or
without systolic expansion, by noninvasive imaging techniques such as echocardiography, CT, MRI, or contrast ventriculography.**

Diseases of the Pericardium

CYSTS

True cysts of the pericardium are coelomic or mesodermal
in origin and are lined by a single layer of cuboidal cells.
These may be completely separated from the pericardial
cavity or may communicate as a cystic diverticulum.
More rarely, bronchial, teratomatous, or angiomatous
cysts may occur. Cysts usually manifest themselves as
radiologic abnormalities—a rounded paracardiac mass
(most commonly in the regions of the right or left cardiophrenic angles). Mediastinal and pulmonary tumors must
be excluded. Demonstration of clear fluid on needle aspiration of a paracardiac mass strongly suggests pericardial cyst.

**ONE OF THE FOLLOWING CRITERIA IS REQUIRED FOR THE
DIAGNOSIS OF PERICARDIAL CYST.**
1. **Demonstration of pericardial cyst by echocardiography.**
2. **Demonstration of the characteristic histopathologic le-
    sion on biopsy of the cyst.**

FIBROSIS OR CALCIFICATION

Pericarditis may lead to fibrosis of the pericardium.
When tuberculosis is the etiologic factor, or when the
pericarditis has a large hemorrhagic component, calcification may ensue. When there is extensive involvement of
pericardium and epicardium by fibrinous inflammation,

healing may result in partial or complete obliteration of the pericardial cavity by fibrous adhesions. This usually has no functional significance. When healing of pericarditis results in the encasement of the heart in a thick, rigid fibrous coat, with or without calcification, pericardial restriction may result. This functional abnormality is dependent on the presence of widespread involvement of the pericardium.

ONE OF THE FOLLOWING CRITERIA IS REQUIRED FOR THE DIAGNOSIS OF FIBROSIS OR CALCIFICATION OF THE PERICARDIUM.
1. **Evidence of pericardial thickening with or without calcification by echocardiography, MRI, or CT.**
2. **Hemodynamic evidence of myocardial restriction in the absence of diffuse myocardial or endocardial fibrosis, neoplastic disease, or pericardial fluid.**

HEMOPERICARDIUM

Blood in the pericardial sac may be caused by trauma or may follow rupture of a myocardial infarct or of a dissecting hematoma of the aorta. Rupture of coronary arteries may also produce hemopericardium. Hemorrhagic pericardial fluid may also be present in the postpericardiotomy and postmyocardial infarction syndromes. Perforation of a cardiac chamber during cardiac catheterization can lead to hemopericardium. Hemopericardium may also result from blood dyscrasias, anticoagulant therapy, tumor, or pericarditis. Considerable bleeding into the pericardial sac may cause cardiac tamponade.

THE CRITERIA REQUIRED FOR THE DIAGNOSIS OF HEMOPERICARDIUM ARE THE SAME AS THOSE REQUIRED FOR THE DIAGNOSIS OF PERICARDIAL EFFUSION (SEE PAGE 121) EXCEPT THAT BLOOD WILL BE FOUND ON ASPIRATION.

NEOPLASM

Primary neoplasms of the pericardium are extremely rare. All varieties of connective tissue tumors have been described, some of which, however, probably arise in the myocardium or other neighboring structures and extend into the pericardium. They may cause abnormal cardiac shadows on radiologic examination. Primary mesothelioma of the pericardium produces pericardial effusions that are usually hemorrhagic.

Secondary neoplasms involve the pericardium by direct extension from the myocardium, lung, mediastinum, and mediastinal lymph nodes. Blood- or lymph-borne metastatic nodules can also reach the pericardial connective tissues. Secondary tumors frequently evoke a hemorrhagic pericardial effusion. Echocardiography, CT, and MRI are the most reliable techniques for demonstrating pericardial tumors.

ONE OF THE FOLLOWING CRITERIA IS REQUIRED FOR THE DIAGNOSIS OF NEOPLASM OF THE PERICARDIUM.
1. **Evidence for neoplasm as demonstrated by presence of tumor cells in pericardial fluid.**
2. **Pericardial effusion or restriction not otherwise explained in the presence of advanced metastatic disease.**

PERICARDIAL EFFUSION (HYDROPERICARDIUM)

Pericardial effusion may be caused by pericarditis, tumor, or trauma. Chronic effusions are seen in patients with uremia undergoing dialysis, thoracic tumors undergoing chemotherapy or radiation, rheumatoid arthritis, systemic lupus erythematosus, progressive systemic sclerosis, and myxedema. In myxedema, pericardial effusion may contribute to the syndrome of myxedema heart disease. It may also occur in diseases in which extracellular fluid volume is increased, as in combined ventricular failure.

Pericardial fluid can muffle heart sounds or be associated with a pericardial friction rub. Serial chest x-rays can demonstrate a rapid change in the cardiac silhouette due to the accumulation of fluid. Fluid often causes a symmetric enlargement of the cardiac silhouette, with obliteration of the outlines of individual cardiac chambers and great vessels.

Gradual accumulation of large quantities of fluid may be accommodated by a slowly distending pericardium, with evidence of pericardial restriction appearing late. Rapid accumulation of fluid leads to cardiac tamponade, which is manifested clinically by falling arterial pressure, rising venous pressure, dyspnea, tachypnea, restlessness, obtundation, and typically a pulsus paradoxus (respiratory decline of arterial pressure). The severity of the clinical manifestations varies directly with the rate of accumulation of pericardial fluid and the volume of fluid, and inversely with the compliance characteristics of the pericardium.

While pericardial effusion may be demonstrated by a variety of techniques, the method of choice is echocardiography because it is noninvasive, simple, and accurate. Cardiac tamponade is also most reliably demonstrated by echocardiography. The effusion is manifested by an echo-free space between the epicardium and parietal pericardium. A localized echo-free space suggests loculation of fluid. Tamponade causes diastolic compression or collapse of any of the four cardiac chambers. The finding of respiration-related reciprocal changes in the size of the two ventricles is associated with a pulsus paradoxus.

ONE OF THE FOLLOWING CRITERIA IS REQUIRED FOR THE DIAGNOSIS OF PERICARDIAL EFFUSION.

1. **Echocardiographic demonstration of pericardial effusion or tamponade as above.**
2. **Demonstration of pericardial fluid by direct aspiration.**

PERICARDITIS

Inflammation of the pericardium results in a localized or widespread deposition of fibrin, which may be scant or dense. The quality of the cellular reaction depends on the inciting organism. The pericardial sac may contain little fluid. However, there may be sufficient serous, purulent, or sanguineous fluid to alter the cardiac silhouette or produce pericardial restriction. The most superficial layers of the subepicardial myocardium may be involved in the disease process and give rise to ECG abnormalities.

Specific causes of pericarditis include viruses, bacteria, and fungi. Bacterial infection may be secondary to septicemia or regional inflammation (pulmonary, pleural, or mediastinal). Penetrating chest wounds, perforation of the esophagus, or descending infection originating in the neck may result in bacterial pericarditis. Infection of the pericardium by bacteria can result in a purulent pericarditis. Tuberculous pericarditis results from extension of pulmonary or pleural foci, from caseous mediastinal lymph nodes, or in the course of miliary tuberculosis. The manifestations of tuberculous pericarditis may vary from a few scattered miliary tubercles to extensive pericardial thickening, caseation, and obliteration of the pericardial sac by tuberculous granulation tissue. Large effusions may be encountered. Healing is often accompanied by calcification and may result in pericardial restriction.

Viral pericarditis, which is not associated with other demonstrable heart disease, occurs chiefly in young adults and is commonly associated with pneumonitis and pleuritis. In infants, children, and young adults, the Coxsackie B virus has been isolated from pericardial fluid and from stools. Death from this infection is rare in adults and children, but in newborn infants, in whom myocarditis usually also occurs, it is not uncommon.

Noninfective pericarditis is seen in rheumatic fever, systemic lupus erythematosus, rheumatoid arthritis, progressive systemic sclerosis, uremia, and following myocardial infarction.

In rheumatic fever, pericarditis almost always occurs in conjunction with myocardial and endocardial lesions. The pericarditis is usually fibrinous, but it may be serofibrinous. In rheumatic fever, systemic lupus erythematosus, and rheumatoid arthritis, the lesion ranges from fibrinous exudate to obliterative fibrosis.

Uremic pericarditis occurs terminally in chronic renal disease in the form of a mild fibrinous inflammation. It has, however, been shown to be reversible in the course of treatment of uremic patients by dialysis. In more severe lesions, the exudate may be hemorrhagic and may show partial organization. The lesion is nonspecific histologically, and the identification of its uremic origin depends on the demonstration of renal disease sufficient to cause renal failure.

Pericarditis may occur following myocardial infarction. It usually is more or less limited to the epicardial surface overlying the zone of infarction but may occasionally be diffuse. It is generally fibrinous in character. In extensive myocardial infarction, a hemorrhagic exudate may cover the entire pericardium. Local adhesions or more widespread obliteration of the pericardial sac may follow healing.

Inflammatory reactions of the pericardium may occur in the absence of identifiable cause: idiopathic (benign) pericarditis, following pericardiotomy (postpericardiotomy syndrome) or as a late consequence of myocardial infarction (postmyocardial infarction syndrome). In these conditions, fluid accumulation in the pericardium is rarely large.

The onset of pericarditis may be insidious or abrupt and marked by fever and dull or sharp precordial or substernal pain radiating to the neck or shoulders. Characteristically, the pain is relieved by sitting up and leaning forward. In the more indolent forms, such as tuberculous and uremic pericarditis, the patient may be free of pain. The characteristic physical finding is a friction rub, which may be heard throughout the cardiac cycle or may be present only in systole or in diastole. Leukocytosis and a rapid erythrocyte sedimentation rate are common findings.

ECGs recorded early in the course may show elevation of the S–T segments in two or three of the standard leads and in some or all of the V leads. Often in association with limb lead S–T segment deviation, the P–R segment is depressed (prominent atrial T wave).

Echocardiography is the most reliable method for demonstrating pericardial fluid.

ONE OF THE FOLLOWING CRITERIA IS REQUIRED FOR THE DIAGNOSIS OF PERICARDITIS.

Initial
Chest pain, pericardial friction rub, and characteristic ECG changes.

Definitive
1. **Demonstration of pericardial fluid by echocardiography or other imaging techniques.**
2. **Direct aspiration of fibrinous, serofibrinous, or purulent fluid.**

PNEUMOPERICARDIUM

Air in the pericardial sac, demonstrable by radiography, is the result of communication with the lung or gastrointestinal tract or, rarely, may result from infection of the pericardium by gas-forming organisms. Fistula formation between the esophagus and pericardial sac may result from peptic ulceration, traumatic rupture, or perforation by tumor. Only rarely will mediastinal emphysema be associated with pneumopericardium. This occurs almost exclusively following pericardiotomy or in infants after forced positive-pressure breathing. Pericardial tap may introduce air into the pericardial space. Pneumopericardium may also be observed following open heart surgery.

THE FOLLOWING CRITERION IS REQUIRED FOR THE DIAGNOSIS OF PNEUMOPERICARDIUM.
X-ray demonstration of gas within the pericardial space.

CONGENITAL ABSENCE OF THE LEFT PERICARDIUM

Most congenital pericardial defects are left-sided; complete absence of the left pericardium is commoner than partial left-sided defects. The anomaly may be isolated or occur with other cardiovascular malformations or with pectus excavatum. Usually, there are no symptoms associated with absent left pericardium; occasionally, chest pain occurs with changing posture or respiratory infection.

In complete absence of the left pericardium, the chest x-ray in the frontal view shows the heart displaced into the left chest, usually with its right border overlying the spine. The pulmonary artery segment is slightly prominent, and an unusually sharp cleft is seen separating the main pulmonary artery from the aortic arch. With partial left-sided defects, which are usually located just inferior and anterior to the left hilus, herniation of the left atrial appendage through the defect often produces an unusually pulsatile mass density in the left infrahilar region. Occasionally, bronchogenic cysts are associated with these partial defects. Echocardiography and other imaging techniques may assist in the diagnosis.

ONE OF THE FOLLOWING CRITERIA IS REQUIRED FOR THE DIAGNOSIS OF CONGENITAL ABSENCE OF THE LEFT PERICARDIUM.

1. **Characteristic findings on chest x-ray.**
2. **Characteristic findings on echocardiography or other imaging techniques.**

Anomalies of Cardiac Position

DEXTROCARDIA

Dextrocardia is an anomaly in which the heart lies predominantly in the right chest. It may be a primary developmental anomaly, or it may result from congenital or acquired abnormalities of the chest wall, spine, lungs, or diaphragm.

The nomenclature used to describe the various types of primary congenital positional abnormalities is related to (1) the position of the right atrium and abdominal viscera and (2) the direction of the bending of the bulboventricular loop during embryologic development, which determines the position of the ventricles relative to each other. For example, the normal rightward bending of this loop (concordant bending relative to atrial and visceral situs) determines that the right ventricle is on the right of the left ventricle.

In normal development, the liver, great veins, and right atrium lie on the right side of the body; this position is termed situs solitus. The bulboventricular loop, which lies distal to the atria, initially bends to the right (concordant dextro [D] loop), and then the entire ventricular region of the heart later shifts to the left to form the normal left-sided heart.

When the liver and right atrium develop on the left, situs inversus, a mirror image of normal relationships is present. The bulboventricular loop initially bends to the left (concordant levo [L] loop), and the entire ventricular region later shifts to the right to produce mirror-image dextrocardia.

When bulboventricular loop formation is discordant to visceroatrial situs (L-loop in situs solitus and D-loop in situs inversus), transposition of the great arteries is regularly present (this combination of anomalies is usually called corrected transposition of the great arteries); additional intracardiac malformations are common. Abdominal heterotaxy, or the development of visceroatrial sinus ambiguus, is often associated with complex intracardiac defects as well as dextrocardia. Midline liver, asplenia, polysplenia, and bilateral lung symmetry are common in this circumstance.

Echocardiography accurately defines apex orientation to the right. The apex or subcostal positions of the transducer can be used as well as parasternal and short-axis views.

Dextrocardia with Situs Inversus

Dextrocardia with situs inversus most commonly results from concordant L-loop bulboventricular development with situs inversus of the abdominal viscera (liver and great veins on the left and stomach on the right). This form of dextrocardia (mirror-image), which represents the normal cardiac position for situs inversus, is infrequently associated with intracardiac defects. Since the right atrium and sinoatrial node are on the left (on the same side as the liver) and the left ventricle is on the right, the ECG characteristically shows a negative P, QRS, and T in lead I.

Dextrocardia with situs inversus occasionally results from discordant D-loop bulboventricular development. In this circumstance, complex intracardiac malformations associated with cyanosis or venoarterial shunting are usually encountered. Ectopic atrial rhythms are often noted on the ECG.

Echocardiography in the abdominal horizontal/coronal view demonstrates the central or right-sided aorta, the left-sided vena cava, and the malpositions of the liver and stomach. Dextrocardia with situs inversus and discordant D-loop bulboventricular development can be identified using segmental anatomic echocardiographic imaging.

THE FOLLOWING CRITERIA ARE REQUIRED FOR THE DIAGNOSIS OF DEXTROCARDIA WITH SITUS INVERSUS.
Radiologic or echocardiographic evidence of the heart in the right chest and evidence of complete abdominal situs inversus.

Dextrocardia with Situs Solitus

Dextrocardia with situs solitus may result from either (1) failure of expected leftward shift of the normal concordant bulboventricular D-loop in situs solitus or (2) inappropriate initial development, that is, discordant L-loop bending of the bulboventricular region, with expected late shift of the ventricular region into the right chest. When the latter mechanism is present, intracardiac defects are frequently encountered.

Echocardiographic imaging demonstrates that the aorta is central or slightly to the left of the spine, and the inferior vena cava is right-sided. Bulboventricular looping will either be normally concordant or occasionally discordant (L-loop). Subcostal or apical views delineate this relationship.

THE FOLLOWING CRITERIA ARE REQUIRED FOR THE DIAGNOSIS OF DEXTROCARDIA WITH SITUS SOLITUS.
Radiologic or echocardiographic evidence of the heart in the right chest and evidence of abdominal situs solitus.

LEVOCARDIA WITH SITUS INVERSUS

A left-sided heart represents a positional abnormality when it is associated with situs inversus of the abdominal viscera. It may result from failure of rightward shift of a concordant L-loop of the bulboventricular region or from an inappropriate discordant D-loop bulboventricular de-

velopment. The right atrium, like the liver, is on the left.
The P wave in the ECG is frequently inverted in lead I.
Using echocardiographic techniques previously described,
situs and the left-sided position of the heart can be
demonstrated.

**THE FOLLOWING CRITERIA ARE REQUIRED FOR THE
DIAGNOSIS OF LEVOCARDIA WITH SITUS INVERSUS.**
**Radiologic and echocardiographic evidence of the heart in
the left chest and evidence of complete abdominal situs
inversus.**

Anomalies of the Aorta and Aortic Arch System

COARCTATION OF THE AORTA

Congenital, localized narrowing of the aorta most often
occurs at the junction of the arch and descending aorta. It
may lie proximal, opposite, or distal to the ductus arteriosus, which may be patent or closed. The aortic obstruction appears to be caused by a curtain-like infolding of
the media toward the lumen, which is thereby narrowed
and eccentrically located.

A systolic pressure gradient develops across the obstruction, causing the blood pressure in the upper extremities to be significantly higher than that in the lower
extremities. Femoral pulses may be weak or absent, and
recordings of femoral pulses show a delayed systolic up-
stroke. Arterial hypertension in the upper extremities
may be progressive with advancing age; its absolute level
may be modified by the development of collateral vessels
that bypass the obstructed segment from proximal to
distal aorta.

Characteristically, there is a harsh systolic murmur in
the back overlying the site of coarctation. Additional
murmurs may be heard over the anterior chest, which are
caused by commonly associated lesions, such as a bicuspid aortic valve.

Chest x-rays in the frontal view with the esophagus
filled with barium may show indentations of the esophagus simulating the letter E, which are caused by irregu-
larities and post-stenotic dilatation of the aorta. Beyond
early childhood, notching of the inferior margins of the

ribs from collateral circulation may be seen on chest films.

Echocardiographic imaging of aortic coarctation is best accomplished from the suprasternal notch and demonstrates long or short segment narrowing. Doppler color flow study indicates a turbulent jet in the area of constriction.

ONE OF THE FOLLOWING CRITERIA IS REQUIRED FOR THE DIAGNOSIS OF COARCTATION OF THE AORTA.

1. **A significant difference in systolic blood pressure between the upper and lower extremities, with higher pressure in the arms.**
2. **Echocardiographic or angiocardiographic demonstration of aortic narrowing.**

RIGHT AORTIC ARCH

A right aortic arch is frequently associated with congenital intracardiac defects; it occurs in about one-third of the patients with tetralogy of Fallot. The ascending aorta and aortic arch normally pass anterior to the right pulmonary artery and right main stem bronchus but instead of crossing to the left in front of the trachea, as with left aortic arch, remain to the right of the trachea and esophagus, leading to a right upper descending aorta. The aorta often descends on the right to the level of the diaphragm, then crosses the midline to the left, and passes through a left-sided hiatus, resulting in an abdominal aorta in the expected position. Most commonly, the branches of the arch are a mirror image to normal; the first branch is a left innominate artery, after which the right common carotid and right subclavian arteries arise separately. The majority of patients have a left ductus arteriosus connecting the left innominate artery with the left pulmonary artery.

A right aortic arch by itself does not produce symptoms. However, when right aortic arch occurs in the absence of associated congenital heart disease, an aberrant left subclavian artery is nearly always present. This combination typically causes a large retroesophageal defect, with considerable anterior displacement of both the esophagus and trachea. The retroesophageal component, including the distal arch, the aberrant left subclavian artery, and a ligamentum arteriosum (from the aorta or left subclavian artery) to the left pulmonary artery, forms a vascular ring that may cause tracheal or esophageal obstruction.

The right aortic arch produces an indentation or indentations on the right of the esophagus and displaces the trachea to the left. Echocardiographic demonstration of a right aortic arch requires use of suprasternal images in the long-axis plane. If the scan plane is tilted leftward and images the tracheal air column, a right aortic arch is present.

ONE OF THE FOLLOWING CRITERIA IS REQUIRED FOR THE DIAGNOSIS OF RIGHT AORTIC ARCH.

1.   **X-ray evidence that the aortic arch is to the right of the trachea or barium-filled esophagus.**
2.   **Demonstration of a right aortic arch by echocardiography, MRI, or CT.**

VASCULAR RING

Variations in the development and arrangement of the aortic arch system may result in the encirclement of the trachea and esophagus. In all these anomalies, the trachea and esophagus, which normally lie posterior to the vascular structures, are surrounded by vessels. Two common patterns are (1) a double aortic arch, consisting of a right and left aortic arch, which unite and continue as the descending aorta, and (2) a right aortic arch with retroesophageal segment, a left ligamentum arteriosum, and left-sided descending aorta.

Symptoms may occur if the ring is "tight," with respiratory distress, stridor, and brassy cough noted in early infancy. Dysphagia may first become apparent in early adult life.

Echocardiographic demonstration of vascular rings requires the use of suprasternal long-axis views and initial determination of the side of the aorta arch.

ONE OF THE FOLLOWING CRITERIA IS REQUIRED FOR THE DIAGNOSIS OF VASCULAR RING.

1.   **Demonstration of the vascular anomalies by echocardiography or other imaging techniques.**
2.   **Evidence on chest x-ray of an indentation on the posterior wall of the barium-filled esophagus in the lateral view. In the frontal projection, appropriate lateral indentation(s) on the barium-filled esophagus made by the aortic arches or possibly by the ligamentum arteriosum.**

Anomalies of the Pulmonary Arteries

PULMONARY ARTERIOVENOUS FISTULA

Congenital pulmonary arteriovenous fistula results from the persistence of fetal anastomotic capillaries, which divert pulmonary arterial blood to the pulmonary veins along a path that fails to traverse the alveolar capillary bed. Such communications tend to increase in size, and the walls of the supplying artery become thin, tortuous, and dilated as an increasing volume of blood flows through this path of least resistance. The veins draining the anastomoses distend and become varicose. The walls separating varicosities atrophy, leaving large, blood-filled cavities partly divided by septa, which are the original walls. When such fistulas exist between a large artery and vein, anastomotic arteries also contribute flow to the "feeder" artery and themselves tend to become dilated. Hence a large arteriovenous anastomosis, once established, is a slowly expanding lesion. These malformations may be solitary or multiple, involving one or both lungs, and may represent but one manifestation of generalized hereditary telangiectasia (Osler-Rendu-Weber disease). On occasion, these fistulas occur as a fine microscopic network of capillaries rather than as the large cavernous lesions previously described. Subpleural fistulas may rupture into the pleural cavity, while intrapulmonary lesions frequently rupture and cause hemoptysis. Pulmonary arteriovenous fistulas may be identified on routine chest x-ray.

The clinical consequences of this disorder depend on the magnitude of total shunt flow across the lungs, regardless of the size of individual lesions. Systemic arterial blood oxyhemoglobin unsaturation, cyanosis, clubbing, and secondary polycythemia appear when shunt flow exceeds approximately 20 percent of total pulmonary blood flow. Overall resistance to pulmonary blood flow is not increased in the presence of these lesions, and right ventricular hypertrophy is rare. Infective angiitis occasionally develops within the lesion and can result in metastatic cerebral and other systemic abscesses. These lesions may also permit systemic embolization or may manifest themselves solely as abnormal densities in the chest x-ray.

Direct echocardiographic identification of this lesion is not possible. Two-dimensional imaging supports the diagnosis by displaying large dilated pulmonary artery branches. Doppler study may demonstrate increased flow velocity in the pulmonary veins, and the diagnosis is confirmed by peripheral venous contrast echocardiography.

ONE OF THE FOLLOWING CRITERIA IS REQUIRED FOR THE DIAGNOSIS OF PULMONARY ARTERIOVENOUS FISTULA.

1. **Angiographic demonstration of the arteriovenous fistula during the stage of pulmonary arterial filling.**
2. **Demonstration of right-to-left intrapulmonary shunt by appropriate indicator-dilution techniques in the presence of normal levels of pulmonary blood flow and pulmonary arterial pressure.**
3. **Specialized echocardiographic study as above.**

PULMONARY VASCULAR SLING

In this anomaly the left pulmonary artery takes origin from the right pulmonary artery and crosses the mediastinum between the trachea (just above its bifurcation) and esophagus to enter the left lung.

Evidence of respiratory distress and frequent pulmonary infections, especially of the right lung, may occur in infancy.

The echocardiographic parasternal short-axis view and subcostal coronal views demonstrate the abnormal origin of the left pulmonary artery from the right.

A chest x-ray in the lateral view with a barium-filled esophagus shows a persistent anterior indentation of the esophagus just above the level of tracheal bifurcation. A selective pulmonary arteriogram outlines the aberrant origin and course of the left pulmonary artery.

ONE OF THE FOLLOWING CRITERIA IS REQUIRED FOR THE DIAGNOSIS OF PULMONARY VASCULAR SLING.

1. **Echocardiographic evidence as above.**
2. **A selective pulmonary arteriogram demonstrating the aberrant origin and course of the left pulmonary artery.**

PERIPHERAL PULMONARY ARTERIAL STENOSIS

Localized constriction may occur at the origin of the right or left pulmonary artery, or multiple sites of narrowing may exist peripherally throughout their distal courses. Both entities are frequently associated with pulmonary valvular stenosis. Multiple peripheral constrictions are common in the postrubella syndrome. Supravalvular aortic stenosis is sometimes associated with these lesions.

Systolic murmurs, and occasionally diastolic ones, may be widely transmitted over the anterior or posterior chest wall. Pressure gradients within the pulmonary vessels may be demonstrated by catheterization. Selective injection of contrast material in the main pulmonary artery reveals the location of the narrowed sites.

Echocardiography with a variety of views can demonstrate both pulmonary arteries, discrete narrowing, and diffuse hypoplasia. When the vascular stenoses cannot be visualized directly, unexplained right ventricular hypertrophy on two-dimensional echocardiography with exaggerated pulsations of the proximal pulmonary artery may indirectly suggest peripheral pulmonary arterial stenosis.

THE FOLLOWING CRITERION IS REQUIRED FOR THE DIAGNOSIS OF PERIPHERAL PULMONARY ARTERIAL STENOSIS.

Angiographic or echocardiographic demonstration of localized or multiple constrictions in right, left, or both pulmonary arteries.

Anomalies of the Coronary Arteries

ANOMALOUS ORIGIN OF THE LEFT CORONARY ARTERY FROM THE PULMONARY ARTERY

In this anomaly the left coronary artery usually arises between the pulmonary valve and the bifurcation of the main pulmonary artery and passes to the myocardium with the same pattern of branching as a "normal" left coronary artery. The direction of blood flow through an anomalously arising left coronary artery usually changes in the first few months of life as the high pulmonary arterial pressure, present at birth, falls toward normal. Initially, blood flows from the main pulmonary artery into the left coronary artery and its distal branches to perfuse the subjacent myocardium. As pulmonary arterial pressure falls and intercoronary anastomotic channels develop between the right and left coronary arteries, blood from the aorta may then flow from the right coronary artery, fill the left coronary in retrograde fashion, and enter the pulmonary artery. This bypass, acting like an arteriovenous fistula, may cause ischemia of the left ventricular myocardium.

The occurrence of symptoms depends on the extent of ischemia resulting from inadequate perfusion of the left ventricular myocardium. Extreme pallor and restlessness may develop in a previously thriving infant and may resemble the pattern seen in angina. Frequently, a shock-like picture occurs around 3 months of age, with the sudden onset of ventricular failure, attributed to myocardial infarction, which may lead to death. Those infants in whom adequate collateral circulation develops may show no symptoms, and the lesion may not be recognized until childhood.

The ECG may show S–T and T-wave changes and the presence of deep Q waves in leads I, aVL, V_5, and V_6 resembling anterolateral myocardial infarction. The chest x-ray shows marked cardiomegaly, predominantly of the left ventricle.

Murmurs are absent in early infancy. An apical systolic murmur compatible with mitral regurgitation may develop in late infancy or childhood secondary to papillary muscle infarction. In children in whom an extensive flow from the aorta to the pulmonary artery has developed, a continuous murmur may be audible over the midprecordium.

Selective retrograde aortography or coronary arteriography will reveal that only the right coronary artery arises from the aorta. Contrast material may be visualized in the anastomotic channels that enter the left coronary artery and drain into the pulmonary artery. Right heart catheterization may demonstrate a left-to-right shunt at the level of the pulmonary artery.

High left parasternal views of the pulmonary artery with anteroposterior tilting may show insertion of the left coronary artery into the posterior wall of the pulmonary artery. Echocardiographic Doppler color flow imaging in the high left parasternal view will show flow from the coronary artery into the main pulmonary artery. The echocardiogram may also demonstrate a dilated, prominent right coronary artery.

ONE OF THE FOLLOWING CRITERIA IS REQUIRED FOR THE DIAGNOSIS OF ANOMALOUS ORIGIN OF THE LEFT CORONARY ARTERY FROM THE PULMONARY ARTERY.

1. **Demonstration by aortography that the normal right coronary artery fills the left coronary artery in retrograde**

fashion via anastomotic channels and contrast material from the left coronary artery enters the pulmonary artery.
2. Demonstration by pulmonary arteriography of the left coronary artery arising anomalously.
3. Echocardiographic data as noted above.

CORONARY ARTERIAL FISTULA TO A
CARDIAC CHAMBER

Either of the coronary arteries, but most commonly the right, arising normally from the aorta may make a direct communication with any one of the cardiac chambers, again usually a right. The artery proximal to the fistulous connection is usually wide and tortuous. The physiologic effect of a communication between a coronary artery and the right heart is that of left-to-right shunt at the level of the right atrium or ventricle. The level of the shunt may be detected during right heart catheterization.

A continuous systolic and diastolic murmur, with the diastolic component frequently the louder, is present over the midprecordium or slightly to the right of the sternum.

The defect is best visualized by selective coronary arteriography or retrograde aortography showing contrast material shunting from an unusually large coronary artery into a particular cardiac chamber.

Multiple two-dimensional echocardiographic views are used to identify coronary artery anatomy in this lesion. In the parasternal short-axis view and subcostal coronal views, one coronary artery is shown to be markedly dilated, while the other is of normal size. Doppler color flow study demonstrates the site of entry of the fistula into the cardiac chamber or vessel.

THE FOLLOWING CRITERION IS REQUIRED FOR THE DIAGNOSIS OF CORONARY ARTERIAL FISTULA TO A CARDIAC CHAMBER.

Demonstration by selective coronary arteriography or aortography or echocardiography of a fistula connecting a coronary artery and a cardiac chamber.

Communications Between the Great Arteries

AORTOPULMONARY WINDOW

Aortopulmonary window, a rare localized defect in the walls of the ascending aorta and main pulmonary artery, permits communication of the great vessels just distal to their respective semilunar valves. Aortopulmonary window mimics the clinical findings and physiologic derangements of patent ductus arteriosus; however, the left-to-right shunt is frequently larger, and pulmonary hypertension is usually present. The continuous systolic and diastolic murmur may be more intense and widespread than in patent ductus arteriosus. The pulse pressure is usually widened.

At cardiac catheterization, the catheter may pass from the main pulmonary artery to the ascending aorta. Following injection of contrast material into the root of the aorta, the main pulmonary artery is opacified.

With echocardiography, the defect in the aortopulmonary septum can be seen in subcostal coronal or parasternal short-axis views.

ONE OF THE FOLLOWING CRITERIA IS REQUIRED FOR THE DIAGNOSIS OF AORTOPULMONARY WINDOW.

1. **Passage of a catheter from the main pulmonary artery into the ascending aorta.**
2. **Direct opacification of the main pulmonary artery when contrast material is selectively injected into the root of the aorta.**
3. **Echocardiographic demonstration of the communication between the aorta and main pulmonary artery.**

PATENT DUCTUS ARTERIOSUS

This persistent fetal communication between the pulmonary artery and aorta is usually several millimeters in length at birth. It is most commonly a left-sided structure that connects the proximal portion of the left pulmonary artery to the descending aorta just distal to the origin of the left subclavian artery. In the fetus, blood flows from the pulmonary artery into the descending aorta; postnatally, if the channel fails to close spontaneously, blood usually flows from the systemic (aortic) circuit into the pulmonary circuit. Reversal of flow with right-to-left shunting may occur when pulmonary arterial pressures exceed those in the systemic arterial bed.

The mechanism by which the ductus normally closes after birth involves changes in arterial PO_2 with production of prostaglandins, which stimulate contraction, endothelial proliferation, and fibrosis.

Symptoms and signs vary with the size of the ductus and the volume and direction of the extracardiac shunt. Although in a small number of infants left ventricular failure may develop from a large shunt from the aorta into the pulmonary artery, the majority grow and develop normally and are asymptomatic in childhood and early adult life. Infective endocarditis is a potential complication.

The characteristic continuous murmur is maximal in the second left intercostal space and is crescendo during systole and decrescendo during diastole. When severe pulmonary hypertension is present, and flow through the ductus is small, one or both components of the murmur may be absent.

The ECG and the chest x-ray may be normal when the shunt is small. With a large left-to-right shunt, the ECG may indicate left or combined ventricular hypertrophy. In this circumstance, the chest x-ray may show prominence of the main and left pulmonary artery segments and increased peripheral pulmonary vascular markings. The heart size is usually increased due to left atrial and left ventricular enlargement.

Echocardiographic demonstration of the patent ductus arteriosus is made with left parasternal and suprasternal views. Doppler color flow mapping facilitates identification of the ductus by detecting turbulent flow across the lesion and diastolic flow in the pulmonary artery from the aorta.

During right heart catheterization, the catheter may be manipulated through the ductus into the descending aorta, a left-to-right shunt demonstrated at the level of the pulmonary artery, or both. Selective retrograde aortography reveals opacification of the pulmonary arteries when contrast material is injected just below the arch of the aorta.

ONE OF THE FOLLOWING CRITERIA IS REQUIRED FOR THE DIAGNOSIS OF PATENT DUCTUS ARTERIOSUS.

1. **Passage of a catheter from the left pulmonary artery into the descending aorta.**
2. **Opacification of the pulmonary arteries via a patent ductus arteriosus following selective retrograde aortography.**
3. **Echocardiographic demonstration of the patent ductus arteriosus.**

TRUNCUS ARTERIOSUS

A single large arterial vessel, truncus arteriosus, gives rise to the coronary, pulmonary, and aortic arch branches and continues as the descending aorta. The truncus takes origin from both ventricles. A common semilunar valve and a large ventricular septal defect are integral parts of the malformation. Variations occur in the site of origin and size of the pulmonary arteries that emerge from the lateral or posterior walls of the truncus. The right and left pulmonary arteries arise either from a common pulmonary trunk immediately above the truncal valve or separately from the ascending portion of the truncus.

When one or both pulmonary arteries are absent, the blood supply to the lungs sometimes may be asymmetric and derived from branches of the brachiocephalic vessels or from the descending aorta through bronchial collateral vessels.

The physiologic derangements and clinical picture depend on the magnitude of the aortic-to-pulmonary shunt, the presence of anatomic changes in the pulmonary vascular bed, and the relation between the systemic and pulmonary blood flow. Although systemic arterial oxyhemoglobin unsaturation is always present, it may be minimal when pulmonary blood flow is markedly increased.

A loud systolic murmur is usually present along the left sternal border. A high-pitched, decrescendo diastolic murmur may be heard in the same area when there is truncal valve dilatation and regurgitation. A loud second sound, often single, may be present. The ECG and chest x-ray offer no specific clues to the diagnosis of truncus arteriosus.

Right heart catheterization usually permits passage of the catheter from the right ventricle to the ascending truncus and frequently into each of the pulmonary arteries. The blood pressure in the right ventricle and frequently in the pulmonary arteries reaches levels encountered in the systemic arterial bed. A left-to-right shunt may be detected at the ventricular level or in the pulmonary arteries. Truncal or systemic arterial oxyhemoglobin unsaturation varies from mild to severe.

Contrast visualization studies are essential to the delineation of the anomaly. Although right ventricular injection of contrast material may establish the diagnosis of truncus arteriosus, additional selective injections into the ascending truncus are frequently required to localize clearly the sites of origin of the pulmonary arteries.

Two-dimensional long-axis parasternal echocardiographic views identify the deficiency in the infundibular septum and overriding aorta. The parasternal short-axis view is best for imaging the pulmonary arteries as they arise from the truncal vessel. The ventricular septal defect can be imaged with apical and subcostal four-chamber views.

THE FOLLOWING CRITERION IS REQUIRED FOR THE DIAGNOSIS OF TRUNCUS ARTERIOSUS.

Demonstration by selective aortic root aortography, right ventriculography, or echocardiography of a single large ascending vessel, or truncus, which gives origin to both the aorta and the pulmonary arteries.

AORTIC ORIGIN OF THE RIGHT PULMONARY ARTERY

In this vascular malformation, the right lung receives its sole arterial blood supply from a large vessel arising from the ascending aorta, and the left lung receives the entire right ventricular output. It is probably derived from embryologic failure of migration of the right sixth aortic arch to join its counterpart on the left before the truncus is divided into the aorta and pulmonary artery. The lesion is not infrequently complicated by a coexisting patent ductus arteriosus.

Although this anomaly may be accompanied by ventricular failure and death in infancy, it may also occur in asymptomatic adults. Clinical findings are not distinctive, although they may suggest truncus arteriosus.

Selective injection of contrast material into the right ventricle delineates a single pulmonary artery going to the left lung; following opacification of the ascending aorta, the anomalous large vessel going to the hilus of the right lung will be visualized at about the same time as the left pulmonary artery. Retrograde aortography provides optimal visualization of the origin and course of the right pulmonary artery.

THE FOLLOWING CRITERIA ARE REQUIRED FOR THE DIAGNOSIS OF AORTIC ORIGIN OF THE RIGHT PULMONARY ARTERY.

Angiographic demonstration of a single large vessel arising from the ascending aorta passing to the hilus of the right lung, with the left pulmonary artery arising from the right ventricle.

Transposition Complexes

COMPLETE TRANSPOSITION OF THE GREAT ARTERIES

The most common transposition complex, referred to as complete transposition of the great arteries (or vessels), designates the aorta arising anteriorly from the right ventricle and the pulmonary artery arising relatively posteriorly from the left ventricle. Because the origins of the great arteries are transposed, the systemic and pulmonary circuits are basically separate: systemic venous blood is directed into the aorta, and pulmonary venous blood is directed into the pulmonary artery. Postnatal survival depends on the presence of other anomalies that, alone or in combination, permit flow of oxygenated blood into the systemic circulation; that is, communications at the atrial or ventricular level or through a patent ductus arteriosus. A variety of additional malformations may coexist, such as pulmonary valvular stenosis, coarctation of the aorta, or single ventricle.

Cyanosis appears early and becomes progressively more intense in the first few weeks of life, especially when the ventricular septum is intact. Most infants with complete transposition of the great arteries succumb in the first 6 months of life from hypoxemia and ventricular failure unless therapeutic enlargement of an atrial communication has been accomplished. The prognosis for immediate survival is improved in those with an associated ventricular septal defect, although progressive pulmonary vascular disease is a liability in this group.

Systolic murmurs are usually present but are not specific. The ECG is abnormal and may show right, left, or combined ventricular enlargement. The chest x-ray may be of diagnostic importance and usually reveals the following: an ovoid, or egg-shaped, cardiac contour (in about 70%), often with a narrow superior mediastinal (vascular) pedicle, progressive cardiac enlargement in early infancy, and increased pulmonary vascular markings.

Severe systemic arterial hemoglobin unsaturation may occur in infants with an intact ventricular septum. Injection of contrast material into the right ventricle permits visualization, particularly in the lateral view, of the anteriorly arising aorta and identifies the relationship between the great arteries, their semilunar valves, and their respective ventricles. Anatomic details of associated malformations, such as ventricular septal defect or pulmonary valvular stenosis, may be enhanced by additional selective injection of contrast material into the left ventricle.

Two-dimensional echocardiography is diagnostic. It demonstrates the abnormal spatial orientation of the aorta and pulmonary artery as well as the associated lesions.

ONE OF THE FOLLOWING CRITERIA IS REQUIRED FOR THE DIAGNOSIS OF COMPLETE TRANSPOSITION OF THE GREAT ARTERIES.

1. **Echocardiographic demonstration of the transposition complex.**
2. **Angiocardiographic demonstration of the aorta arising from the right ventricle and receiving the systemic venous return, while the pulmonary artery arises from the left ventricle.**

CONGENITALLY CORRECTED TRANSPOSITION OF THE GREAT ARTERIES

This entity consists of ventricular inversion and transposition of the pulmonary artery and aorta in their anteroposterior relations. Ventricular inversion results in the right-sided venous ventricle having the morphologic structure of the left ventricle and the left-sided systemic ventricle resembling the right ventricle; it derives from discordant L-loop bulboventricular development in the presence of a normal, or situs solitus, position of the abdominal viscera. Typically, the pulmonary artery arises medially and posteriorly from the right-sided venous ventricle, and the aorta ascends anteriorly and laterally from the left-sided systemic ventricle. The atrioventricular valves are inverted in concert with the ventricles. Hence the valve on the right is bicuspid and resembles a mitral valve, and that on the left is tricuspid. Intracardiac blood flows and pressures are normal unless there are additional malformations such as ventricular septal defect.

The clinical course and findings depend on the associated intracardiac defects. In the absence of other malformations, bradycardia at birth or developing childhood may be the only clue to the underlying anomaly. Murmurs are not present unless there is left-sided atrioventricular valvular regurgitation. A loud second sound at the left base represents aortic valve closure.

The ECG frequently shows atrioventricular conduction defects, including complete atrioventricular heart block. A Q wave is often present in right precordial leads and absent in the left precordial leads.

Echocardiographically, subcostal views are especially useful because they provide in a single view imaging of all cardiac chambers, great vessels, and their connections. The smooth-walled left ventricle with two papillary muscles and the right ventricle with marked trabeculation and moderator band are seen in the apical four-chamber view. The great arteries can be identified in a short-axis view as "double circles."

THE FOLLOWING CRITERION IS REQUIRED FOR THE DIAGNOSIS OF CONGENITALLY CORRECTED TRANSPOSITION OF THE GREAT ARTERIES.

Echocardiographic or angiocardiographic demonstration of ventricular morphology, with the pulmonary artery arising medially and posteriorly from a smooth-walled, right-sided (anatomic left) ventricle and the aorta arising on the left and anteriorly from a trabeculated, left-sided (anatomic right) ventricle.

DOUBLE-OUTLET RIGHT VENTRICLE

In double-outlet right ventricle, both the aorta and pulmonary artery take origin from the morphologic right ventricle. Neither semilunar valve is in fibrous continuity with the mitral valve. A ventricular septal defect is an integral part of the anomaly and is the only outlet for blood from the left ventricle. Variations in the anomaly may be identified by the position of the ventricular defect relative to the semilunar valves and the location of the conus or infundibulum. The Taussig-Bing malformation is a form of transposition of the great arteries complicated by a double-outlet right ventricle with a subpulmonary ventricular septal defect.

The hemodynamic and clinical picture of double-outlet right ventricle resembles that of ventricular septal defect. If, however, there is associated obstruction to pulmonary blood flow, the lesion may mimic tetralogy of Fallot. The ECG frequently shows a left or superior QRS axis in the range of -30 to -170 degrees.

Cardiac catheterization may reveal a left-to-right shunt at the ventricular level and increased pulmonary artery pressure; the aortic or systemic arterial oxyhemoglobin saturation may be normal from direct streaming of left ventricular blood into the aorta. In right ventricular infundibular stenosis or pulmonary vascular disease, systemic arterial hemoglobin unsaturation may be present.

The diagnosis rests on filling of both great arteries by contrast material following injection into the right ventricle and visualization of an aortic valve that lies abnormally high and at the same level as the pulmonary valve. Additional selective injections of contrast material into the aorta or left ventricle may be needed to clarify the relationship and origin of the great arteries.

Two-dimensional echocardiography is diagnostic for this lesion, demonstrating both great arteries connected to the right ventricle. The malalignment of the interventricular septum, associated septal defects, and the spatial relationships of the semilunar valves can be identified in parasternal and apical four-chamber views.

THE FOLLOWING CRITERION IS REQUIRED FOR THE DIAGNOSIS OF DOUBLE-OUTLET RIGHT VENTRICLE.

Echocardiographic or angiocardiographic demonstration that both great arteries arise from the right ventricle, with the aortic valve lying in an abnormally high position, and with both semilunar valves separated from the anterior leaflet of the mitral valve by muscular (or conal) tissue.

Defects at the Atrial Level

PATENT FORAMEN OVALE

A patent foramen ovale may be significant as a conduit permitting "paradoxical" emboli from the right side to the systemic circulation. It is an important aperture during fetal life, permitting shunting of inferior vena caval blood, which has a high oxygen content, from the right atrium to the left atrium. At or soon after birth, the left atrial pressure rises, and the flap, or valve, is pushed tightly against the septum, functionally closing the foramen ovale. Anatomic or probe patency usually occurs for several months and may persist into adult life in 20 to 30 percent of persons. Occasionally, a cardiac catheter advanced through the inferior vena cava may cross the atrial septum through the foramen ovale and enter the left atrium.

An isolated patent foramen ovale is of no clinical significance. If, however, right atrial pressure is increased because of associated malformations, such as tricuspid atresia or severe pulmonary valvular stenosis with an intact ventricular septum, a right-to-left shunt may occur through the foramen ovale into the left atrium.

Excellent transthoracic echocardiographic images of the atrial septum can be obtained with subcostal four-chamber or sagittal views, which demonstrate the patent foramen. In some patients the transesophageal approach is necessary.

ONE OF THE FOLLOWING CRITERIA IS REQUIRED FOR THE DIAGNOSIS OF PATENT FORAMEN OVALE.

1. **Echocardiographic visualization of the patent foramen ovale.**
2. **Passage of a catheter from the right to the left atrium or angiographic demonstration of a right-to-left shunt at the atrial level in the absence of specific findings compatible with the diagnosis of an atrial septal defect of an ostium secundum or primum type.**

ATRIAL SEPTAL DEFECT (OSTIUM SECUNDUM)

Atrial septal defect (ostium secundum), a common type of interatrial communication, usually occurs in the region of the fossa ovalis and is separated from the atrioventricular valves by a rim of septal tissue. The size of the defect may range from 0.5 to 3.0 cm or more. It is usually a single opening, although bands of septal tissue may divide it into multiple apertures. When the location of the defect is high (near the superior vena cava–sinus venosus defect), some of the pulmonary veins, particularly from the right lung, may drain anomalously into the right atrium or the proximal portion of the superior vena cava. Blood is usually shunted through the defect from the left to the right atrium in the presence of normal, or only slightly elevated, right heart pressure.

Symptoms and signs vary with the size of the defect and the volume and direction of intracardiac shunting. A left-to-right shunt at the atrial level may not occur in early infancy until the pulmonary vascular resistance falls toward normal because of maturation of the pulmonary vascular bed. Slow weight gain may be noted in children in whom extremely large left-to-right atrial shunts develop. The majority of children and young adults have moderate shunts and are asymptomatic. In those few in whom increased pulmonary vascular resistance develops in late childhood or adult life, right-to-left shunting may occur and cyanosis ensues.

Murmurs characteristic of atrial septal defect are related to increased blood flow across the tricuspid and pulmonic valves: a mid-diastolic murmur at the lower left sternal border and a more prominent systolic ejection murmur at the upper left sternal border. The second sound in the pulmonic area is widely split and usually fixed. With right-to-left shunting at the atrial level, the pulmonic component of the second sound is very loud and may be followed by a decrescendo diastolic murmur of pulmonary valvular regurgitation.

The ECG usually reveals right-axis deviation and right ventricular conduction delay of the right bundle branch type, with an rsR′ pattern in the right precordial leads. Prolongation of the P–R interval is occasionally noted. Atrial arrhythmias, notably atrial fibrillation, may occur in older children and adults.

The chest x-ray may show mild to moderate cardiac enlargement, particularly involving the right atrium and right ventricle, and prominent pulmonary vascular markings.

Echocardiography in the four-chamber subcostal view demonstrates the septal defect, and Doppler examination identifies the left-to-right shunt. A dilated right ventricle and abnormal septal motion can also be demonstrated.

Right heart catheterization reveals a left-to-right shunt at the atrial level, with normal or elevated pulmonary arterial pressure. A transesophageal approach may sometimes be necessary.

ONE OF THE FOLLOWING CRITERIA IS REQUIRED FOR THE DIAGNOSIS OF ATRIAL SEPTAL DEFECT (OSTIUM SECUNDUM).

Initial

A systolic ejection murmur in the pulmonary area, followed by a widely split and fixed second sound, ECG evidence of right axis deviation and rsR′ in the right precordial leads, and radiologic evidence of increased pulmonary vascular markings.

Definitive

1. **Documentation of a left-to-right shunt at the atrial level, with one or both of the following: a systolic ejection**

murmur in the pulmonary area, followed by a widely split second sound, or normal or right axis deviation.
2. Angiocardiographic demonstration of a right-to-left shunt at the atrial level, with markedly elevated pulmonary vascular resistance.
3. Echocardiographic demonstration of the defect and the dilated right ventricle and pulmonary artery.

ENDOCARDIAL CUSHION DEFECT (OSTIUM PRIMUM AND ATRIOVENTRICULAR CANAL DEFECTS)

Abnormalities in the development of the endocardial cushions and the regions immediately adjacent produce characteristic defects of the atrial septum, ventricular septum, and atrioventricular valves. These defects may occur together or singly and range in complexity from the so-called partial form of atrioventricular canal, or persistent ostium primum atrial defect with cleft mitral valve, to the complete form of atrioventricular canal, in which there is a common atrioventricular valve (formed by contiguity of the mitral and tricuspid apparatus), with an ostium primum defect above and a subjacent ventricular defect. The ostium primum defect occupies the lowermost portion of the atrial septum, so that no rim of tissue exists below it. A cleft of the anterior leaflet of the mitral valve is almost always present, and the septal leaflet of the tricuspid valve is frequently deformed. These atrioventricular valvular malformations also occur when no atrial septum is present, as in single, or common, atrium.

The ostium primum defect permits a left-to-right shunt at the atrial level. Often, though not invariably, mitral regurgitation occurs through the cleft anterior leaflet. In the complete form of atrioventricular canal, additional left-to-right shunting may occur at the ventricular level or from left ventricle to right atrium. Pulmonary hypertension and increased pulmonary vascular resistance may develop early in the complete forms of atrioventricular canal and result in bidirectional or right-to-left shunting.

The majority of patients with ostium primum defect and cleft mitral valve without mitral regurgitation have a clinical course similar to that of ostium secundum atrial septal defect. Ventricular failure may occur in infancy or early childhood in those with severe mitral regurgitation or in those with a common atrioventricular valve. Survival beyond childhood is uncommon with the complete forms of atrioventricular canal. The incidence of trisomy 21, or mongolism, is high in all varieties of endocardial cushion defect.

The murmurs associated with ostium primum defect are similar to those found in secundum atrial defect, but an apical systolic murmur may also be heard in the presence of mitral regurgitation.

The ECG is valuable in the diagnosis of endocardial cushion defects, since it characteristically shows left axis deviation or a superior QRS axis, usually between -40 and -180 degrees, with vectorcardiographic display of a counterclockwise loop in the frontal plane. Right bundle branch block is usually seen. Prolongation of the P–R interval is common. In addition, right, left, or biventricular enlargement may be present.

Selective left ventriculography shows specific deformity of the left ventricular outflow tract related to the abnormality of insertion of the anterior leaflet of the mitral valve.

Echocardiographic study can define the extent of the atrial and ventricular communication, the anatomy of the atrioventricular valves, the degree of atrioventricular valve insufficiency, and chamber size as well as associated lesions, if present. Multiple planes of two-dimensional imaging are required for complete analysis, and Doppler color flow mapping is especially useful for evaluation of atrioventricular valve insufficiency.

THE FOLLOWING CRITERIA ARE REQUIRED FOR THE DIAGNOSIS OF ENDOCARDIAL CUSHION DEFECT (OSTIUM PRIMUM AND ATRIOVENTRICULAR CANAL DEFECTS).

Initial

Typical systolic murmur(s) and ECG evidence of a left or superior QRS axis.

Definitive

1. **Evidence of a left-to-right shunt at the atrial level and echocardiographic demonstration of the complex of septal and valvular abnormalities.**
2. **Angiocardiographic demonstration of the characteristic left ventricular outflow tract deformity.**

SINGLE (COMMON) ATRIUM

In single atrium, the atrial septum is absent, but there are two atrial appendages. A left superior vena cava, as well as a right superior vena cava, is frequently present. A single sinoatrial node is usually present on the right but may be bilateral. Functionally, a left-to-right shunt predominates, the magnitude being dependent on the relationship of the pulmonary-to-systemic resistance.

A single atrium is encountered mainly in two circumstances: (1) abnormalities of cardiac position associated with discordant visceroatrial situs and bulboventricular looping and (2) endocardial cushion defects with the cleft mitral valve or common atrioventricular valve.

The clinical picture resembles that of large atrial septal defects of the secundum or primum types. Ectopic atrial rhythms are occasionally noted.

The echocardiographic subcostal four-chamber and sagittal views identify complete absence of the atrial septum except for a rim of superior tissue.

ONE OF THE FOLLOWING CRITERIA IS REQUIRED FOR THE DIAGNOSIS OF SINGLE (COMMON) ATRIUM.
1. **Echocardiographic demonstration of a single atrium.**
2. **Angiocardiographic demonstration of a single large atrial chamber receiving both systemic and pulmonary venous blood, usually in association with a diagnosis of anomalous cardiac position or endocardial cushion defect.**

COR TRIATRIATUM

Cor triatriatum is an unusual congenital anomaly in which there is failure of the pulmonary veins to be directly incorporated into the definitive left atrium, emptying instead to an atrium-like chamber above the left atrium. The two chambers communicate through an opening that, if narrow, causes obstruction to pulmonary venous flow, with altered dynamics simulating those of mitral obstruction. An atrial septal defect with communication between the right atrium and the left atrium sometimes coexists.

Tachypnea and evidences of respiratory distress may be the major findings in infancy or early childhood. An apical systolic or diastolic murmur may be audible. ECGs usually indicate right ventricular enlargement. Chest x-rays may show pulmonary venous congestion.

During right heart catheterization, the catheter may pass across the atrial septum to the left atrium. If the atrial defect is above the level of the obstructing membrane, a high atrial pressure will be recorded; if the defect is between the membrane and the mitral valve, the left atrial pressure will be normal. Pulmonary arterial hypertension is usually severe, with the systolic pressure sometimes exceeding that in the systemic arterial bed.

Angiocardiography, best performed by injection into the pulmonary artery, reveals drainage of the pulmonary veins into an accessory left atrial chamber and a linear filling defect, indicating a ledge or diaphragm between the chamber and the more distal true left atrium.

Two-dimensional echocardiography identifies the membranes in the left atrial cavity that divide the left atrium into two chambers. Pulsed Doppler echocardiography and Doppler color flow study can be used to quantify degrees of left ventricular inflow obstruction.

ONE OF THE FOLLOWING CRITERIA IS REQUIRED FOR THE DIAGNOSIS OF COR TRIATRIATUM.

1. **Echocardiographic demonstration of the two-chambered left atrium, the posterior superior chamber receiving the pulmonary veins and the anteroinferior chamber giving rise to the left atrial appendage and communicating with the mitral valve.**
2. **Angiocardiographic demonstration of the pulmonary veins draining into an accessory atrial chamber, which is separated by a linear filling defect from the more distal true left atrium.**

Defects at the Ventricular Level

CONGENITAL VENTRICULAR SEPTAL DEFECT

Ventricular septal defects are among the most common of all congenital heart lesions, alone or in combination with other malformations. The size of an isolated ventricular septal defect is probably the most important feature in determining the hemodynamic derangements that ensue. However, the anatomic location, whether in the membranous or muscular portion of the septum or above or below the crista supraventricularis, also may influence the clinical course and surgical management. The most common defect, usually referred to as the membranous type, lies inferior to the crista and is in part overhung by the septal leaflet of the tricuspid valve. Muscular defects may occur in any portion of the muscular part of the septum; they are frequently small and may be multiple.

A ventricular septal defect may decrease in size with advancing age or even close completely.

Symptoms vary with the magnitude of left-to-right shunting through the defect, which is dependent on its size and the level of pulmonary vascular resistance. When defects are large, ventricular failure may develop during the first few months of life. When shunts are moderate in size, reduced exercise tolerance and growth impairment may occur. When shunts are small, no symptoms ensue. Pulmonary vascular resistance may increase when shunts are large; high pulmonary vascular resistance in children and young adults may cause reversal of the shunt and the appearance of cyanosis.

The physical signs usually include a harsh holosystolic murmur and thrill along the lower left sternal border. An apical mid-diastolic murmur accompanies large left-to-right shunts, which markedly increase the pulmonary venous flow traversing the mitral valve into an enlarged left ventricular chamber. The intensity of the pulmonic valve closure sound varies directly with the pulmonary arterial pressure. In the presence of cyanosis due to right-to-left shunting at the ventricular level, a decrescendo diastolic murmur may indicate pulmonary valvular regurgitation.

When the left-to-right shunt through the ventricular septal defect is small, the ECG and chest x-ray may be normal. However, with moderate and large shunts, there is usually increased left ventricular QRS voltage in the ECG. The chest film may show enlargement of the left atrium and ventricle, a dilated pulmonary arterial segment, and increased pulmonary vascular markings. With right-to-left shunting, right ventricular hypertrophy is noted on the ECG, and the central pulmonary arteries may appear enlarged, with sparse peripheral vascular markings.

Two-dimensional echocardiography can assess the number, location, and size of the defects, which may occur in the various portions of the interventricular septum (membranous, inlet, trabecular, outlet). Multiple views and Doppler color flow examination are required for complete anatomic definition and physiologic evaluation of transeptal flows, pulmonary artery pressure, and ventricular function.

Right heart catheterization indicates the presence of a left-to-right shunt at the ventricular level, with normal or elevated pulmonary arterial pressure. No shunt will be detected if pulmonary vascular resistance is markedly increased. Occasionally, a catheter in the right ventricle will traverse the ventricular defect and enter the aorta.

Injection of contrast material into the left ventricle demonstrates a left-to-right shunt and the size and location of the defect. Following right ventricular injection, there may be reopacification of the right ventricle or pulmonary artery after the left ventricle fills. If there is severe pulmonary hypertension, selective injection into the right ventricle may demonstrate a right-to-left ventricular shunt.

ONE OF THE FOLLOWING CRITERIA IS REQUIRED FOR THE DIAGNOSIS OF CONGENITAL VENTRICULAR SEPTAL DEFECT.

Initial

A loud systolic murmur along the lower left sternal border.

Definitive

1. **Echocardiographic demonstration of the defect.**
2. **Demonstration of the defect and a left-to-right shunt at the ventricular level with an elevated pulmonary artery pressure and normally related great vessels.**
3. **Demonstration of a right-to-left shunt at the ventricular level with severe pulmonary hypertension and in the absence of other malformations.**

CONGENITAL VENTRICULAR SEPTAL DEFECT WITH OBSTRUCTION TO RIGHT VENTRICULAR OUTFLOW

Mild or Moderate Obstruction to Right Ventricular Outflow

A ventricular septal defect, usually one of moderate or large size, may be complicated by obstruction to right ventricular outflow either at the subvalvular or valvular level. There may be hypertrophy of the crista supraventricularis or occasionally pulmonary valvular stenosis. The presence of mild to moderate obstruction to right ventricular outflow effects a rise in right ventricular pressure and a reduction in the flow from left to right through the ventricular septal defect. In some instances, the muscular hypertrophy is progressive and may develop into severe obstruction, presenting the clinical picture of tetralogy of Fallot.

The signs differ from those of isolated ventricular septal defect due to the associated right ventricular obstruction. A loud, coarse, ejection systolic murmur may be heard along the entire left sternal border and may be well transmitted under the clavicles. The murmur is usually associated with a thrill. The second heart sound at the pulmonic area is usually of normal intensity. The ECG usually shows a right ventricular hypertrophy pattern; the chest x-ray shows only a modest increase in pulmonary vascularity.

In addition to a left-to-right shunt at the ventricular level, a systolic pressure gradient usually in excess of 20 mm Hg is recorded across the right ventricular outflow tract, the pulmonary valve, or both.

Angiocardiography permits visualization of the narrowed right ventricular outflow tract or pulmonary valvular obstruction.

Echocardiographic assessment of the septal defect is described in the previous section. Right ventricular outflow tract obstruction at the infundibular level is evaluated with subcostal coronal or sagittal views. Doppler study allows calculation of the outflow tract pressure gradient.

ONE OF THE FOLLOWING CRITERIA IS REQUIRED FOR THE DIAGNOSIS OF CONGENITAL VENTRICULAR SEPTAL DEFECT WITH MILD OR MODERATE OBSTRUCTION TO RIGHT VENTRICULAR OUTFLOW.

1. **Echocardiographic demonstration of the anatomic and physiologic components of the anomaly.**
2. **Documentation of a left-to-right shunt at the ventricular level and measurement of a systolic pressure gradient between the body of the right ventricle and the pulmonary artery or angiographic demonstration of obstruction.**

Severe Obstruction to Right Ventricular Outflow (Tetralogy of Fallot)

The combination of a ventricular septal defect, usually of large size, and severe obstruction to right ventricular outflow comprises the two critical anatomic components of tetralogy of Fallot. The ventricular defect usually lies below the crista supraventricularis. Obstruction to right ventricular outflow is most frequently due to narrowing of the infundibulum associated with muscular hypertrophy and may be progressive. In addition, there may occasionally be pulmonary valvular stenosis, hypoplasia of the pulmonary annulus, or constriction at the origin of the right or left pulmonary artery.

The two other features included in the designation of tetralogy of Fallot are overriding of the aorta and right ventricular hypertrophy, both of which are of secondary importance. The aorta arises from both ventricles above the large ventricular defect, with considerable variation in the degree of its dextroposition or overriding of the right ventricle. Since the systolic pressures in the body of the right ventricle and aorta are always equal, and the right ventricular outflow tract is obstructed, the direction of the right-to-left shunt is determined physiologically rather than anatomically. Additional anomalies encountered in tetralogy of Fallot include a right aortic arch, present in about one-third of patients, and an aberrant branching of the right coronary artery, with a large anterior descending vessel crossing the outflow tract of the right ventricle. The coexistence of a patent ductus arteriosus permits survival in those with pulmonary atresia.

Signs and symptoms vary with the severity of obstruction of the right ventricular outflow tract. Cyanosis may be present at birth or develop sometime after infancy. Clubbing of the digits eventually accompanies the cyanosis. Breathlessness with exertion may be manifested in infancy by distress during crying. Hypoxic "spells" with loss of consciousness may ensue. Breathlessness or extreme fatigue with exercise in childhood may be relieved by a squatting posture. Ventricular failure does not occur except in infants with associated pulmonary atresia. Cerebral complications, which include thrombosis or profound hypoxia, may be life-threatening or cause death.

A systolic thrill and harsh systolic murmur are usually present at the mid and upper left sternal border. The murmur is related to the systolic pressure gradient at the site or sites of right ventricular outflow obstruction. When pulmonary atresia exists, no systolic murmur is audible. The pulmonic component of the second sound is diminished or absent; the aortic valve closure sound may be prominent along the left sternal border.

Echocardiographic study, using various views, delineates all the major elements of this complex lesion, including deviation of the right infundibular septum, dextroposition and overriding of the aorta, right ventricular outflow tract narrowing, septal defect, and right ventricular hypertrophy.

The ECG shows right axis deviation and moderate to severe right ventricular hypertrophy. The chest x-ray reveals a small or normal-sized heart, usually with uplifted apex (boot-shaped contour) due to right ventricular hypertrophy and a relatively concave pulmonary artery segment. The pulmonary arteries are small, and the peripheral vascular markings are usually diminished. The aortic knob may be seen to the right.

A systolic pressure gradient exists between the body of the right ventricle and the outflow tract, and an additional distal gradient may occasionally be found at the level of the pulmonary valve. The pulmonary arterial pressure may be normal but is usually reduced. The systolic pressure in the right ventricle equals that in the aorta, which is frequently entered by passage of a catheter through the large ventricular septal defect. Systemic arterial oxyhemoglobin saturation is always reduced.

Angiocardiography with selective injection into the right ventricle demonstrates early opacification of the aorta as contrast material passes directly from the right ventricle into the aorta. It also indicates the site or sites of right ventricular outflow tract obstruction and the size of the pulmonary arteries.

ONE OF THE FOLLOWING CRITERIA IS REQUIRED FOR THE DIAGNOSIS OF CONGENITAL VENTRICULAR SEPTAL DEFECT WITH SEVERE OBSTRUCTION TO RIGHT VENTRICULAR OUTFLOW (TETRALOGY OF FALLOT).

1. **Echocardiographic demonstration of the anatomic and physiologic components of the anomaly.**
2. **Angiocardiographic demonstration, following selective right ventricular injection, of early opacification of the left ventricular outflow tract and aorta in addition to the site of right ventricular outflow tract obstruction.**

CONGENITAL LEFT VENTRICULAR TO RIGHT ATRIAL COMMUNICATION

Left ventricular to right atrial communication is an uncommon defect. Two types occur: (1) a defect in that part of the membranous portion of the ventricular septum that enters into the formation of the floor of the right atrium and (2) a defect in the ventricular septum posterior to the crista supraventricularis, associated with a cleft or a double orifice of the tricuspid valve. In the latter situation, left ventricular blood may be ejected through the right ventricle directly into the right atrium. An extra opening of the tricupsid valve or adhesions between the edges of the ventricular septal defect and those of the cleft often permit a direct channel from left ventricle to right atrium.

The clinical picture, including a systolic thrill and murmur along the left sternal border, is identical with that noted with a ventricular septal defect, usually one of small or moderate size.

The ECG often shows tall P waves, suggesting right atrial enlargement. The chest x-ray may show prominence of the right atrium. The pulmonary vascular markings are increased. Right heart catheterization documents a left-to-right shunt at the atrial level. Selective left ventriculography demonstrates shunting from the left ventricle to the right atrium.

THE FOLLOWING CRITERION IS REQUIRED FOR THE DIAGNOSIS OF CONGENITAL LEFT VENTRICULAR TO RIGHT ATRIAL COMMUNICATION.
Demonstration by left ventriculography or echocardiography of a normal left ventricular outflow tract and direct communication or shunt into the right atrium.

SINGLE (COMMON) VENTRICLE

Morphologically, single ventricle usually resembles a large left ventricle into which both atrioventricular valves empty; the outflow tract of the underdeveloped right ventricle is represented by the infundibulum. The aorta and pulmonary artery are usually transposed, with the aorta arising anteriorly above the infundibular chamber. In the circumstances of ventricular inversion, single ventricle may also occur.

As a result of admixture of right and left atrial blood in the single ventricle, there may be evidence of a left-to-right shunt at the ventricular level and of a right-to-left shunt as revealed by a reduction in oxyhemoglobin saturation in the systemic arterial circulation. The relative magnitude and direction of the shunt depend on the pulmonary vascular resistance and the presence or absence of obstruction at the outlet of either the aorta or pulmonary artery.

The clinical features are variable, depending on the relative magnitude of pulmonary blood flow and associated defects. Cyanosis is usually obvious, since the most frequently encountered form is that of single ventricle with transposition of the great arteries and increased pulmonary vascular resistance. Auscultation, ECG, and x-ray are not helpful in differential diagnosis.

Specific diagnosis can be made by angiocardiography. Particularly valuable is the selective injection of contrast media into the left atrium through the usually present atrial communication. Opacification of the common ventricular chamber reveals a large, relatively smooth, finely trabeculated ventricle, which resembles the left ventricle. Following opacification of the large ventricular chamber, there may be dense opacification of an anterior infundibular chamber, from which the aorta may arise in a transposed position.

Various views in two-dimensional echocardiography diagnose the principal chamber with left ventricular trabeculation, associated atrioventricular connections, and transposition of the aorta and pulmonary artery. The rudimentary right ventricle can be identified and separated from the main chamber. The less common univentricular heart of the right ventricular type can also be recognized echocardiographically.

ONE OF THE FOLLOWING CRITERIA IS REQUIRED FOR THE DIAGNOSIS OF SINGLE (COMMON) VENTRICLE.

1. **Echocardiographic demonstration of the univentricular heart.**
2. **Selective angiocardiographic demonstration of a ventricular chamber receiving both atrioventricular valves.**

Congenital Malformations of the Aortic Valve

AORTIC LEAFLET, ANNULAR, OR COMMISSURAL DEFORMITIES CAUSING REGURGITATION

Congenital defects of the aortic valve resulting in regurgitation are less frequently observed than those causing obstruction. Bicuspid aortic valves may become incompetent with advancing age, due to cusp distortion. Aortic regurgitation may occur with ventricular septal defect, most often due to prolapse of the right coronary cusp. In rare instances, distortion of a single leaflet or commissure may impair cusp apposition.

The symptoms and signs will be affected by the associated defects and by the degree of regurgitation. A high-pitched, decrescendo diastolic murmur is heard at the right base and transmitted down the left sternal border. An aortic ejection sound is frequently present. Echocardiography demonstrates dilatation of the left ventricle, exaggerated wall motion, and fine fluttering of the anterior leaflet of the mitral valve. In addition, echocardiography, especially by the transesophageal route, may demonstrate a bicuspid or prolapsing valve. Doppler color flow study identifies transvalvular reflex from aorta to left ventricle.

Retrograde aortography with selective injection at the aortic root best demonstrates the degree of regurgitation and may outline the precise type of valve deformity present.

THE FOLLOWING CRITERIA ARE REQUIRED FOR THE DIAGNOSIS OF CONGENITAL AORTIC LEAFLET, ANNULAR, OR COMMISSURAL DEFORMITIES CAUSING REGURGITATION.

A decrescendo diastolic murmur at the right base or left sternal border, dating either from infancy or early childhood or noted in association with another congenital defect, and demonstration of aortic valvular regurgitation by echocardiography or selective aortography.

AORTIC ATRESIA

With aortic atresia, a fibrous membrane without an orifice constitutes the valve area; the ascending aorta is almost invariably hypoplastic. The mitral valve is small but structurally normal and communicates with a diminutive blind left ventricular cavity. An interatrial communication permitting a left-to-right shunt is essential for survival. The right ventricle therefore supplies both the pulmonary circulation and, through a patent ductus arteriosus, the systemic circulation. Atresia of the aortic valve is one of the variants in the so-called hypoplastic left heart syndrome. This designation refers to a group of lesions that include varying degrees of mitral and aortic valve obstruction, a small left ventricle, and a hypoplastic ascending aorta.

Symptoms and signs are usually severe and progressive and result from pulmonary venous congestion and right ventricular failure, with inadequate systemic arterial perfusion and shock. Respiratory distress, pallor, and poor peripheral pulses are striking. Death almost invariably occurs during the first 2 weeks of life. Murmurs are nonspecific and unimpressive. The pulmonic component of the second heart sound is very loud.

The ECG shows right axis deviation and right ventricular hypertrophy. The chest x-ray may show cardiac enlargement due to right atrial and right ventricular dilatation; the pulmonary artery may be dilated. Pulmonary venous congestion is prominent. Multiple echocardiographic views, particularly parasternal and apical four-chamber, delineate the large right ventricle, the small left ventricle and ascending aorta, and the abnormal aortic valve.

Cardiac catheterization demonstrates a left-to-right shunt at the atrial level, systemic pressure in the right ventricle, and patency of the ductus arteriosus by passage of a catheter through it.

After selective left atrial injection, angiocardiography demonstrates the blind left ventricular cavity and the passage of contrast material into the right atrium. Additional right ventricular or pulmonary artery injection permits visualization of retrograde aortic flow to the level of the atretic valve through a patent ductus arteriosus.

ONE OF THE FOLLOWING CRITERIA IS REQUIRED FOR THE DIAGNOSIS OF AORTIC ATRESIA.

1. **Echocardiographic demonstration of the ventricular and valvular components of the anomaly.**
2. **Angiocardiographic demonstration of a small left ventricular chamber that does not opacify the aorta and retrograde aortic flow to the level of the aortic valve.**

CONGENITAL AORTIC VALVULAR STENOSIS

Congenital aortic valvular stenosis is a common type of valve defect that may occur in three major anatomic forms according to the nature of commissural fusion and the number of apparent leaflets present: (1) a dome-shaped malformation due to varying degrees of fusion of the three commissures, producing a central orifice; (2) a unicuspid valve resulting from complete fusion of two commissures, usually leaving a single commissure, which produces an eccentric orifice; and (3) a bicuspid valve, which may be only mildly obstructive in early childhood but may become progressively narrowed by thickening and calcification and cause obstruction in adult life.

Severe obstruction in early infancy may be associated with left ventricular failure. Mild or moderate stenosis in early life may cause few or no symptoms. However, progression to severe obstruction in later years may result in fatigue, chest pain, or syncope. Sudden death may be preceded by ECG evidence of severe left ventricular hypertrophy, with S–T segment and T-wave changes.

A loud, harsh ejection systolic murmur accompanied by a thrill may be present at the right base and is transmitted to the brachiocephalic vessels. An ejection click is frequently audible. A narrow pulse pressure may be noted with moderate or severe obstruction.

The ECG usually is normal in mild obstruction. Evidence of left ventricular hypertrophy and S–T segment and T-wave changes in the left precordial leads may occur with increasing obstruction.

The chest x-ray shows a normal heart size, with some dilatation of the ascending aorta. Left ventricular enlargement may be apparent with severe obstruction or left ventricular failure.

A systolic gradient is present across the aortic valve. This may range from 10 mm Hg with minimal obstruction to over 200 mm Hg with extreme obstruction.

Echocardiographic examination identifies the morphology and number of aortic valve cusps. Ventricular size, thickness, and function can also be assessed. Physiologic evaluation by Doppler techniques allows quantitative evaluation of the transvalvular gradient and valve area.

Selective left ventriculography permits visualization of the nature and the site of obstruction.

THE FOLLOWING CRITERIA ARE REQUIRED FOR THE DIAGNOSIS OF CONGENITAL AORTIC VALVULAR STENOSIS.

Initial

A harsh systolic murmur at the right base dating from infancy or early childhood.

Definitive

Demonstration of aortic valve obstruction by echocardiography or cardiac catheterization.

CONGENITAL SUBVALVULAR AORTIC STENOSIS

A fibrous ridge or diaphragm may be present a few millimeters to several centimeters below a normal aortic valve. Clinically, this type of discrete obstruction may be indistinguishable from that due to valvular stenosis, except that no ejection click is audible, and dilatation of the ascending aorta is not prominent. Discrete subvalvular aortic stenosis must be distinguished from diffuse, fixed, tunnel-like obstruction of the left ventricular outflow tract and from diffuse obstruction caused by a hypertrophied septum abutting the anterior leaflet of the mitral valve during systole.

Echocardiographic examination reveals the discrete subvalvular fibrous membrane as a thin linear echo in the outflow tract of the left ventricle. Subcostal and apical four-chamber views are also informative. Doppler study quantifies the magnitude of the left ventricular outflow tract obstruction. Echocardiography will also differentiate discrete subvalvular obstruction from an obstruction due to a hypertrophied septum.

Left ventriculography may demonstrate that the stenotic site is below a normally moving valve. However, when the fibrous diaphragm is close to the valve, it may be difficult to distinguish it from valvular stenosis.

THE FOLLOWING CRITERION IS REQUIRED FOR THE DIAGNOSIS OF CONGENITAL SUBVALVULAR AORTIC STENOSIS.

Evidence of a localized obstruction below the valve demonstrated by echocardiography, MRI, CT, or angiography.

CONGENITAL SUPRAVALVULAR AORTIC STENOSIS

Supravalvular aortic stenosis is a localized or diffuse narrowing of the aorta originating just above the level of the coronary arteries at the superior margin of the sinuses of Valsalva. It may occur with or without peripheral pulmonary arterial stenosis in a familial or sporadic form. The anomaly may be identified with idiopathic infantile hypercalcemia when associated defects include mental retardation, elfin facies, strabismus, dental abnormalities, and peripheral pulmonary and systemic arterial stenoses.

The symptoms are similar to those of aortic valvular stenosis. Although the systolic thrill and ejection murmur at the right base may be indistinguishable from those of valvular or subvalvular stenosis, the aortic closure sound is frequently accentuated, and an ejection click is uncommon. Inequality in the brachial arterial pressures may be noted, the right more often being higher than the left.

The ECG and chest x-ray resemble those of aortic valvular stenosis. A systolic pressure gradient is present above the valve. Left ventriculography permits visualization of the supravalvular aortic obstruction. The coronary arteries, located proximal to the stenosis, are usually prominent vessels. Selective injection of contrast material into the main pulmonary artery may permit demonstration of associated peripheral pulmonary arterial stenosis.

Echocardiographic study discloses the small diameter of the supravalvular aorta, and an hourglass deformity may be noted. The narrowed segment may be quite long, extending from the aortic sinuses to the origin of the innominate artery. Aortic valve thickening may also be found, and coronary ostial narrowing should be excluded.

THE FOLLOWING CRITERION IS REQUIRED FOR THE DIAGNOSIS OF CONGENITAL SUPRAVALVULAR AORTIC STENOSIS.

Echocardiographic or angiographic demonstration of obstruction distal to the aortic valve.

Congenital Malformations of the Mitral Valve

MITRAL LEAFLET, ANNULAR, OR COMMISSURAL DEFORMITIES CAUSING REGURGITATION

Isolated congenital malformations of the mitral valve are uncommon; more often, these malformations are associated with other defects, such as endocardial cushion defect with a cleft in the anterior leaflet, congenitally corrected transposition of the great arteries with abnormality of the left-sided atrioventricular valve, or anomalous origin of the left coronary artery from the pulmonary artery, causing infarction of a papillary muscle. The rare isolated deformities of the mitral valve causing regurgitation include clefts in the anterior or posterior leaflet, separation of the commissures with dilatation of the annulus, an accessory orifice in one of the cusps, anomalies of the chordae tendineae or their insertion, and prolapsing of a cusp associated with papillary muscle dysfunction.

The symptoms and signs vary with the severity of the valvular defect. Left ventricular failure with pulmonary edema may occur early in severe cases; milder cases have exertional breathlessness. A blowing apical systolic murmur present from early infancy usually distinguishes these lesions from acquired mitral valvular deformity, notably that secondary to rheumatic valvulitis. At the apex, a prominent systolic click is heard when papillary muscle dysfunction permits billowing of a leaflet.

The ECG shows a broad P wave, with usually a normal QRS axis and left ventricular hypertrophy. Progressive T-wave changes may develop in papillary muscle dysfunction with inversion in leads II, III, and aVF and over the left precordium.

The chest x-ray displays left atrial and left ventricular enlargement. The left atrium may be enormous in severe cases. The pulmonary arterial wedge pressure is usually elevated, and there is a tall V wave in the left atrial pressure tracing.

Significant regurgitation into the left atrium may be demonstrated by injection of contrast material into the left ventricle. Cineangiocardiography permits precise identification of the valve dysfunction. Doppler color flow echocardiography can be used for definite diagnosis and physiologic evaluation of the severity of mitral regurgitation.

THE FOLLOWING CRITERIA ARE REQUIRED FOR THE DIAGNOSIS OF CONGENITAL MITRAL LEAFLET, ANNULAR, OR COMMISSURAL DEFORMITIES CAUSING REGURGITATION.

Initial

A blowing apical systolic murmur first noted in infancy or early childhood.

Definitive

Echocardiographic or angiocardiographic demonstration of mitral regurgitation in the absence of congenitally corrected transposition of the great arteries and anomalous origin of the left coronary artery.

MITRAL ATRESIA

With mitral atresia, only a blind dimple is seen at the site of the mitral valve. It is usually associated with aortic valvular hypoplasia or atresia and an atrial septal defect. Usually, the interatrial communication is small, so that the left-to-right shunt is limited, and pulmonary venous congestion occurs. When the great arteries are normally related, some of the blood from the pulmonary artery may pass through a patent ductus arteriosus to the systemic arterial bed or through a ventricular septal defect to the left ventricle and then to the aorta. Occasionally, mitral atresia may coexist with single ventricle and complete transposition of the great arteries.

Severe respiratory distress, present from birth, is the dominant finding. Pallor or mild to moderate cyanosis may develop. Pulmonary venous congestion and right ventricular failure are usually progressive. Death usually occurs in infancy or childhood.

Murmurs are nonspecific. When present, they are related to the associated defects. The pulmonic valve closure sound is usually very loud. The ECG reveals marked right-axis deviation and right ventricular hypertrophy. The chest x-ray shows enlargement of the right heart chambers and pulmonary venous congestion. Left atrial pressure is elevated, and there is severe pulmonary hypertension. There is failure of the left ventricle to opacify after selective injection of contrast material into the left atrium.

Two-dimensional echocardiography is diagnostic of mitral atresia. Both parasternal and apical four-chamber views demonstrate the atretic mitral valve, and Doppler color flow imaging confirms lack of flow from the left atrium to the left ventricle.

ONE OF THE FOLLOWING CRITERIA IS REQUIRED FOR THE DIAGNOSIS OF MITRAL ATRESIA.

1. **Echocardiographic demonstration of an abnormal mitral valve and left ventricle.**
2. **Angiocardiographic demonstration of failure to opacify the left ventricle after injection of contrast material into the left atrium.**

CONGENITAL MITRAL STENOSIS

Mitral stenosis, an uncommon congenital lesion, may result from a fusion of the two leaflets at the commissures and a shortening of the chordae tendineae, often creating a funnel-shaped mitral valve. Malformation of the mitral valve causing obstruction must be considered in the differential diagnosis of cor triatriatum. Congenital mitral stenosis is frequently associated with other defects, particularly aortic stenosis, coarctation of the aorta, and patent ductus arteriosus.

Symptoms of respiratory distress dominate the clinical picture. An apical diastolic murmur, usually with presystolic accentuation, is audible from early infancy. The loud pulmonary valve closure sound reflects the severe pulmonary hypertension that is commonly present.

The ECG shows broad P waves, right axis deviation, and right ventricular hypertrophy. The chest x-ray shows left atrial enlargement, a prominent pulmonary arterial segment, and right ventricular enlargement. Pulmonary venous congestion may be present.

There is a diastolic pressure gradient across the mitral valve, and the pressures in the left atrium and pulmonary circulation are elevated. There may be a prominent A wave in the left atrial pressure curve.

Selective angiocardiography with injection of contrast material into the pulmonary artery shows delayed emptying of an enlarged left atrium.

The major forms of congenital mitral stenosis may be demonstrated by echocardiography: supramitral ring, hypoplastic mitral valve, congenital mitral stenosis, and parachute mitral valve. Doppler flow studies permit quantification of the mitral valve area and transvalvular gradient.

THE FOLLOWING CRITERIA ARE REQUIRED FOR THE DIAGNOSIS OF CONGENITAL MITRAL STENOSIS.

Initial

An apical diastolic murmur dating from infancy or early childhood.

Definitive

Demonstration by echocardiography or cardiac catheterization of mitral valve obstruction.

Congenital Malformations of the Pulmonary Valve

ABSENT PULMONARY VALVE

In absent pulmonary valve, the sinuses of Valsalva or cusps have not developed, and only a rim of irregular

fibrous tags exists. The hypoplastic valve ring is frequently obstructive. This may occur as an isolated lesion
but is more often associated with a ventricular septal
defect and right ventricular outflow tract obstruction.
Pulmonary regurgitation invariably results.

Evidence of respiratory distress and right ventricular
failure often dominate the picture in early infancy. A
medium- to low-pitched diastolic murmur along the upper left sternal border is usually present. Additional
murmurs vary, depending on the frequently associated
ventricular septal defect and the presence or absence of
right ventricular outflow tract obstruction.

The ECG demonstrates right ventricular hypertrophy.
The chest x-ray frequently shows striking enlargement
of the pulmonary arterial trunk and its main branches.
Sometimes these vessels may be aneurysmally dilated
and cause bronchial compression.

There is low diastolic pressure in the pulmonary artery,
with a normal or low systolic pressure and an elevated
end-diastolic pressure in the right ventricle.

Injection of contrast material into the pulmonary artery demonstrates the pulmonary valvular regurgitation. Most commonly seen with tetralogy of Fallot, the
fibrous remnants of the pulmonic valve are shown as
linear echoes without evidence of valve leaflet. Doppler
study and two-dimensional echocardiography also display severe pulmonic regurgitation and dilated pulmonary arteries.

**THE FOLLOWING CRITERIA ARE REQUIRED FOR THE
DIAGNOSIS OF ABSENT PULMONARY VALVE.**

Echocardiographic or angiocardiographic demonstration of
the abnormal pulmonic valve and pulmonic regurgitation.

PULMONARY ATRESIA WITH INTACT
VENTRICULAR SEPTUM

In pulmonary atresia with intact ventricular septum,
there is no patency of the valve, which is represented by a
fibrous diaphragm, from the upper aspect of which three
equidistant raphes radiating to the pulmonary arterial
wall may be visible. The pulmonary trunk distal to the
atretic valve may be somewhat narrower than normal,
but its two major branches are usually of normal size. The
size of the right ventricular cavity is usually small, and
the wall is markedly hypertrophied. If, however, the tri-

cuspid valve is of normal size, the right ventricular chamber may be either normal in size or enlarged. In all instances of pulmonary atresia, an interatrial communication is present, permitting a right-to-left shunt. The lungs are perfused via a patent ductus arteriosus.

The symptoms and signs are severe. Marked cyanosis and difficulty in breathing are present soon after birth. The absence of a murmur in the presence of ischemic lung fields suggests the diagnosis.

The ECG shows high voltage of QRS and left-axis deviation. Both the ECG and chest x-ray may be similar to those seen with tricuspid atresia; differentiation between the two conditions can be made only by further laboratory studies. Passage of a catheter from the right atrium into the right ventricle distinguishes this lesion from tricuspid atresia.

Angiocardiography demonstrates the size of the right ventricular lumen, the atretic pulmonic valve, and the right-to-left atrial shunt.

Two-dimensional echocardiography is of great value in demonstrating the thick right ventricle, which ends blindly, and tricuspid valve abnormalities, if present. Doppler study confirms the absence of antegrade flow from the right ventricle.

THE FOLLOWING CRITERION IS REQUIRED FOR THE DIAGNOSIS OF PULMONARY ATRESIA WITH INTACT VENTRICULAR SEPTUM.

Angiographic or echocardiographic demonstration of a blind right ventricular outflow tract with an intact ventricular septum.

CONGENITAL PULMONARY VALVULAR STENOSIS WITH INTACT VENTRICULAR SEPTUM

Pulmonary valvular stenosis with intact ventricular septum is a common lesion that, in mild form, usually shows a partial fusion of one or more commissures of a bicuspid or tricuspid valve. In severe stenosis, the commissures are poorly developed, and the valve cusps form a dome-shaped diaphragm with a small central orifice. Right ventricular hypertrophy is present, varying directly with the severity of the obstruction. Subvalvular hypertrophy of the crista supraventricularis develops with the more severe degrees of stenosis. Right atrial enlargement may occur, and a right-to-left shunt through a patent foramen ovale may develop with severe obstruction.

No symptoms may be present with mild and even moderate stenosis. However, with severe obstruction, breathlessness and cyanosis with exertion are common, and right ventricular failure may ensue. The physical signs include a prominent left parasternal impulse, a systolic thrill at the left base, a loud, harsh ejection systolic murmur maximal in the first and second left intercostal spaces, and a delayed, low-intensity pulmonic valve closure sound. A systolic click is frequently audible in the pulmonic area.

With mild stenosis, the ECG may be normal. With moderate obstruction, the ECG usually shows right-axis deviation and evidence of right atrial and right ventricular hypertrophy. With very severe obstruction, extreme R-wave voltage in the right precordial leads may be accompanied by deep T-wave inversion.

The chest x-ray is normal with mild stenosis but may show evidence of right ventricular enlargement with the more severe lesions. Post-stenotic dilatation of the main or left pulmonary artery or both is common.

The hypertrophied right ventricle, including concomitant infundibular stenosis, and thickened pulmonic valve are accurately demonstrated by two-dimensional echocardiography. Doppler study allows physiologic evaluation of the magnitude of the transvalvular gradient.

Cardiac catheterization documents right ventricular hypertension and a systolic pressure gradient across the pulmonary valve, with normal or low pulmonary arterial pressure.

Selective angiocardiography from the right ventricle allows precise visualization of the site of obstruction and absence of shunting at the ventricular level.

THE FOLLOWING CRITERIA ARE REQUIRED FOR THE DIAGNOSIS OF PULMONARY VALVULAR STENOSIS WITH INTACT VENTRICULAR SEPTUM.

An ejection systolic murmur at the upper left sternal border and echocardiographic or angiocardiographic evidence of pulmonary valvular obstruction and an intact ventricular septum.

Congenital Malformations of the Tricuspid Valve

TRICUSPID ATRESIA

With tricuspid atresia, no valve elements are visible, and only a dimple may be seen in the floor of the right atrium.

Survival demands that an interatrial communication exist, which may be either a secundum atrial defect or, more frequently, a patent foramen ovale. Right atrial blood is shunted to the left atrium and mixes with the pulmonary venous blood, which flows to the left ventricle; its subsequent course varies with the associated anomalies. Most often, the great arteries are normally related (in 70%), and blood is shunted through a small ventricular septal defect into a hypoplastic right ventricle and out through a small pulmonic valve and trunk to the lungs. When the great arteries are transposed (in 30%) so that the pulmonary artery arises from the left ventricle, blood flow to the lungs is increased unless subpulmonic stenosis is present.

Cyanosis usually exists from birth. A systolic murmur at the left sternal border is audible if pulmonary valvular stenosis or a ventricular septal defect is present.

Echocardiographic examination demonstrates the relative increase in the size of the left ventricle and diminutive size of the right ventricular cavity. The ventricular septal defect is also noted, as well as transposition of the great vessels, if present. The apical four-chamber and subcostal views allow examination of the right ventricular outlet and the structure of the tricuspid valve remnants or membrane. The interatrial communication is also demonstrated.

The ECG is helpful, showing left axis deviation, tall peaked P waves, and increased left ventricular QRS voltage for the age level.

The chest x-ray usually shows a small or normal-sized heart with a prominent right atrial border and an enlarged left ventricle. Pulmonary vascular markings are usually diminished, since pulmonary valvular stenosis or right ventricular outflow obstruction is commonly present.

The right atrial pressure is elevated. A cardiac catheter cannot be passed into the right ventricle but may enter the left atrium.

Selective angiocardiography from the right atrium demonstrates all the contrast material passing from the right atrium to the left atrium and into the left ventricle. Its course thereafter is determined by the associated lesions.

ONE OF THE FOLLOWING CRITERIA IS REQUIRED FOR THE DIAGNOSIS OF TRICUSPID ATRESIA.

1. **Echocardiographic demonstration of the valvular and ventricular components of the anomaly.**

2. **Failure of a cardiac catheter to enter the right ventricle from the right atrium, and angiocardiographic demonstration of the entire right atrial contents flowing into the left atrium and left ventricle.**

DOWNWARD DISPLACEMENT OF THE TRICUSPID VALVE (EBSTEIN'S MALFORMATION)

In downward displacement of the tricuspid valve, portions of the valve, usually the septal and posterior leaflets, may be attached to the right ventricular wall at varying distances between the annulus fibrosus and the apex. The downwardly displaced leaflets divide the right ventricle into a large proximal atrialized portion and a small-volume distal portion, which functions as the ejectile chamber. The right atrium is usually large. The pulmonary valve is normal, and the pulmonary artery is of normal or small caliber. A patent foramen ovale is usually present, although a secundum atrial septal defect may occur.

The symptoms and signs vary with the severity of the tricuspid regurgitation and the capacity of the distal portion of the right ventricle. When the small right ventricular ejectile chamber causes an obstruction to forward flow, a rise in right atrial pressure results, and blood is shunted from right to left at the atrial level, producing cyanosis. Right ventricular failure may occur when considerable tricuspid regurgitation exists.

A blowing systolic murmur and often an early, low-pitched diastolic murmur may be heard over the lower precordium. Prominent third and fourth heart sounds are common.

The ECG usually shows tall, peaked P waves and right ventricular conduction delay, with low voltage in the right precordial leads. The Wolff-Parkinson-White syndrome may occur. Atrial arrhythmias are common.

The chest x-ray may show a relatively normal to massively enlarged cardiac silhouette. Echocardiography establishes the diagnosis. The pulmonary vascularity is normal or reduced. The echocardiographic four-chamber view is best for visualization of the leaflets of the tricuspid valve and their apical displacement in the right ventricle. The size of the right atrium and atrialized right ventricle is also evaluated in this view. Tricuspid regurgitation is easily assessed by Doppler color flow mapping.

Right atrial pressure is usually elevated; the right ventricular and pulmonary arterial systolic pressures are either normal or low. Cardiac catheterization shows the tricuspid valve displaced to the left of the spine.

Angiocardiography demonstrates an enlarged right atrium and an abnormal division of the right ventricle into an "atrialized" segment proximal to the displaced tricuspid leaflets and a small ejectile chamber distal to them.

THE FOLLOWING CRITERION IS REQUIRED FOR THE DIAGNOSIS OF DOWNWARD DISPLACEMENT OF THE TRICUSPID VALVE (EBSTEINS'S MALFORMATION).

Echocardiographic or angiocardiographic demonstration of the displaced tricuspid valve in the right ventricle.

CONGENITAL TRICUSPID STENOSIS

Isolated stenosis resulting from congenital fusion of the tricuspid leaflets is an uncommon malformation. More often, a narrowing of the tricuspid valve orifice is associated with hypoplasia of the right ventricle, pulmonary valvular obstruction, or both. The elements of the valve are identifiable, but smaller than normal or even diminutive.

When tricuspid stenosis occurring as an isolated lesion is mild, symptoms are usually absent. With severe stenosis, increasing right atrial pressure may cause systemic venous congestion and hepatomegaly or a right-to-left shunt through a patent foramen ovale. When pulmonary valvular obstruction coexists, its signs dominate the clinical picture.

A low-pitched diastolic murmur may be heard along the lower sternal border. The ECG usually shows peaked P waves, decreased right ventricular voltage, and left ventricular hypertrophy. The chest x-ray shows right atrial enlargement and sometimes diminished pulmonary vascularity.

The echocardiographic apical four-chamber view is best for visualization of the narrowed tricuspid valve as well as assessing by Doppler the degree of stenosis and presence of tricuspid regurgitation.

A diastolic pressure gradient is present across the tricuspid valve, and the right atrial pressure is elevated. There is delayed emptying of a dilated right atrial chamber through a small tricuspid orifice into the right ventricular cavity, which is usually small.

**THE FOLLOWING CRITERION IS REQUIRED FOR THE
DIAGNOSIS OF CONGENITAL TRICUSPID STENOSIS.**
Echocardiographic demonstration of a narrowed tricuspid
orifice.

Anomalies of Venous Drainage

ANOMALOUS PULMONARY VENOUS DRAINAGE

Total

In total anomalous pulmonary drainage, the pulmonary
veins from the right and left lungs may terminate directly in the right atrium or coronary sinus, enter a common
pulmonary vein and drain via a vertical vein into the left
innominate vein, or drain below the diaphragm into a
tributary of the inferior vena cava. These locations are
sometimes referred to as cardiac, supracardiac, or infra-
cardiac to designate respectively the anatomic type of
total anomalous pulmonary venous drainage. An atrial
septal defect, or patent foramen ovale, is an integral part
of the anomaly, permitting some of the admixed pulmonary and systemic venous blood in the right atrium to flow
into the left atrium. Systemic arterial oxyhemoglobin
unsaturation is always present and ranges from minimal
to severe. Pulmonary hypertension is frequent. In occasional circumstances, the pulmonary venous pressure is
elevated because of anatomic obstruction or compression
of the pulmonary veins.

Tachypnea and signs of right ventricular failure may
occur in the neonatal period, especially when the drainage of the pulmonary veins is below the diaphragm or in
other locations when there is obstruction of the pulmonary veins. Cyanosis may be present. Systolic murmurs
are frequently heard along the left sternal border but are
nonspecific. The second sound in the pulmonic area is
usually widely split and fixed.

The ECG usually reveals tall P waves and right ventricular hypertrophy. Atrial tachycardia or flutter may
occur. The chest x-ray shows markedly increased pulmonary vascular markings, occasionally with pulmonary
venous engorgement. Prominent convex vascular shadows are present bilaterally at the base of the heart in the
supracardiac type of anomalous drainage, in which the
pulmonary veins enter a left vertical vein, which in turn

drains into the left innominate vein, the right superior vena cava, and the right atrium.

Right heart catheterization reveals an elevated oxygen content in the right atrium or in one of the venae cavae. Pulmonary arterial pressure may approximate that in the systemic arterial tree, particularly in early infancy. Selective angiocardiography performed from the pulmonary artery delineates the pathways of anomalous pulmonary venous return.

Echocardiography is diagnostic for the variety of forms of total anomalous pulmonary venous return. Multiple views are required to demonstrate the principal forms of the anomaly: drainage into the right atrium or coronary sinus, drainage into the superior vena cava or a left vertical vein, and drainage into the hepatic veins or the hepatic portal system.

THE FOLLOWING CRITERION IS REQUIRED FOR THE DIAGNOSIS OF TOTAL ANOMALOUS PULMONARY VENOUS DRAINAGE.

Echocardiographic or angiocardiographic visualization of anomalous pathways of pulmonary venous drainage from the right and left lungs.

Partial

In partial anomalous pulmonary drainage, some of the pulmonary veins from one or more lobes, usually of the right lung, may drain directly into the right atrium, superior vena cava, innominate vein, or inferior vena cava. Frequently, an ostium secundum atrial defect is present; with a sinus venosus type of atrial defect, partial anomalous pulmonary vein drainage into the right superior vena cava is common.

The clinical and laboratory findings, including echocardiographic signs, are similar to those of an ostium secundum atrial septal defect. Right heart catheterization may reveal an elevated oxygen content in the superior or inferior cava in addition to a left-to-right shunt at the atrial level. Selective angiocardiography from the pulmonary artery may delineate the sites of partial anomalous pulmonary vein drainage.

ONE OF THE FOLLOWING CRITERIA IS REQUIRED FOR THE DIAGNOSIS OF PARTIAL ANOMALOUS PULMONARY VENOUS DRAINAGE.

1. **Echocardiographic or angiocardiographic visualization of partial anomalous pulmonary vein drainage.**

2. **Elevated oxygen content in the superior or inferior vena cava or in the right atrium.**

PERSISTENT LEFT SUPERIOR VENA CAVA

The most common malformation involving the major central systemic veins is the presence of bilateral superior venae cavae, usually called persistent left superior vena cava. The latter vein usually terminates in the coronary sinus, through which blood is delivered to the right atrium. A venous bridge in the superior mediastinum commonly exists between the left and right upper venous systems. Occasionally, the right superior vena cava is absent. Persistent left superior vena cava may occur with any other cardiovascular defect and is particularly frequent with tetralogy of Fallot.

The chest x-ray may reveal a vertical shadow at the upper left border of the cardiac silhouette lateral to the aorta and pulmonary artery.

Echocardiography in the parasternal long-axis view demonstrates the enlarged coronary sinus as a round structure lying posterior to the posterior leaflet of the mitral valve. The coronary sinus may also be visualized in other views. Doppler study shows typical vena cava patterns in this structure. The persistent left superior vena cava can be imaged directly from suprasternal views.

THE FOLLOWING CRITERION IS REQUIRED FOR THE DIAGNOSIS OF PERSISTENT LEFT SUPERIOR VENA CAVA.
Echocardiographic or angiographic visualization of a left-sided superior vena cava.

AZYGOS CONTINUATION OF THE INFERIOR VENA CAVA

The inferior vena cava may fail to take a normal position with respect to the liver and becomes continuous with the azygos vein, which drains into the superior vena cava and thence into the right atrium. It may occur without heart disease, though more frequently it is associated with lesions such as ventricular septal defect or complex abnormalities of cardiac position and abdominal visceral situs, especially as seen in the polysplenia syndrome.

The chest x-ray in the frontal projection may show a right-sided mediastinal mass in the angle between the trachea and the right main stem bronchus. This shadow is produced by the azygos vein, the lateral margin of which can often be followed inferiorly in the right paravertebral region.

In this anomaly, echocardiographic examination in subcostal sagittal views demonstrates continuation of the abdominal portion of the inferior vena cava at the azygos vein, which connects posteriorly to the right superior vena cava. The intrathoracic segment of the inferior vena cava connecting the hepatic veins and the abdominal portion of the inferior vena cava to the right atrium is absent.

When a venous catheter is passed from a lower extremity to the right atrium, it can be seen on fluoroscopy in the lateral view to pass behind the heart and then bend forward as it enters the superior vena cava; the configuration of the catheter resembles that of a "candy cane."

THE FOLLOWING CRITERION IS REQUIRED FOR THE DIAGNOSIS OF AZYGOS CONTINUATION OF THE INFERIOR VENA CAVA.

Echocardiographic or angiocardiographic visualization of the abnormal venous channel.

3

The Physiologic Cardiac Diagnosis

Nomenclature

Complete Trifascicular Block
Incomplete Trifascicular Block
Nonspecific Intraventricular Block
Aberrant Ventricular Conduction
Ventricular Preexcitation
Disorders of Supravalvular, Valvular, or
Subvalvular Function
Aortic Stenosis (Supravalvular, Valvular, or
Subvalvular Obstruction)
Aortic Regurgitation
Mitral Stenosis
Mitral Regurgitation
Pulmonic Stenosis (Valvular or Subvalvular
Obstruction)
Pulmonic Regurgitation
Tricuspid Stenosis
Tricuspid Regurgitation
Malfunction of Prostheses and Homografts
Prolapse of Valves
Prolapse of the Aortic Valve
Prolapse of the Mitral Valve
Disorders of Myocardial Function
Ventricular Failure and Congestive Heart
Failure
Left Ventricular Failure
Right Ventricular Failure
Diastolic Dysfunction
Ventricular Asynergy
Pericardial Constriction
Myocardial Restriction
Cardiogenic Shock
Disorders of Intravascular Pressure
Pulmonary Arterial Hypertension
Pulmonary Venous Hypertension
Systemic Arterial Hypertension
Pulmonary or Systemic Circulatory Congestion
Abnormal Communications in the Heart or Great
Vessels
Intracardiac Shunts
Left-to-Right Shunts
Right-to-Left Shunts
Extracardiac Shunts
Left-to-Right Shunts
Right-to-Left Shunts
Anginal Syndrome

Normal and Ectopic Impulse Formation

MECHANISMS OF ECTOPIC IMPULSE FORMATION

Ectopic rhythms are disorders of impulse formation in which the site of origin of the pacemaker or rhythm lies outside the sinoatrial node. They are subdivided into two main groups:

1. Automatic rhythms, which are manifestations of the inherent capacity of potential sites of impulse formation (latent, subsidiary, or secondary pacemakers) to form manifest rhythms if they are not prematurely depolarized by the faster primary or dominant pacemaker. Such rhythms have previously been called homogenetic, escape, nonparoxysmal, and passive, and are currently named automatic.
2. Reentrant rhythms, which are linked to or caused by the preceding dominant (primary) pacemaker. Such rhythms have previously been labeled heterogenetic, extrasystolic, active, paroxysmal, and coupled and are currently named reentrant.

Automatic ectopic rhythms occur when there is a change in the rate relationship between primary and secondary pacemakers such that the effective rate of the secondary pacemaker exceeds the effective rate of the primary pacemaker. This may occur if (1) there is deceleration of the primary pacemaker, (2) there is acceleration of the secondary pacemaker, (3) the effective rate of the primary pacemaker is reduced by the presence of atrioventricular block, or (4) nonpacemaker cells acquire the capacity to become pacemakers (abnormal automaticity). While different models of reentrant rhythms have been postulated, all require an initiating impulse, an anatomic or functional circuit that allows the impulse to depolarize tissue in only one direction (unidirectional block), travels slowly enough in the circuit so that excitable tissue always precedes the impulse (excitable gap), and allows the initiating impulse to return to its site of origin and reenter the circuit. Extensive laboratory and clinical electrophysiologic data support the concept of reentry.

Recently a third mechanism for ectopic impulse formation has been identified, related to the occurrence of early
and late afterdepolarizations in transmembrane action
potentials recorded from single myocytes. Occurring during the relative refractory period or early in diastole,
such afterdepolarizations may, under certain circumstances, reach threshold and cause premature beats or
bursts of paroxysmal tachycardia. Such arrhythmias have
been named triggered rhythms. Their relevance to clinical disorders of impulse formation is not completely understood, but they may be involved in certain rhythms
due to digitalis toxicity, acute myocardial ischemia, and
the ventricular tachycardia associated with the long Q–T
syndromes. While automaticity, reentry, and triggering
are the current dominant theories of ectopic impulse
formation, other less well-defined mechanisms have been
proposed (anisotropy, reflection).

SINUS RHYTHMS

Sinus rhythms originate within the sinoatrial node, presumably from specialized pacemaker (P) cells. Depolarization of the atria by impulses arising in the sinoatrial
node causes the P wave of the electrocardiogram (ECG). If
atrioventricular conduction occurs, the P wave is followed
by a P–R interval, which represents the time required for
impulse transmission in the atrioventricular junction,
and the QRS and ST–T complexes, which constitute the
initial (depolarization) and final (repolarization) ventricular deflections. However, sinus rhythm refers only to
the atrial rhythm, and the presence of sinus rhythm
should be noted in the physiologic diagnosis whether or
not there are coexisting disorders of atrioventricular
conduction (e.g., atrioventricular dissociation, atrioventricular block, ventricular preexcitation). The rate of
impulse formation in the sinoatrial node varies widely in
response to physiologic and pathophysiologic stimuli. In
the adult, it does not usually exceed 170 beats per minute or fall below 40 beats per minute. In infants and
young children and in adults under unusual stress faster
rates may occur. The mean frontal plane P wave axis is
usually between + 30 and + 90 degrees, and the spatial P
axis is oriented inferiorly, to the left and slightly anteriorly, causing upright P waves in leads I, II, III, aVF, V_4,
V_5, and V_6 and an inverted P wave in lead aVR. Uncom-
monly, however, the P axis may lie between + 29 and 0

degrees, causing an inverted deflection in leads III and aVF.

THE FOLLOWING CRITERIA ARE REQUIRED FOR THE DIAGNOSIS OF SINUS RHYTHM.
1. **P waves are present.**
2. **The P wave is a downward deflection in lead aVR.**
3. **The atrial rate does not exceed 170 beats per minute.**

Normal Sinus Rhythm

Normal sinus rhythm is a sinus rhythm at a rate of 60 to 100 beats per minute, and the cycle length (P–P interval) does not vary by more than 10 percent or 120 msec.

THE FOLLOWING CRITERIA ARE REQUIRED FOR THE DIAGNOSIS OF NORMAL SINUS RHYTHM.
1. **Sinus rhythm is present.**
2. **The atrial rate is 60 to 100 beats per minute.**

Sinus Tachycardia

Sinus tachycardia is a regular sinus rhythm at a rate exceeding 100 beats per minute. It may be induced by any condition or agent that abolishes or decreases vagal tone, stimulates sympathetic tone, or both. Emotion, anxiety, exercise, thyrotoxicosis, hypotension, hypoxia, hyperthermia, anemia, hemorrhage, infections, certain neuroses, and neurocirculatory asthenia (vasomotor instability) are frequent causes. Ventricular failure and diseases of the pericardium, myocardium, or endocardium are often accompanied by sinus tachycardia. Certain drugs, such as atropine, epinephrine, isoproterenol, nicotine, lysergic acid diethylamide (LSD), marijuana, cocaine, heroin, and morphine can elicit sinus tachycardia.

THE FOLLOWING CRITERIA ARE REQUIRED FOR THE DIAGNOSIS OF SINUS TACHYCARDIA.
1. **Sinus rhythm is present.**
2. **The atrial rate exceeds 100 beats per minute.**

Reentrant Sinus Tachycardia

Reentrant sinus tachycardia is an unusual arrhythmia thought to be due to reentry within the sinoatrial node. It begins with a premature beat (possibly of sinoatrial origin) and terminates with a relatively long pause. The P waves during the tachycardia are identical in morphology to the sinus P wave, and the rate is usually between

110 and 140 beats per minute. It resembles ordinary sinus tachycardia and cannot be differentiated from it unless the onset and termination of the arrhythmia are recorded.

THE FOLLOWING CRITERION IS REQUIRED FOR THE DIAGNOSIS OF REENTRANT SINUS TACHYCARDIA.

The onset with a premature P wave, and termination with a pause, of a sinus tachycardia with an average rate of 100 to 140 beats per minute.

Sinus Bradycardia

Sinus bradycardia is a regular sinus rhythm at a rate less than 60 beats per minute. The cause is usually an increase in vagal tone, but it may also result from primary depression of the sino-atrial node. The vagus center may be stimulated by central nervous system diseases such as meningitis, by increased intracranial pressure due to tumor or hemorrhage, or reflexly by pain, gastrointestinal disturbances, pressure on the carotid sinus or the eyeballs, or stimulation of the posterior pharynx. Prolonged hypotension or severe hypothermia may cause bradycardia. Certain inhalation anesthetics and beta-adrenergic blocking agents can also cause bradycardia. Sinus bradycardia can occur during normal rest or sleep, in young athletes, in persons convalescing from infectious diseases, and in patients with jaundice.

The hemodynamic and clinical consequences of sinus bradycardia depend on heart rate and the adequacy of the compensatory increase in stroke volume. The stroke volume, in turn, is related to the overall effectiveness of ventricular systolic function. Thus, many subjects with normal ventricular function remain symptom free at sinus rates as slow as 40 to 50 beats per minute. At rates substantially below 40 beats per minute, symptoms of end organ hypoperfusion (dizziness, breathlessness, fatigue, oliguria, anginal syndrome, syncope) are likely even when ventricular function is normal. When ventricular function is impaired, symptoms may occur even at rates as fast as 70 to 80 beats per minute.

THE FOLLOWING CRITERIA ARE REQUIRED FOR THE DIAGNOSIS OF SINUS BRADYCARDIA.

1. **Sinus rhythm is present.**
2. **The atrial rate is less than 60 beats per minute.**

Sinus Arrhythmia

Sinus arrhythmia is a sinus rhythm with variations in the P–P intervals that exceed 10 percent or 120 msec. It occurs in three forms. Phasic or respiratory sinus arrhythmia, the most common form, seen especially in infants and young children and mediated by physiologic variations in vagal tone, is characterized by an increase in sinus rate at the end of inspiration and a decrease in rate at the end of expiration. The changes in P–P interval are progressive and disappear during voluntary apnea. Nonphasic sinus arrhythmia, an uncommon arrhythmia, is a random variation in sinus rate, not related to the respiratory movements. It is usually a manifestation of sinus node disease or digitalis toxicity. Ventriculophasic sinus arrhythmia is a variation in sinus cycle length seen most typically during 2 : 1 atrioventricular block. Alternating longer and shorter P–P intervals are structured in relation to the QRS complexes. Usually the P–P interval that contains the QRS complex is 10 to 20 msec shorter than the P–P interval without the intervening QRS complex. The mechanism for this uncommon arrhythmia is uncertain but may be related to the vagal effect on sinoatrial rate of the arterial pulse wave following ventricular contraction.

THE FOLLOWING CRITERIA ARE REQUIRED FOR THE DIAGNOSIS OF SINUS ARRHYTHMIA.
1. **Sinus rhythm is present.**
2. **P–P intervals vary by more than 10 percent or 120 msec.**
3. **Phasic, nonphasic, and ventriculophasic forms are recognized as noted above.**

Sinus Arrest

Sinus arrest can result from digitalis, quinidine, reserpine, excess potassium, vagotonia, or intrinsic disease of the sinoatrial node. During sinus rhythm there is periodic failure of impulse formation within the primary pacemaker, the sinoatrial node. The P wave and its accompanying QRS–T complex fail to appear at the expected time. The resulting pause is usually slightly shorter than two normal cardiac cycles and is not an exact multiple of the P–P cycle length. If the sinus pause is long, escape beats may appear.

If the pause is long and no escape rhythm takes over, the symptoms of hypoperfusion of vital organs similar to those seen with sinus bradycardia occur. Such long pauses are seen in the carotid sinus syndrome, in which a very sensitive carotid sinus is mechanically stimulated and produces sinus arrest.

THE FOLLOWING CRITERIA ARE REQUIRED FOR THE DIAGNOSIS OF SINUS ARREST.

1. **A sinus rhythm is interrupted by a sudden lengthening of the P–P cycle.**
2. **The long P–P interval varies in duration and is not a whole-number multiple of the basic sinus cycle, and the shortest of such intervals is usually slightly less than twice the basic sinus cycle.**

Dysfunction of the Sinoatrial Node (Sick Sinus Syndrome)

Disordered function of the sinoatrial node often occurs in the absence of identifiable disease, presumably on the basis of fibrotic or sclerotic lesions localized in the nodal area. It may also occur during the course of atherosclerotic heart disease with or without myocardial infarction, rheumatic and congenital heart disease, and a variety of inflammatory conditions, pericarditis, cardiomyopathies, or surgical injury to nodal tissue. Digitalis and excessive vagal discharge may disturb the function of the sinoatrial node, but since their effects are temporary, the resulting disturbances are excluded from the syndrome.

Malfunction of the sinoatrial node may be manifested by

1. Sinus bradycardia, which is severe ($\leq$50 beats/min) or unexpected (often the earliest sign of a failing sinoatrial node) or is intermittent and resistant to atropine and exercise.
2. Sinus arrest for short periods with supervening atrial or atrioventricular junctional or occasionally ventricular escape rhythms.
3. Sinus arrest for long periods without escape rhythms (implying coexistent infranodal disease), which can produce asystolic periods leading to cardiac arrest.
4. Inability of the heart to resume sinus rhythm after cardioversion from atrial fibrillation or flutter.
5. Chronic atrial fibrillation with a slow ventricular rate that cannot be related to drugs; atrial fibrillation permanently replaces sinus rhythm, which cannot be generated by the sinoatrial node, and the slow ventricular rate is due to coexisting atrioventricular block.
6. Sinoatrial exit block not related to drug therapy.

This syndrome is often characterized by periods of sinus bradycardia or sinus arrest that immediately follow bursts of ectopic tachycardias such as atrial tachycardia, atrial flutter, atrial fibrillation, or atrioventricular junctional tachycardia (tachycardia-bradycardia syndrome). The symptoms of such periods are dizziness, faintness, syncopal attacks, and palpitations, and if the episodes of slow or fast rate are frequent, ventricular failure may appear. Sudden death can occur if asystole is prolonged. Prolonged ECG monitoring may be necessary to establish the periodic abnormalities that together make up the syndrome of dysfunction of the sinoatrial node.

In some patients, electrophysiologic study may demonstrate a prolonged sinus node recovery time (SNRT) in response to rapid atrial pacing (a manifestation of excessive overdrive suppression of the diseased sinus node) and prolonged sinoatrial conduction time (SACT) determined by programmed stimulation of the atria.

THE FOLLOWING ARRHYTHMIAS ARE THE MOST SPECIFIC MANIFESTATIONS OF SINUS NODE DYSFUNCTION.

1. **Marked sinus bradycardia not due to negative chronotropic drugs or excessive vagal tone.**
2. **Sinoatrial exit block or sinus arrest.**
3. **Tachycardia-bradycardia syndrome.**

ATRIAL RHYTHMS

Ectopic atrial rhythms (nonsinus) may be due to enhanced automaticity or different forms of reentry. Such rhythms probably originate in true pacemaker cells that are scattered throughout the atria, especially in the region of the opening of the coronary sinus.

Atrial Premature Depolarization

Atrial premature depolarizations (also known as atrial premature complexes, atrial premature systoles, atrial premature beats, or atrial extrasystoles) can be found in normal hearts, in inflammatory or degenerative myocardial diseases, especially rheumatic and atherosclerotic, in ventricular failure, and in conditions stimulating the release of endogenous catecholamines such as anxiety, fatigue, and disturbed psychologic states.

The symptom of these and indeed of all premature contractions is usually a sensation in the chest of an irregular heartbeat in the form of a choking sensation or thump.

The atrial premature depolarization is manifested by a premature P wave that is different in morphology from the sinus P wave. The P–R interval is usually longer than that of the sinus beat. The QRS complex of the atrial premature depolarization may be similar in configuration to the sinus QRS, or it may be different (aberrant ventricular conduction). If the premature atrial impulse reaches the atrioventricular node when it is refractory, no QRS complex follows the P wave (nonconducted or blocked atrial premature depolarization). If the premature beats have P waves of different form, they are termed multifocal atrial premature depolarizations. A succession of such variable P waves with at least three distinctly different morphologies at a rate greater than 100 beats per minute is termed multifocal atrial tachycardia.

THE FOLLOWING CRITERION IS REQUIRED FOR THE DIAGNOSIS OF THE ATRIAL PREMATURE DEPOLARIZATION.

A premature P wave that differs in morphology from the sinus P wave.

Ectopic Atrial Rhythm

Ectopic atrial rhythm is a relatively slow and regular rhythm usually between 50 and 80 beats per minute. It is an automatic rhythm that becomes manifest when its rate exceeds that of the sinus node.

The P wave differs in morphology from the sinus P wave and most typically is inverted in leads II, III, and aVF and upright in lead aVR, indicating retrograde excitation of the atria. Pacemaker cells near the coronary sinus in the right atrium are thought to be the site of origin of this arrhythmia. The P–R interval exceeds 0.11 second. This automatic rhythm may occur at rates over 100 beats per minute (ectopic atrial tachycardia).

THE FOLLOWING CRITERIA ARE REQUIRED FOR THE DIAGNOSIS OF ECTOPIC ATRIAL RHYTHM.

1. **Inverted P waves in leads II, III, and aVF and upright in lead aVR.**
2. **Rate range of 50 to 80 beats per minute.**
3. **Gradual onset and termination, often with fusion P waves.**

Reentrant Atrial Tachycardia

This arrhythmia is thought to be caused by a functioning microreentry circuit within atrial myocardium. It may occur in subjects with structurally normal hearts as well as in those with virtually any type of heart disease.

The symptoms of this tachycardia are usually limited to a feeling of palpitation but may include faintness, nausea, and rarely chest pain. In infants, rapid atrial tachycardia may be a serious disturbance initiating ventricular failure and may be fatal if untreated.

The arrhythmia begins with an atrial premature beat and ends with a pause. In the ECG, there is a rapid and regular succession of uniform P waves, the morphology of which differs from the P wave of sinus rhythm. The P waves are usually upright in the bipolar limb leads but occasionally are inverted. The P–R interval is normal but sometimes difficult to measure if the P wave is superimposed on the T wave. The R–P interval is usually longer than the P–R interval. The QRS complex may be normal or aberrant. There is an isoelectric baseline between P waves. The rate range of reentrant atrial tachycardia is 120 to 250 beats per minute with a 1 : 1 atrioventricular response.

THE FOLLOWING CRITERIA ARE REQUIRED FOR THE DIAGNOSIS OF REENTRANT ATRIAL TACHYCARDIA.

1. **Onset of the arrhythmia with an atrial premature depolarization and termination with a pause.**
2. **A regular succession of P waves differing in morphology from sinus P waves, usually upright in leads I and II and inverted in lead aVR, at a rate of 120 to 250 beats per minute with 1 : 1 atrioventricular conduction.**

Atrial Tachycardia with Atrioventricular Block

This arrhythmia is thought to be due to enhanced automaticity rather than reentry. It occurs most frequently in subjects with serious underlying heart disease and is a common manifestation of digitalis toxicity. The atrial rate ranges between 120 and 250 beats per minute, and various forms of atrioventricular nodal block are present, including 2 : 1 atrioventricular block. The P waves are upright in leads I and II and differ in morphology from the sinus P waves. In contrast to reentrant atrial tachycardia, the P waves may vary somewhat in form and cycle length from beat to beat.

THE FOLLOWING CRITERIA ARE REQUIRED FOR THE DIAGNOSIS OF ATRIAL TACHYCARDIA WITH ATRIOVENTRICULAR BLOCK.

1. **Atrial rate of 120 to 250 beats per minute.**
2. **P wave morphology different from sinus P waves.**

3. **First degree, second degree or third degree atrioventricu-lar block.**

Atrial Flutter

Atrial flutter is usually associated with organic heart disease and is most frequently seen in rheumatic or atherosclerotic heart disease or conditions that cause atrial enlargement. It can also occur in the Wolff-Parkinson-White syndrome, hyperthyroidism, and atrial septal defect. It may complicate acute myocardial infarction, pulmonary embolization, acute pericarditis, restrictive pericardial disease, or severe hypoxia or may develop after intrathoracic operations. Infiltration of the atria by tumor tissue is another cause for this arrhythmia.

The symptoms are related to the fall in cardiac output that occurs with the onset of atrial flutter and to the rapid ventricular rate. These include nausea, faintness, fatigue, palpitations, and occasionally chest pain and ventricular failure.

Atrial flutter is felt to be due to a specialized form of reentry in the right atrium. In classic type 1 atrial flutter, atrial activity is represented in the ECG by regular oscillations (F waves), instead of P waves, that are of uniform shape and cycle length and occur at rates between 200 and 400 beats per minute, usually 300 beats per minute. In the majority of patients with untreated atrial flutter, there is 2 : 1 atrioventricular conduction. Varying degrees of atrioventricular block are common and produce an irregular ventricular rhythm. One-to-one atrioventricular conduction is rare. The F waves are largest in amplitude in the inferior leads II, III, and aVF, where they are predominantly inverted but have a continuous, periodic, or "sawtooth" appearance without an isoelectric baseline separating successive deflections. In lead V_1, however, where the F waves are small, they often resemble P waves, and an isoelectric baseline may separate successive deflections. Vagal stimulation does not terminate atrial flutter but may increase the atrioventricular block and allow the flutter waves to become clearly visible. It is rare for atrial flutter to become a chronic arrhythmia.

Type 2 atrial flutter is much less common than type 1, with faster atrial rates and predominantly upright F waves in leads II, III, and aVF.

THE FOLLOWING CRITERIA ARE REQUIRED FOR THE DIAGNOSIS OF ATRIAL FLUTTER.

1. **P waves are absent.**
2. **F (flutter) waves are present.**
3. **F waves have rates of 200 to 400 per minute and are homogeneous in morphology and cycle length and lack an isoelectric baseline between consecutive atrial deflections in leads II, III, and aVF.**

Atrial Fibrillation

In contrast to atrial flutter, atrial fibrillation may occur in otherwise normal hearts in paroxysmal form. In diseased hearts, however, it often becomes a chronic arrhythmia. The causes and symptoms are similar to those of atrial flutter.

Atrial fibrillation is thought to be caused by multiple, small, functioning reentrant circuits in the atria that are perpetuated by local areas of refractoriness and excitability. Cancellation of wave fronts and varying degrees of concealed conduction into the atrioventricular junction cause the ventricular rhythm to be irregular unless atrioventricular dissociation with an atrioventricular junctional rhythm or complete atrioventricular block with an idioventricular rhythm is present. P waves are absent and replaced by f waves (fibrillation deflections), which are of low voltage and variable in morphology and cycle length. They occur at a rate of 450 to 600 per minute and are largest in leads II, III, and especially V_1. The average ventricular rate varies widely, ranging from 40 to over 200 beats per minute, depending on the presence or absence of spontaneous or drug-induced atrioventricular block.

THE FOLLOWING CRITERIA ARE REQUIRED FOR THE DIAGNOSIS OF ATRIAL FIBRILLATION.

1. **P waves are absent.**
2. **f (fibrillation) deflections are present.**
3. **f waves have rates of 450 to 600 per minute and are heterogeneous in morphology and cycle length.**
4. **While an irregular ventricular rhythm is usually present, it is not an obligatory criterion for the recognition of atrial fibrillation.**

ATRIOVENTRICULAR JUNCTIONAL RHYTHMS

Anatomically, the atrioventricular junction includes the atrioventricular node, the common bundle of His, the bundle branches, and the Purkinje system. However, only ectopic impulse formations in the atrioventricular node and the common bundle are described as atrioventricular junctional rhythms. Separation of atrioventricular nodal from intra-Hisian rhythms can be made only with the aid of intracardiac electrography. For clinical purposes, the inclusive term *atrioventricular junctional* is used. Ectopic impulses taking origin in the atrioventricular junction are simultaneously transmitted antegrade to the ventricles and retrograde to the atria. The QRS complex of atrioventricular junctional rhythms is normal (supraventricular) in duration and configuration unless aberrant ventricular conduction is present. Retrograde excitation of the atria occurs (unless retrograde block is present), and the P waves are upright in lead aVR and inverted in leads II, III, aVF. The position of the P wave in respect to the QRS complex is determined by the duration of antegrade conduction to the ventricles and retrograde conduction to the atria. If the former exceeds the latter, the P waves precede the QRS complexes, but the P–R interval is less than 0.12 sec and; if the latter exceeds the former, the P waves follow the QRS complexes. If the bidirectional impulses reach the atria and ventricles simultaneously, the P waves and QRS complexes are superimposed; the P wave is then obscured by the QRS complex and can be identified only with intracardiac electrograms.

Atrioventricular Junctional Escape Beat

An atrioventricular junctional escape beat occurs when the rate of the sinoatrial node falls below the rate of a secondary pacemaker in the atrioventricular junction or when sinoatrial exit block, sinus arrest, or second-degree atrioventricular block reduces the rate of the ventricles below the rate of a secondary pacemaker. Thus, it usually terminates a pause or an R–R interval longer than the sinus R–R interval. The morphology of the QRS complex and the position of the P wave are as noted above.

THE FOLLOWING CRITERIA ARE REQUIRED FOR THE DIAGNOSIS OF AN ATRIOVENTRICULAR JUNCTIONAL ESCAPE BEAT.

1. **A QRS complex of supraventricular morphology terminates an interval that exceeds the sinus cycle.**

2. **The P wave is upright in lead aVR and inverted in leads II, III, and aVF and may precede, succeed, or superimpose on the QRS complex.**

Atrioventricular Junctional Rhythm

A succession of atrioventricular junctional escape beats constitutes atrioventricular junctional rhythm. The usual rate of this automatic rhythm is 40 to 60 beats per minute, but faster rates may occur, up to 120 to 140 beats per minute (accelerated atrioventricular junctional rhythm). The accelerated form of this rhythm may be seen in a variety of diseases, particularly digitalis toxicity, acute myocarditis and acute myocardial ischemia. The position of the P wave and its frontal plane axis are as noted above.

THE FOLLOWING CRITERIA ARE REQUIRED FOR THE DIAGNOSIS OF ATRIOVENTRICULAR JUNCTIONAL RHYTHM.

1. **A regular succession of supraventricular QRS complexes at a rate of 40 to 60 beats per minute.**
2. **The P wave is upright in lead aVR and inverted in leads II, III and aVF and may precede, succeed, or superimpose on the QRS complex.**

Atrioventricular Junctional Premature Depolarization

This reentrant premature beat is manifested by a premature QRS complex of supraventricular form and duration. The retrograde P wave may precede, succeed, or superimpose on the QRS complex.

THE FOLLOWING CRITERIA ARE REQUIRED FOR THE DIAGNOSIS OF THE ATRIOVENTRICULAR JUNCTIONAL PREMATURE DEPOLARIZATION.

1. **A premature supraventricular QRS complex.**
2. **The retrograde P wave precedes, succeeds, or superimposes on the QRS complex.**

Reentrant Atrioventricular Nodal Tachycardia

This common ectopic rhythm is due to a reentry mechanism within or near the atrioventricular node. It begins abruptly with a premature beat and ends with a pause. The QRS complexes are supraventricular in form and duration ("narrow complex"), and the retrograde P wave usually occurs at the same time as the QRS complex and is not identifiable. The rate range is 120 to 250 beats per minute. Electrophysiologic studies have identified, localized, and characterized the antegrade and retrograde pathways within and near the atrioventricular node that constitute the reentry circuit.

Reentrant atrioventricular nodal tachycardia may occur in subjects without structural heart disease as well as in those with any type of heart disease.

THE FOLLOWING CRITERIA ARE REQUIRED FOR THE DIAGNOSIS OF REENTRANT ATRIOVENTRICULAR NODAL TACHYCARDIA.

1.   **Onset with a premature beat and termination with a pause.**
2.   **A regular supraventricular rhythm with rate range 120 to 250 beats per minute.**
3.   **The retrograde P waves are usually not identifiable but may occur early in the S–T segment.**

PAROXYSMAL SUPRAVENTRICULAR TACHYCARDIA

The term *paroxysmal supraventricular tachycardia* designates a group of reentrant ectopic tachycardias that have supraventricular QRS morphology ("narrow complex tachycardias"). Included within this group are the previously discussed rhythms, reentrant sinus tachycardia, reentrant atrial tachycardia, reentrant atrioventricular nodal tachycardia, and the two forms of atrioventricular reciprocating tachycardia (orthodromic and antidromic) that occur in the ventricular preexcitation syndromes (see page 218). Separation of these arrhythmias electrocardiographically is theoretically based on the position and polarity of the P waves. However, there is much overlap among the various rhythms in regard to the P waves, which may be difficult to characterize because of superimposition of QRS and T deflections, and precise differentiation of the rhythms requires intracardiac electrophysiologic study. When accurate rhythm diagnosis is not possible, the more general term *paroxysmal supraventricular tachycardia* may be used. Reentrant atrioventricular nodal tachycardia is, by far, the most common form of paroxysmal supraventricular tachycardia.

THE FOLLOWING CRITERIA ARE REQUIRED FOR THE DIAGNOSIS OF PAROXYSMAL SUPRAVENTRICULAR TACHYCARDIA.

1.   **A regular succession of QRS complexes with normal duration and configuration at usual rates of 150 to 200 beats per minute.**
2.   **P waves are not identified (superimposed on QRS complex), or they precede or succeed the QRS complexes.**

3. **The P-wave axis indicates antegrade or retrograde excitation of the atria.**

VENTRICULAR RHYTHMS

The automatic rhythms of ventricular origin include the ventricular escape beat, idioventricular rhythm, accelerated idioventricular rhythm, and ventricular parasystole. The reentrant (and perhaps "triggered") rhythms include the ventricular premature depolarization, ventricular tachycardia, and ventricular fibrillation. All ventricular rhythms (except ventricular fibrillation) have abnormal QRS complexes, which are prolonged, notched, slurred, and bizarre ("ventricular form"). They may occur without electrophysiologic relation to P waves (atrioventricular dissociation), or they may be associated with retrograde atrial excitation.

Ventricular Premature Depolarization

Ventricular premature depolarizations (ventricular premature complexes, ventricular premature systoles, ventricular premature beats, and ventricular extrasystoles) often occur in normal subjects, but they are more frequent and more frequently complex (multifocal, pairs, short bursts of nonsustained ventricular tachycardia) in patients with structural heart disease, especially atherosclerotic heart disease and cardiomyopathy. Palpitation may or may not be experienced by the patient. In patients with atherosclerotic heart disease, ventricular premature depolarizations increase the risk of sudden and nonsudden cardiac death.

Ventricular premature depolarizations are premature QRS complexes with ventricular form not preceded by premature P waves. Impulses causing ventricular premature depolarizations enter the atrioventricular junction but usually do not reach and depolarize the atria. Consequently, the atrial rhythm is undisturbed. Thus, a sinus impulse will reach the atrioventricular junction and ventricles during their effective refractory periods, transmission of impulse to the ventricles will not occur, and the ensuing pause will be terminated by the next scheduled sinus P wave (fully compensatory pause). Frequently, however, retrograde excitation of atria by the ventricular premature depolarization does occur, with premature depolarization and resetting of the sinus node. The post extrasystolic sinus P wave then occurs earlier (less than fully compensatory pause). If the sinus impulse coinciding with the ventricular premature depolarization reaches the atrioventricular junction and ventricles after their effective refractory periods have ended, excitation of the ventricles can occur, and there will be no pause following the ventricular premature depolarization (interpolated ventricular premature depolarization). Because of retrograde excitation of the atrioventricular junction and residual partial refractoriness, the P–R interval of the post extrasystolic impulse is usually longer than the sinus P–R interval. Interpolated ventricular premature depolarizations are more likely to occur when the sinoatrial rate is slow and the premature beat very early.

When multiple ventricular premature depolarizations are present and are uniform in morphology (unifocal), the coupling time of the premature beat to the preceding sinus beat is usually fixed, presumably representing the constant physiologic properties of the reentry circuit linked to the sinus impulse. When multiple ventricular premature depolarizations display varying morphology (multifocal), the coupling intervals also vary.

THE FOLLOWING CRITERIA ARE REQUIRED FOR THE DIAGNOSIS OF VENTRICULAR PREMATURE DEPOLARIZATION.

1. A premature QRS complex of ventricular form.
2. Retrograde excitation of the atria may or may not occur.
3. Interpolated, unifocal, and multifocal forms as noted.

Ventricular Escape Beat

The ventricular escape beat is the unit form of automatic rhythm of ventricular origin. Like the atrioventricular junctional escape, it terminates a pause equal to or longer than the basic sinus cycle, and as in the case of the atrioventricular junctional escape, the initiating pause may be due to deceleration of the sinoatrial node, sinus arrest, sinoatrial exit block, or second-degree atrioventricular block. It is often difficult to differentiate the ventricular escape from the atrioventricular junctional escape with aberrant ventricular conduction except with intracardiac electrography.

THE FOLLOWING CRITERION IS REQUIRED FOR THE DIAGNOSIS OF VENTRICULAR ESCAPE BEAT.

A QRS complex of ventricular form that terminates an R–R interval longer than the sinus cycle.

Idioventricular Rhythm

Idioventricular rhythm is an automatic rhythm that takes origin in pacemaker cells located distal to the bifurcation of the common bundle of His. Such pacemakers are very slow (20–45 beats/min) and unstable. Their rates may change, the pacemaker site may shift, and the pacemaker may cease functioning unpredictably, causing ventricular standstill.

Ventricular tachycardia and ventricular fibrillation may also interrupt idioventricular rhythm. The QRS complexes of idioventricular rhythm are ventricular in form, and the rhythm is regular, although slight variations in cycle length may occur. Atrioventricular dissociation is usually present. The most common cause of idioventricular rhythm is complete atrioventricular block. An accelerated form of idioventricular rhythm (rate 70–90 beats/min) not related to atrioventricular block may occur, most often during acute myocardial infarction.

THE FOLLOWING CRITERIA ARE REQUIRED FOR THE DIAGNOSIS OF IDIOVENTRICULAR RHYTHM.

1. **A succession of QRS complexes ventricular in form at a regular rate of 20 to 45 beats per minute.**
2. **Atrioventricular dissociation.**

Ventricular Tachycardia

Ventricular tachycardia is usually a reentrant rhythm, but it may be caused by enhanced automaticity and afterdepolarizations. While it may occasionally occur in structurally normal hearts, it is most often associated with atherosclerotic heart disease or cardiomyopathy. The hemodynamic consequences of this arrhythmia vary in relation to the degree of impairment of ventricular contractile function. If preexisting ventricular function is significantly decreased, ventricular tachycardia may precipitate pulmonary edema, shock, or loss of consciousness. If ventricular function is relatively normal, only minimal symptoms may be present. In addition, ventricular tachycardia may be the predecessor of ventricular fibrillation.

The arrhythmia begins with a ventricular premature beat—sometimes superimposed on the T wave of the preceding sinus beat or sometimes after a slight pause—and continues as a succession of abnormal QRS complexes that are either similar in morphology (monomorphic ventricular tachycardia) or variable (polymorphous ventricular tachycardia). An arbitrary distinction is made between nonsustained ventricular tachycardia (a succession of three or more premature beats lasting not more than 30 seconds) and sustained ventricular tachycardia (arrhythmia lasting more than 30 seconds). Atrioventricular dissociation is usually present, but retrograde excitation of the atria may occur with varying ventriculoatrial conduction ratios (e.g., 1 : 1, 2 : 1, 3 : 2).

A distinct form of polymorphous ventricular tachycardia is characterized by cyclic progressive changing of the polarity of the QRS complexes (torsades de pointes). This arrhythmia, thought to be initiated by early afterdepolarizations, occurs in subjects with congenital or acquired prolongation of the Q–T interval. Other rare forms of ventricular tachycardia include bundle branch reentrant tachycardia, bidirectional ventricular tachycardia, and left bundle branch type ventricular tachycardia seen in normal subjects or those with right ventricular dysplasia.

Differentiation of ventricular tachycardia from paroxysmal supraventricular tachycardia or sinus tachycardia with bundle branch block or aberrant ventricular conduction may be difficult or impossible in the surface ECG. If P waves and atrioventricular dissociation are demonstrated, ventricular tachycardia is almost certainly present. However, since superimposition of P waves on QRS or ST–T complexes occurs very commonly at the rapid rates of ventricular tachycardia, atrioventricular dissociation is recognizable in less than 50 percent of cases of true ventricular tachycardia. Other ECG criteria that may be helpful in the diagnosis of ventricular tachycardia are a markedly prolonged QRS interval (>0.14 second), marked right axis or left axis deviation, and absence of biphasic QRS complexes in precordial leads.

THE FOLLOWING CRITERIA ARE REQUIRED FOR THE DIAGNOSIS OF VENTRICULAR TACHYCARDIA.

1. **A succession of predominantly regular QRS complexes, ventricular in form, at a rate of 130 to 250 beats per minute.**
2. **Atrioventricular dissociation.**
3. **Special forms as noted above.**

Ventricular Parasystole

Ventricular parasystole is an uncommon form of automatic ectopic rhythm in which a slow subsidiary or latent ventricular pacemaker is not depolarized by the dominant faster (usually sinus) pacemaker and continues to initiate rhythmic electrical impulses that are capable of depolarizing the ventricles whenever they are excitable. Thus, this arrhythmia violates one of the most fundamental electrophysiologic properties of the mammalian heart, premature depolarization of subsidiary potential pacemakers by the dominant fastest pacemaker. The cause for this "protection" of the lower pacemaker, sometimes referred to as "entrance block," is unknown. Electrocardiographically, ventricular parasystole is characterized by QRS complexes that are of uniform ventricular form, with variable coupling intervals to preceding dominant QRS complexes, and with interectopic intervals that are exactly or nearly exactly a whole number multiple of the cycle length of the parasystolic pacemaker, which is usually the shortest manifest interectopic interval. Fusion beats of parasystolic and nonparasystolic QRS complexes are common.

Although classic parasystole possesses the form described above, more detailed ECG, electrophysiologic, and experimental observations have demonstrated important variations from the typical arrhythmia, including intermittent parasystole, parasystolic ventricular tachycardia, parasystole with fixed coupling, and modulation of the rate of a parasystolic pacemaker by sinus impulses.

Most parasystolic pacemakers are located in the ventricles distal to the bifurcation of the common bundle. Rarely, however, parasystolic rhythms may originate in the atria or atrioventricular junction and very rarely in two foci simultaneously.

THE FOLLOWING CRITERIA ARE REQUIRED FOR THE DIAGNOSIS OF VENTRICULAR PARASYSTOLE.
1. **Multiple QRS complexes of uniform ventricular form.**
2. **Variable coupling to preceding sinus QRS complexes.**
3. **Interectopic intervals that are whole-number multiples of the shortest interectopic interval.**
4. **Fusion beats.**

Ventricular Fibrillation

Ventricular fibrillation is characterized by the absence of QRS complexes and T waves and the presence of ECG wave forms that vary in amplitude, cycle length, and

morphology. Atrial deflections usually cannot be identified. Sometimes ventricular fibrillation is initiated by a
short run of ventricular flutter, a more regular series of
ventricular deflections that resemble a periodic function
curve. Organized ventricular contraction is replaced by
quivering and twitching movements of the ventricles
incapable of expelling blood. Occasionally, ventricular
fibrillation is initiated by a ventricular premature depolarization superimposed on the T wave of the preceding
QRS complex (R on T phenomenon). Ventricular fibrillation is the predominant arrhythmia causing sudden cardiac death.

**THE FOLLOWING CRITERIA ARE REQUIRED FOR THE
DIAGNOSIS OF VENTRICULAR FIBRILLATION.**
1. **Absence of QRS and T complexes.**
2. **Presence of irregular oscillations in the ECG that vary in
   cycle length, amplitude, and morphology.**

ELECTRONIC PACEMAKER RHYTHMS

Cardiac Rhythms from Electronic Pacemakers

Cardiac pacemakers are electronic instruments capable
of electrically stimulating atrium or ventricle and sensing electrical events of either chamber and of physiologic
or non-physiologic sensors of body need. Circuits within
the pulse generator can be programmed to change electrical output, repetition (stimulation) rate, and sensitivity of the system to sensed spontaneous or paced physiologic events. Some pacemakers incorporate sensors that
respond to specific physiologic events such as activity,
body temperature, Q–T interval, and minute ventilation
and trigger metabolically appropriate changes in the
pacemaker stimulation rate (rate responsive, rate modu-
lated, adaptive rate). Because of the operational, programmable, and rate-modulated complexity of pacemaker systems, a universally used five-position letter code is
used to categorize the functional properties of different
pacemakers (Table 3-1). Pacemaker rhythms may involve
atria, ventricles, or both chambers and may be classified
as single chamber (atrial or ventricular) or dual chamber
(atrioventricular).

Atrial Rhythm from Electronic Pacing

Electrical stimulation of the atrium is via electrode contact with the atrial wall, and a pacemaker artifact will, if

Table 3-1. The NASPE/BPEG generic (NBG) code

Position	I*	II*	III*	IV	V
Category	Chamber(s) paced	Chamber(s) sensed	Response to sensing	Programmability, rate modulation	Antitachyarrhythmia function(s)
	O = none	O = none	O = none	O = none	O = none
	A = atrium	A = atrium	T = triggered	P = simple programmable	P = pacing
	V = ventricle	V = ventricle	I = inhibited	M = multiprogrammable	S = shock
	D = dual (A + V)	D = dual (A + V)	D = dual (T + I)	C = communicating	D = dual (P + S)
				R = rate modulation	
Manufacturers' designation only	S = single (A or V)	S = single (A or V)			

NASPE = North American Society of Pacing and Electrophysiology; BPEG = British Pacing and Electrophysiology Group.
*Positions I through III are used exclusively for antibradyarrhythmia function.
Source: Bernstein, A. D., et al. The NASPE/BPEG generic code for antibradyarrhythmia and adaptive-rate pacing and antitachyarrhythmia devices. *PACE*, Vol. 10, July–Aug. 1987. Pp. 794–799.

stimulation is effective, be followed immediately by a P wave. If atrioventricular conduction occurs, a QRS complex follows. If atrioventricular conduction is prolonged or impaired, atrial pacing can form part of a dual-chamber pacing system in which the atrioventricular sequence is provided by the pacemaker. Atrial pacing may also be part of an antitachycardia pacing mode.

Single-Chamber Ventricular Rhythm from
Electronic Pacing

A ventricular rhythm results from direct stimulation of the ventricle without regard to atrial activity. The normal atrioventricular sequence is lost, and ventriculo-atrial conduction may occur.

VENTRICULAR INHIBITED (VVI). Ventricular stimulation occurs at the programmed lower rate limit, and the ECG shows a pacemaker stimulus artifact followed by a wide QRS complex of the left bundle branch block pattern when stimulation is from the right ventricular apex. If a spontaneous QRS complex occurs before the elapse of the lower rate limit, which can be abbreviated by sensor driven rate modulation, the pacemaker stimulus is inhibited and a new timing cycle is begun. The lower rate limit interval is commonly identical between two paced events and a sensed event followed by a paced event. It is possible to set two different intervals, one between two paced events and another between a sensed event followed by a paced event. This is termed hysteresis.

VENTRICULAR TRIGGERED (VVT). The VVT mode is similar to the VVI except that when a spontaneous ventricular event is sensed before the end of the lower rate limit a stimulus artifact is emitted into the QRS complex without delay between sensing and stimulation and without physiologic effect. This mode cannot be inhibited, with possible resultant asystole, by electromagnetic or electromyographic interference (EMI).

Atrioventricular Rhythms from Electronic Pacing
(Dual-Chamber Pacing)

This group of pacing modes involves sensing the atrium and pacing the ventricle or pacing the atrium and ventricle. Ventricular pacing may be at the atrial rate, at the lower rate limit, or at a sensor-driven rate for both atrium and ventricle. Both chambers, atrium and ventricle, should be sensed so that pacemaker stimuli are not competitive with spontaneous events in either chamber. Modes that do not sense both atrium and ventricle are obsolete and are used only in special circumstances.

VENTRICULAR SYNCHRONOUS (VDD). The atrium is sensed and the ventricle paced at the atrial rate, after a programmed atrioventricular delay. If the atrial rate is less than the ventricular rate, which may be sensor driven, pacing will be at the ventricular rate only.

ATRIOVENTRICULAR SEQUENTIAL (DVI). The atrium is paced but not sensed. The ventricle is paced after a programmed atrioventricular interval following the atrial paced event. In the noncommitted version, a spontaneous ventricular event will inhibit ventricular output; in the committed version, the atrial stimulus is always followed by a ventricular stimulus. Because of the absence of atrial pacing and the risk of competitive induction of atrial arrhythmia, this mode is obsolete.

ATRIOVENTRICULAR SEQUENTIAL (DDI). The atrium is sensed and may be paced at the lower rate interval. An atrial event inhibits the atrial stimulus and the ventricle is paced at the lower rate limit unless a spontaneous event occurs and inhibits output. The atrial and ventricular rates are at a programmed single rate and atrioventricular interval, which may be prolonged. The ECG appearance is of paced atrium and ventricle with programmed atrioventricular interval, or unpaced P wave, programmed atrioventricular interval, and ventricular stimulus at the lower rate limit.

ATRIOVENTRICULAR UNIVERSAL (DDD). The atrium is sensed and paced if the spontaneous atrial rate is less than the lower rate limit. The ventricle is paced after the programmed atrioventricular interval unless inhibited by a spontaneous ventricular event. The atrioventricular interval is as programmed until modified by the upper rate limit. The ECG appearance is of a paced or unpaced P wave, the programmed atrioventricular interval followed by a paced or pacer-inhibiting ventricular event.

ONE OF THE FOLLOWING CRITERIA IS REQUIRED FOR THE RECOGNITION OF ELECTRONIC PACEMAKER RHYTHMS.

1. ECG demonstration of atrial or ventricular stimulation artifacts or both.
2. Initiation of a P wave or QRS complex by the stimulus.
3. Stimulation and sensing patterns in accord with the specific pacing modes.

Malfunction of Electronic Pacemaker Systems

Pacemaker malfunction may be due to depletion of the pulse generator power source, which is usually gradual and orderly and is manifested by a reduction in the magnetic rate of the generator (the stimulation rate when sensing has been disabled by placing a magnet over the generator); electronic failure because of circuit deterioration, which may also cause sudden no-output failure; lead malposition resulting in improper contact of the electrode with myocardium; excessively high sensing or pacing thresholds; or lead deterioration, with fracture of the metal conductor or deterioration of the insulation as a result of contact with body fluids.

ONE OF THE FOLLOWING CRITERIA IS REQUIRED FOR DIAGNOSIS OF MALFUNCTION OF ELECTRONIC PACEMAKER SYSTEMS.

1. **Reduction in the magnetic rate of the pulse generator or absence of pacemaker stimulus artifacts when sensing function has been disabled by magnet application.**
2. **Failure of pacing or sensing in accord with programmed parameters and modes.**
3. **Loss of sensing or capture at any pulse generator setting.**
4. **Muscle stimulation at the site of the lead in the subcutaneous tissue.**
5. **Radiologic evidence of electrode or lead malposition (e.g., in the coronary sinus, posterior cardiac vein, left ventricle, or superior or inferior vena cava).**

Pacemaker Syndrome

Pacemaker syndrome is the result of single-chamber ventricular pacing with hypotension, reduction of cardiac output, or activation of cardiopulmonary reflexes resulting from increase of intra-atrial pressure. Symptoms may include pounding in the neck or chest synchronous with the heartbeat, dyspnea, weakness, fatigue, syncope, precordial distress, congestive heart failure, and ventricular arrhythmias. Pacemaker syndrome is caused by single-chamber ventricular pacing and retrograde excitation of the atria, resulting in their contraction against closed atrioventricular valves; variations in stroke volume and atrial contribution to stroke volume; single rate pacing inadequate for physiologic needs; or an excessively prolonged atrioventricular interval during atrial or dual-chamber pacing in which the atrial contraction occurs soon after the preceding ventricular contraction.

Defibrillation by Implantable Device

The implantable cardioverter defibrillator (ICD) is intended for the termination of ventricular tachycardia or fibrillation. Tachyarrhythmia detection is by one or a combination of techniques based on rapidity of rate, sudden rate acceleration, rate stability (at a rapid rate), and the probability density function (PDF), a measure of the duration of the isoelectric interval during ventricular depolarization and repolarization. This interval is relatively longer during normal sinus rhythm, sinus tachycardia, or supraventricular tachycardia and briefer during ventricular tachycardia and ventricular fibrillation.

The ICD can deliver a shock of full amplitude (approximately 35 joules), which will be seen on ECG, Holter, or monitor as a single event 8 to 15 seconds after onset of ventricular fibrillation, in response to detection of ventricular fibrillation. It is also capable of antitachycardia pacing in a variety of modes in response to ventricular tachycardia, usually by rapid single stimuli or burst pacing at stimuli coupling intervals briefer than the tachycardia coupling interval (the reciprocal of rate). Following antitachycardia pacing four results are possible: termination, no effect, acceleration, and ventricular fibrillation. If tachycardia is not terminated or accelerated, additional bursts of the same or a different antitachycardia pacing mode may be delivered or a lower or progressively greater amplitude shock, all referred to as tiered therapy. If the steps in the tier are ineffective, a full-output rescue shock is delivered. In the presence of initial or post-treatment ventricular fibrillation, a full-output shock is promptly delivered. If tachycardia termination is followed by significant bradycardia of sinus origin or due to atrioventricular block, antibradycardia ventricular pacing continues at conventional pacemaker output and rate until a spontaneous cardiac rate inhibits output. Engineering and clinical characteristics of the device and technique are under intensive investigation.

Antitachycardia Pacing

Pacing of the atrium or ventricle with discrete stimuli of 0.5- to 2.0 msec duration and energy of 5 to 50 microjoules may be used for management of an ectopic reentrant tachyarrhythmia. Underdrive stimuli at a fixed slower rate than the tachycardia, and out of phase with it, randomly change the timing relationship to atrial and ventricular depolarization with a single stimulus falling into a portion of the cardiac cycle that can terminate the arrhythmia. Overdrive stimuli are at a more rapid rate than the tachycardia and capture and drive the ventricle or atrium; at the conclusion of stimulation the tachycardia may have ended. Scanning single stimuli follow each depolarization, progressively changing the timing interval until one of the stimuli terminates the tachycardia. Antitachycardia pacing may accelerate, terminate or convert the tachycardia to fibrillation. Ventricular antitachycardia pacing is used only with an implantable cardioverter-defibrillator system.

Normal and Abnormal Impulse Transmission

Normal transmission of the sinoatrial impulse to the atria and ventricles is accomplished in an orderly sequence: sinus node to atria (perinodal fibers to right atrium and rapid conduction to left atrium via the anterior internodal tract), atria to atrioventricular node (possible functional rapid conduction pathways), atrioventricular node and bundle of His to its bifurcation (intra-Hisian conduction), bifurcation of common bundle to ventricular myocytes (via bundle branches and Purkinje fibers), and myocyte to myocyte transmission (intraventricular conduction). Thus, standard ECG can identify sinoatrial block, intra-atrial block, atrioventricular block, bundle branch block, and intraventricular block. More precise localization of sites of conduction delay can be made using intracardiac electrography.

SINOATRIAL EXIT BLOCK

Since impulse formation in the sinus node is not manifested in the standard ECG, normal sinoatrial conduction time cannot be measured. Both normal sinoatrial conduction and sinoatrial exit block can be measured indirectly (or directly if electrograms from the sinus node are recorded) using intracardiac recording techniques. Although sinoatrial exit block, like atrioventricular block, can be classified as first degree, second degree, and third degree (complete), only second-degree sinoatrial exit block can be diagnosed using conventional ECG. It is recognized by intermittent complete failure of sinoatrial conduction causing dropped beats (absence of P waves when expected). Like second-degree atrioventricular block, second-degree sinoatrial block can be further subdivided into type I and type II. In type I, the S–P intervals (sinus node to atria) progressively increase until the dropped beat occurs. In type II, the S–P intervals of the conducted beats remain constant. Thus, in type II sinoatrial exit block, a sinus P and QRS–T fail to appear at the expected time. The dropped beats may occur sporadically or in regularly recurring patterns after every second, third, or fourth normal beat. The resulting pause is an exact multiple of the P–P cycle length, representing 2 : 1 sinoatrial exit block. Occasionally, two or more consecutive sinus impulses fail to reach the atria, causing higher degrees of sinoatrial exit block. Escape beats from the atrioventricular junction or ventricle may interrupt the long pause.

In type I sinoatrial exit block, the P–P intervals progressively shorten until a long P–P interval occurs (containing the dropped beat). The long P–P cycle is shorter than the sum of any two contiguous P–P intervals. This arrhythmia closely resembles phasic sinus arrhythmia except that the longest P–P interval follows the shortest P–P cycle, whereas in sinus arrhythmia the longest P–P interval follows "the next to the longest interval."

THE FOLLOWING CRITERIA ARE REQUIRED FOR THE DIAGNOSIS OF SECOND-DEGREE SINOATRIAL EXIT BLOCK.

1. **Periodic absence of a P wave.**
2. **Type I: Progressive shortening of the P–P interval followed by a long P–P cycle that is shorter than the sum of any two consecutive P–P intervals.**
3. **Type II: The long P–P intervals are exact whole-number multiples of the shortest constant P–P interval.**

INTRA-ATRIAL BLOCK

A delay in conduction through the atrial myocardium, an abnormality of the spread of atrial excitation in the interatrial or internodal tracts, or both is manifested by prolongation of the P wave to 0.12 second or longer. The P wave may be widely notched and its amplitude increased or decreased. Enlargement of the left atrium may cause similar changes in P wave duration, amplitude, and morphology. Narrow notching of the P wave alone is not abnormal.

THE FOLLOWING CRITERIA ARE SUGGESTIVE OF, BUT NOT SPECIFIC FOR, INTRA-ATRIAL BLOCK.
1.   P wave duration greater than or equal to 0.12 second.
2.   Wide notching of the P wave.

ATRIOVENTRICULAR BLOCK

The anatomic components of the atrioventricular junction that are involved in the various forms of atrioventricular block include the atrioventricular node, the bundle of His, and the bundle branches. Using intracardiac electrography and the standard ECG, it is possible to localize the area of conduction delay to the atrioventricular node alone, the bundle of His alone, the bundle branches alone, and in various combinations and degrees of conduction delay. Atrioventricular block may be caused by a wide variety of congenital and acquired diseases, drugs, and autonomic stimuli.

First-Degree Atrioventricular Block (Incomplete Atrioventricular Block Without Dropped Beats)

In this arrhythmia, the P–R interval is prolonged (greater than 0.21 second), but 1 : 1 atrioventricular conduction occurs. Electrophysiologic study indicates that, in the absence of intraventricular block, first-degree atrioventricular block is almost always due to dysfunction within the atrioventricular node, with prolongation of the A–H interval of the bundle of His electrogram.

THE FOLLOWING CRITERIA ARE REQUIRED FOR THE DIAGNOSIS OF FIRST-DEGREE ATRIOVENTRICULAR BLOCK.
1.   P–R interval greater than 0.21 second.
2.   One-to-one atrioventricular conduction.

Second-Degree Atrioventricular Block (Incomplete Atrioventricular Block with Dropped Beats)

In this form of atrioventricular block, some of the atrial impulses are transmitted to the ventricles; others are not, resulting in P waves that are not followed by QRS complexes (dropped beats). Second-degree atrioventricular block is subdivided into two types: Mobitz I and Mobitz II.

Mobitz Type I

Type I conduction is characterized by varying P–R intervals of the conducted beats. Usually, but not always, the type of P–R interval variation is in the form of the Wenckebach period. The typical Wenckebach period has three features: The P–R intervals become progressively longer until the dropped beat occurs, the R–R intervals become progressively shorter until the dropped beat occurs (because the increments in P–R interval progressively decrease), and the long R–R interval containing the dropped beat is shorter than the sum of any two contiguous R–R intervals. Typical Wenckebach periods are uncommon. While the first and third features of the Wenckebach period are always present, the second occurs infrequently because the P–P intervals often vary and the increment in P–R interval often varies from beat to beat instead of progressively decreasing. However, the first R–R interval of the Wenckebach period is usually longer than the second, and the last R–R interval is often longer than the penultimate R–R interval. Electrophysiologic study indicates type I block is a manifestation of atrioventricular nodal dysfunction with progressive prolongation in A–H intervals until the His signal is not recorded. However, Wenckebach periodicity may occur in the bundle of His itself or in the bundle branches.

Mobitz Type II

Type II second-degree atrioventricular block, much less common than type I, is characterized by constant P–R intervals of the conducted beats, and the dropped beats often contain two or more nonconducted P waves. Electrophysiologic study demonstrates dysfunction in the distal His-Purkinje system with normal A–H intervals, prolonged H–V intervals, and absence of ventricular signals after the His signals when dropped beats occur. Type II second-degree atrioventricular block is often associated with bundle branch block and is a common predecessor of complete atrioventricular block.

THE FOLLOWING CRITERIA ARE REQUIRED FOR THE DIAGNOSIS OF SECOND-DEGREE ATRIOVENTRICULAR BLOCK.

1. **Presence of sinus rhythm.**
2. **Some P waves are followed by QRS complexes. Others are not.**

3. **Type I: P–R intervals of conducted beats vary according to Wenckebach periodicity.**
4. **Type II: P–R intervals of conducted beats are normal or prolonged but constant.**

Second-Degree Atrioventricular Block with 2 : 1 Atrioventricular Conduction

In this arrhythmia, there is a constant P–R interval, which may be of normal duration or may be prolonged, and a constant degree of atrioventricular block such that every other P wave is completely blocked. The atrioventricular ratio is stable at 2 : 1. This form of incomplete atrioventricular block may become more marked, such that two or more consecutive P waves are not followed by QRS complexes. Two-to-one A–V block may be caused by A–V nodal or infranodal dysfunction.

THE FOLLOWING CRITERIA ARE REQUIRED FOR THE DIAGNOSIS OF 2 : 1 ATRIOVENTRICULAR BLOCK.

1. **Presence of sinus rhythm.**
2. **Alternate P waves are not followed by QRS complexes.**

Third-Degree Atrioventricular Block (Complete Atrioventricular Block)

In complete atrioventricular block, no supraventricular impulses reach the ventricles, and independent pacemakers control the atria and ventricles. There is complete atrioventricular dissociation. The atrial pacemaker may be the sinus node or other atrial foci. The atrial rhythm is faster than the ventricular. The P waves are unrelated to the QRS complexes.

In complete atrioventricular block, His bundle electrograms demonstrate that the most common site of block is distal to the His bundle; there is a normal A–H interval but no H–V interval or H spike preceding the QRS complexes. The block is probably due to complete bilateral bundle branch block. However, in congenital forms of complete atrioventricular block, the block is generally proximal to the His bundle. The His bundle electrogram reveals no H spike after the P waves (absence of A–H interval); the junctional rhythm controlling the ventricles is characterized by a narrow QRS complex preceded by an H spike and a normal H–V interval.

The ventricular pacemaker in complete atrioventricular block may be located above or below the bifurcation of the common bundle. If it is located in the common bundle, the ventricular rate is 40 to 55 beats per minute in adults and 70 to 80 beats per minute in children, and the QRS complexes are normal in duration and morphology. If the idioventricular pacemaker is below the branching of the common bundle, the rate range is 20 to 45 beats per minute, and the QRS complex is prolonged, notched, and slurred. Such pacemakers are unstable.

THE FOLLOWING CRITERIA ARE REQUIRED FOR THE DIAGNOSIS OF COMPLETE ATRIOVENTRICULAR BLOCK.

1. **Atrioventricular dissociation.**
2. **Idioventricular rhythm.**

Morgagni-Stokes-Adams Syndrome

The Morgagni-Stokes-Adams syndrome is an acute neurologic disorder consisting of transient dizziness, loss of consciousness and convulsions due to abrupt reduction in cerebral blood flow. It occurs most typically during the course of complete atrioventricular block. The cerebral ischemia is due to ventricular fibrillation, ventricular standstill, ventricular tachycardia, or a sudden marked reduction in the rate of the idioventricular pacemaker. Other arrhythmias such as marked sinus bradycardia, sinus arrest, or sinoatrial exit block may cause similar symptoms.

THE FOLLOWING CRITERIA ARE REQUIRED FOR THE DIAGNOSIS OF MORGAGNI-STOKES-ADAMS SYNDROME.

Transient dizziness, loss of consciousness, and convulsions associated with ventricular standstill, ventricular tachycardia, or ventricular fibrillation during the course of complete atrioventricular block.

ATRIOVENTRICULAR DISSOCIATION

Atrioventricular dissociation is an abnormality of atrioventricular conduction characterized physiologically by independent beating of atria and ventricles and electrocardiographically by a totally variable P–R distance. It occurs when two pacemakers coexist at similar but not identical effective rates, one exciting the atria (usually the sinoatrial node), the other exciting the ventricles (an atrioventricular junctional or ventricular focus). Dissociation is initiated by acceleration of a junctional or ventricular pacemaker, deceleration of the sinus pacemaker, or atrioventricular block. This dissociation is perpetuated by refractoriness in the atrioventricular node (caused by the near simultaneous arrival of both pacemaker impulses at the atrioventricular node), which prevents each pacemaker from exciting the opposite set of chambers. The atrioventricular node may be in its physiologic refractory period, or its refractory period may be abnormally prolonged (atrioventricular block).

Three forms of atrioventricular dissociation are recognized: complete, incomplete, and isorhythmic. During complete atrioventricular dissociation, the atrioventricular node is continuously refractory to excitation. Thus, the R–R interval is constant, the P–P interval is constant, and the P–R distance is totally variable. During incomplete atrioventricular dissociation, an atrial impulse may reach the atrioventricular node when it is no longer refractory, traverse the atrioventricular junction, and excite opposite chambers ("ventricular capture"). Periodic shortening of the R–R interval then occurs at a fixed P–R interval. During isorhythmic dissociation, a rare arrhythmia, the P waves cluster near or within the QRS complex with very short P–R or R–P distances. The mechanism for this arrhythmia may be variations in vagal tone that modulate the rate of the sinus node so that it is virtually identical to the rate of the lower pacemaker.

THE FOLLOWING CRITERIA ARE REQUIRED FOR THE DIAGNOSIS OF ATRIOVENTRICULAR DISSOCIATION.
1. Totally variable P–R distance.
2. Regular ventricular rhythm if the atria are fibrillating.
3. Complete, incomplete, and isorhythmic variants as noted.

INTRAVENTRICULAR BLOCK

The inclusive term *intraventricular block* comprises conduction delays, complete or incomplete, permanent or transient, in the following anatomic loci, alone or in combination: distal bundle of His, right bundle branch, main trunk of the left bundle branch, the anterosuperior division of the left bundle branch and the posteroinferior division of the left bundle branch. Used in conjunction, the conventional ECG and His bundle intracardiac electrography allow classification of intraventricular block into three broad categories: monofascicular block (intra-Hisian block, right bundle branch block, left bundle branch block, block in the anterosuperior division of the left bundle branch, or block in the posteroinferior division of the left bundle branch); bifascicular block (right bundle branch block and left anterior fascicular block, right bundle branch block and left posterior fascicular block, right bundle branch block and main trunk left bundle branch block, left anterior fascicular block and left posterior fascicular block); and trifascicular block (right bundle branch block, left anterior fascicular block, and left posterior fascicular block).

Monofascicular Block

His Bundle Block

Intra-Hisian block is manifested by a prolonged P–R interval, prolonged H–V interval (>55 msec), and normal QRS complex duration and morphology. This uncommon form of intraventricular block cannot be distinguished from first-degree atrioventricular nodal block without intracardiac electrography. Block in the bundle of His may also cause wide splitting of the His signal.

Right Bundle Branch Block

In right bundle branch block, the QRS complex is prolonged, equalling or exceeding 0.12 second. The QRS complex in precordial lead V_1 has an rSR' configuration or consists of a large notched R wave. The R' deflection is large and prolonged (>40 msec). There are prolonged S waves in leads, I, V_5 and V_6 and a prolonged R wave in lead aVR. The T wave is inverted in leads over the delayed right ventricle (V_1, V_2).

When calculating the position of the mean frontal plane QRS axis in right bundle branch block, it is necessary to ignore the distortion of the mid and terminal portions of the QRS complex caused by the right bundle branch block. The beginning of this portion of the QRS complex can usually be identified by a notch. In general, only the first 40 or 50 msec of the QRS complex should be used to calculate axis. In uncomplicated right bundle branch block, the mean QRS axis varies widely but is not more superior than − 45 degrees or more rightward than + 100 degrees.

In incomplete right bundle branch block, the QRS duration is equal to or greater than 0.10 second but less than 0.12 second. The terminal R' in lead V_1 (and S waves in leads I, V_5, and V_6) is small and often less than 40 msec in duration. The diagnosis of incomplete right bundle branch block is often of questionable validity. Terminal, small upright deflections may occur in lead V_1 in normal subjects and in right ventricular enlargement as well as in bundle branch block.

Right bundle branch block is frequently found in subjects without structural heart disease as well as in those with many forms of congenital and acquired heart disease. Intermittent right bundle branch block is common and may or may not be rate related.

THE FOLLOWING CRITERIA ARE REQUIRED FOR THE DIAGNOSIS OF RIGHT BUNDLE BRANCH BLOCK.
1. **QRS duration is 0.12 second or longer.**
2. **The QRS complex in lead V_1 has rsR′ configuration or is a solitary notched R wave.**

Left Bundle Branch Block

The duration of the QRS complex in left bundle branch block is 0.12 second or longer. Characteristically the midportion of the QRS complex displays prominent notching or splintering. This is usually best seen in leads I, aVL, V_5, and V_6. The QRS complex in lead V_1 is a downward deflection and has a QS or rS configuration. There are no Q waves in leads I, aVL, V_5, or V_6. The S–T segment is depressed in leads V_5 and V_6 and conspicuously elevated in leads V_1–V_3. The T wave is inverted in leads I, aVL, V_5, and V_6. Less marked prolongation of QRS (0.10 second or 0.11 second) and absence of Q waves in leads V_5 and V_6 may suggest incomplete left bundle branch block, but the specificity of these criteria is poor.

While left bundle branch block may occur in normal subjects, it is more likely to be associated with structural heart disease. Like right bundle branch block, it may be intermittent and rate-dependent or non-rate-dependent.

THE FOLLOWING CRITERIA ARE REQUIRED FOR THE DIAGNOSIS OF LEFT BUNDLE BRANCH BLOCK.
1. **QRS duration is 0.12 second or longer.**
2. **The QRS complex is notched and splintered and has a QS or rS deflection in lead V_1.**

Left Anterior Fascicular Block

This form of intraventricular conduction defect consists of complete block in the anterior fascicle of the left bundle, with normal conduction through the posterior fascicle and right bundle branch.

The diagnostic criteria depend largely on the presence of marked left axis deviation. In terms of the frontal plane projection of this QRS vector, marked left axis deviation lies between -30 and -90 degrees. Since there is little or no increase in the QRS duration with anterior fascicular block—an increase of 0.01 to 0.02 second—the diagnosis of anterior fascicular block rests on the presence of this particular axis orientation. It is best to require an axis of -45 to -90 degrees to be certain that anterior fascicular block is present because other causes of left axis deviation may occasionally rotate the QRS vector beyond -30 degrees but do not usually shift it beyond -45 degrees.

Left ventricular excitation in anterior fascicular block occurs over the posterior fascicle (thus the initial forces are directed inferiorly and to the right), then travels through the Purkinje network, and later spreads superiorly, anteriorly, and to the left over the area normally supplied by the anterior fascicle. The terminal forces are directed superiorly and to the left. This results in the mean QRS axis being markedly to the left, with qR in I, aVL, and V_6 and S in leads II, III, and aVF.

The commonest cause of this conduction defect is fibrosis of unknown etiology or myocardial infarction due to atherosclerotic heart disease. However, it is also seen in hypertensive heart disease; in disease of the aortic valve that produces fibrosis or calcification at the valve base in the area of the interventricular septum; in diabetes, obesity, and cardiomyopathies; in myocarditis, especially in chronic Chagas' disease; in sclerosis of the left side of the cardiac conduction system in the elderly; and in some types of congenital heart disease, particularly endocardial cushion defects and tricuspid atresia. Surgical injury during operation for left ventricular outflow tract obstruction also is a cause of anterior fascicular block.

The consequences of anterior fascicular block are negligible from a functional point of view. However, it is known that disease of the ventricular fascicular system can be a slowly progressive one, with one fascicle after another being damaged or being damaged and recovering, only to be blocked once again. This is true of both the acquired form and a newly described congenital hereditary form.

Hence prospective sequential observation of a patient with anterior fascicular block is essential.

Monofascicular block that becomes bifascicular or trifascicular has serious consequences. On the other hand, many patients with anterior fascicular block may live a decade or more without complications.

THE FOLLOWING CRITERIA ARE REQUIRED FOR THE DIAGNOSIS OF LEFT ANTERIOR FASCICULAR BLOCK.

1.   **Frontal plane QRS axis −45 to −90 degrees.**
2.   **Q waves in leads I and aVL that are less than 30 msec in duration.**

Left Posterior Fascicular Block

In this form of intraventricular conduction defect, there is complete block in the posterior fascicle of the left bundle, with normal conduction through the anterior fascicle and right bundle branch.

Isolated posterior fascicular block is rare, and the diagnosis difficult. Of the three pathways to the ventricles (right bundle, anterior fascicle, posterior fascicle), the posterior fascicle is least vulnerable to block, which probably accounts for the rarity of isolated posterior fascicular block. It usually is seen in association with right bundle branch block. The axis in pure posterior fascicular block lies between +90 and +100 degrees and occasionally as far to the right as +120 degrees. There is minimal change in the QRS duration, which is usually 0.09 to 0.10 second. Such subtle alterations—slight right axis deviation with a normal QRS duration—make a definitive diagnosis from the ECG alone almost an impossibility. A normal vertical heart, right ventricular enlargement, emphysema, and extensive lateral wall myocardial infarction must be excluded. A rightward shift in axis that has appeared sequentially, together with large R waves in leads II, III, and aVF, suggests the diagnosis of posterior fascicular block. In posterior fascicular block, left ventricular activation occurs over the normal anterior fascicle, and initial forces are directed anteriorly, superiorly, and to the left. Later, excitation occurs via the Purkinje network to include the area normally served by the posterior fascicle. Thus terminal activation spreads posteriorly, inferiorly, and to the right. The mean QRS thus has a right axis deviation with qR in leads II, III, and aVF. The R waves in leads II, III, and aVF are large.

THE FOLLOWING CRITERIA ARE REQUIRED FOR THE DIAGNOSIS OF LEFT POSTERIOR FASCICULAR BLOCK.

1. **Frontal plane QRS axis is +100 to +110 degrees.**
2. **Q waves in leads II, III, aVF that are less than 30 msec in duration.**

Bifascicular Block

Right Bundle Branch Block and Left Bundle Branch Block

This form of bifascicular block consists of complete block of the right bundle branch and the main stem of the left bundle.

Such complete bilateral bundle branch block produces complete atrioventricular block; complete bilateral bundle branch block, rather than damage to the atrioventricular node, is the commonest cause of complete atrioventricular block. This conclusion is supported by pathologic, clinical, and electrophysiologic evidence. Atrioventricular dissociation is present and an idioventricular pacemaker excites the ventricles. This usually arises below the bifurcation of the His bundle. Intracardiac electrophysiologic study demonstrates a His electrogram (H) following each atrial electrogram (A) but no fixed H–V relation. The body surface ECG and the intracardiac electrogram are indistinguishable from complete trifascicular block.

The most common cause of this arrhythmia is idiopathic fibrosis and sclerosis of the cardiac conduction system (Lenegre's disease). Less common causes are atherosclerotic heart disease, aortic valvular lesions, and cardiomyopathy.

The physiologic and clinical manifestations are similar to those of complete atrioventricular block.

THE FOLLOWING CRITERIA ARE REQUIRED FOR THE DIAGNOSIS OF COMPLETE BILATERAL BUNDLE BRANCH BLOCK.

1. **Atrioventricular dissociation.**
2. **Idioventricular rhythm.**
3. **Abnormal His bundle electrogram as noted above.**

Right Bundle Branch Block and Incomplete Left Bundle Branch Block

In this form of bifascicular block, there is complete block of the right bundle and delayed conduction in the main stem of the left bundle.

The ECG displays right bundle branch block (without abnormal axis deviation) and first-degree atrioventricular block. Intracardiac electrography will demonstrate a prolonged H–V interval rather than a prolonged A–H interval. If block in the left bundle branch is second degree, some of the H signals are not followed by V signals, and the ECG will display second-degree atrioventricular block (Mobitz II). The combination of bundle branch block and Mobitz II second-degree atrioventricular block is an important predecessor of complete atrioventricular block.

THE FOLLOWING CRITERIA ARE REQUIRED FOR THE DIAGNOSIS OF COMPLETE RIGHT BUNDLE BRANCH BLOCK AND INCOMPLETE LEFT BUNDLE BRANCH BLOCK.
1. **ECG criteria for right bundle branch block.**
2. **ECG criteria for first- or second-degree atrioventricular block.**
3. **Intracardiac electrography required to demonstrate H–V prolongation.**

Right Bundle Branch Block and Left Anterior
Fascicular Block

In this common form of bifascicular block, there is complete block in the right bundle branch and the anterosuperior division of the left bundle branch.

The diagnostic criteria are those of right bundle branch block and marked left axis deviation.

This form of intraventricular block may be caused by idiopathic fibrosis of the cardiac conduction system and a variety of other acquired heart diseases. It is also observed in congenital endocardial cushion defects.

The prognostic significance of this conduction abnormality is the risk of developing complete atrioventricular block. Long-term studies have determined this risk to be small, 1 to 2 percent per year over a 5- to 10-year period. When this form of bifascicular block complicates acute myocardial infarction, the risk of developing complete atrioventricular block is substantially higher, 25 to 50 percent.

THE FOLLOWING CRITERIA ARE REQUIRED FOR THE DIAGNOSIS OF RIGHT BUNDLE BRANCH BLOCK AND LEFT ANTERIOR FASCICULAR BLOCK.
1. **ECG criteria for right bundle branch block.**
2. **Abnormal left axis deviation.**

*Right Bundle Branch Block and Left Posterior
Fascicular Block*

In this uncommon conduction abnormality, there is complete block in the right bundle branch and the posteroinferior division of the left bundle branch. It is recognized by the presence of right bundle branch block and right axis deviation. As in the case of monofascicular left posterior fascicular block, other causes for right axis deviation should be excluded (normal variant, chronic obstructive lung disease, right ventricular hypertrophy). The prognosis of this form of bifascicular block is the same as for right bundle branch block with left anterior fascicular block.

THE FOLLOWING CRITERIA ARE REQUIRED FOR THE DIAGNOSIS OF RIGHT BUNDLE BRANCH BLOCK AND LEFT POSTERIOR FASCICULAR BLOCK.

1.   ECG criteria for right bundle branch block.
2.   Right axis deviation.

*Left Anterior Fascicular Block and Left Posterior
Fascicular Block*

Complete block of these two fascicles results in complete left bundle branch block, and some consider all instances of complete left bundle branch block the result of this form of bifascicular block.

THE DIAGNOSTIC CRITERIA FOR LEFT ANTERIOR FASCICULAR BLOCK AND LEFT POSTERIOR FASCICULAR BLOCK ARE THE SAME AS THOSE FOR LEFT BUNDLE BRANCH BLOCK ON PAGE 210.

Trifascicular Block

This arrhythmia includes complete block in the right bundle branch and complete or incomplete block in both divisions of the left bundle branch. It is manifested electrocardiographically by the presence of bifascicular block and atrioventricular block, but it can be accurately identified (i.e., excluding atrioventricular nodal block) only by intracardiac electrography.

*Complete Trifascicular Block (Right Bundle Branch Block,
Complete Left Anterior Fascicular Block and Complete Left
Posterior Fascicular Block)*

Complete block in the three subdivisions of the bundle of His interrupts atrioventricular transmission. The ECG displays complete atrioventricular block with atrioventricular dissociation and an idioventricular pacemaker located below the bifurcation of the common bundle. The intracardiac electrogram demonstrates atrial signals (A) followed by His signals (H). The ventricular signals (V) occur at a constant cycle but independently of the A–H sequence. Most instances of chronic complete atrioventricular block are due to this combination of conduction defects.

THE FOLLOWING CRITERIA ARE REQUIRED FOR THE DIAGNOSIS OF COMPLETE TRIFASCICULAR BLOCK.

1. **Atrioventricular dissociation.**
2. **Idioventricular pacemaker located below branching of the bundle of His.**
3. **Intracardiac electrogram demonstrates no conduction distal to the His electrogram.**

Incomplete Trifascicular Block

The combination of complete block in one or two subdivisions of the common bundle and incomplete block in one or two subdivisions results in ECGs that show both bifascicular block and atrioventricular block. Intracardiac electrography is required to localize the atrioventricular block to the distal His-Purkinje system (prolonged H–V intervals). Combinations of bundle branch block and atrioventricular block that cause the various forms of bifascicular and trifascicular block may also be associated with atrioventricular nodal dysfunction. In such cases, the intracardiac electrogram demonstrates a prolonged A–H interval in addition to prolonged H–V intervals.

THE FOLLOWING CRITERIA ARE REQUIRED FOR THE DIAGNOSIS OF INCOMPLETE TRIFASCICULAR BLOCK.

1. **ECG evidence of monofascicular or bifascicular bundle branch block.**
2. **ECG evidence of first degree or second degree atrioventricular block.**
3. **Prolongation of the H–V interval of the intracardiac electrogram.**

Nonspecific Intraventricular Block

When the duration of the QRS complex exceeds 0.10 second but the QRS morphology is not that of bundle branch block, the rubric "nonspecific intraventricular block" may be used. Diffuse myocardial diseases of many types, especially left ventricular hypertrophy, can prolong intraventricular conduction. Other causes include hypothermia, hyperkalemia, and the class 1 antiarrhythmic drugs.

THE FOLLOWING CRITERIA ARE REQUIRED FOR THE DIAGNOSIS OF NONSPECIFIC INTRAVENTRICULAR BLOCK.
1. **QRS complex duration exceeding 0.10 second.**
2. **Absence of typical ECG characteristics of right bundle branch block and left bundle branch block.**

Aberrant Ventricular Conduction

Aberrant ventricular conduction refers to transient changes in the morphology of the QRS complex during a supraventricular rhythm. The changes vary from minor increases in QRS duration and alterations in the amplitude of the QRS complex to more marked notching, slurring, and prolongation, including typical forms of monofascicular or bifascicular block. The modifications in the time course of ventricular depolarization are due to a change in the timing of the supraventricular impulse or in the duration of refractionness in specialized conduction tissue such that a supraventricular impulse reaches specialized tissue that is refractory to excitation.

Several specific electrophysiologic mechanisms may initiate aberrant ventricular conduction. The most common is an atrial premature depolarization with short coupling interval that reaches specialized tissue during its relative refractory period (phase 3 block). Such atrial premature beats may be erroneously diagnosed as ventricular premature depolarizations. Acceleration of the rate of the supraventricular rhythm may result in ventricular aberration for a similar reason. During supraventricular rhythms that cause an irregular ventricular rhythm (i.e., atrial fibrillation, sinus rhythm, or atrial tachycardia or atrial flutter with varying atrioventricular block), variations in cycle length—which cause corresponding variations in refractory period duration of specialized tissue—may initiate aberrant ventricular conduction when a long cycle is followed by a short cycle. The QRS complex terminating the short cycle may be aberrant. Several such aberrant QRS complexes may occur in succession, simulating ventricular tachycardia (Ashman's phenomenon). Abrupt slowing of the rate of the supraventricular rhythm or escape beats terminating a pause may cause aberrant ventricular conduction (phase 4 block), possibly due to prolonged diastolic depolarization and less negative resting membrane potential. While the mechanisms responsible for aberrant ventricular conduction may not be completely understood, the phenomenon itself is common and important. Differentiation of aberrant conduction from ventricular ectopic rhythms is often difficult or impossible.

THE FOLLOWING CRITERIA ARE REQUIRED FOR THE DIAGNOSIS OF ABERRANT VENTRICULAR CONDUCTION.
1. **Transient change in duration, amplitude, or morphology of a QRS complex of supraventricular origin.**
2. **One or more initiating mechanisms as described previously.**

VENTRICULAR PREEXCITATION

Ventricular preexcitation is an abnormality of atrioventricular conduction in which the atrial impulse (usually arising in the sinus node) bypasses all or part of the atrioventricular junction, thus prematurely exciting the ventricles. In this way, preexcitation is a form of accelerated atrioventricular conduction. The disorder is a congenital anomaly due to the presence of accessory, extranodal, atrioventricular conduction pathways. Such pathways may connect (1) atria and ventricles–atrioventricular pathways–Kent bundles; (2) atria and bundle of His–atrio-Hisian pathway–James fibers; and (3) atrioventricular node and ventricles–nodal ventricular pathway–Mahaim fibers; His bundle or bundle branches and ventricles–His ventricular or fasciculoventricular pathways–Mahaim fibers. The accessory pathways are also classified according to their general location (e.g., left or right posteroseptal, anteroseptal, left lateral, right lateral).

Impulses arising in the atria enter the accessory pathway and normal atrioventricular conduction pathway nearly simultaneously but reach the ventricles first via the accessory pathway, since the atrioventricular node slows conduction in the normal pathway. This initial excitation of the ventricles via the accessory pathway causes the pathognomonic ECG abnormality of preexcitation, the delta wave. The delta wave is a distortion of the initial portion of the QRS complex, appearing as a decrease in slope, notch, or slur. Usually, the remainder of ventricular depolarization—caused by the impulse reaching ventricles via the normal atrioventricular conduction system—is normal. The resulting QRS complex is a fusion beat, and its actual morphology and duration will vary depending on the amount of myocardium depolarized via the accessory pathway compared to the normal atrioventricular pathway. This, in turn, will be a function of conduction velocity and refractoriness in the two pathways. Delay in impulse transmission in the normal pathway will result in a very aberrant, prolonged QRS complex; delay in the accessory pathway will cause a relatively normal QRS complex, even without a delta wave. Secondary ST–T changes occur in proportion to the degree of abnormality of the QRS complex. If the accessory pathway bypasses the atrioventricular node, the P–R segment disappears, the QRS complex has its onset near the end of the P wave, and the P–R interval is shortened.

Precise localization of the accessory pathways and an assessment of their functional state require detailed intracardiac electrography. However, analysis of the polarity of the delta waves in the conventional ECG does provide fairly reliable evidence of the general location of the accessory pathway. For example, left posteroseptal pathways cause upright delta waves in precordial leads V_1 and V_2 and inverted delta waves in standard leads II, III, and aVF; left lateral pathways cause upright delta waves in leads V_1 and V_2 and upright delta waves in leads II, III, and aVF; anterior accessory pathways tend to cause inverted delta waves in leads V_1 and V_2 and upright delta waves in leads II, III, and aVF. The earlier ECG classification of the forms of preexcitation into Types A, B, and C has been replaced by the more detailed localization based on electrophysiologic study and surgical analysis.

The combination of atria, ventricles, accessory pathway, and normal atrioventricular junction constitutes an anatomic circuit that permits reentrant ectopic rhythms, usually initiated by an atrial premature depolarization. The most common of these arrhythmias is termed atrioventricular reciprocating tachycardia, and it occurs in two forms: orthodromic, in which the atrial impulse enters the normal atrioventricular conduction pathway and, after exciting the ventricles, returns to the atria retrogradely via the accessory pathway; and antidromic, in which the direction of impulse transmission is atria to accessory pathway to ventricles and retrogradely to atria via the normal atrioventricular conduction pathway. The former has the general form of paroxysmal supraventricular tachycardia; the latter mimics ventricular tachycardia. Atrial fibrillation is a less common but important ectopic rhythm in ventricular preexcitation. Very rapid ventricular rates during atrial fibrillation may occur if the atrial impulses are transmitted to the ventricles via the accessory pathway, and certain drugs (e.g., digitalis glycosides) which ordinarily slow the ventricular rate in atrial fibrillation when conduction takes place through the atrioventricular node, may parodoxically accelerate the ventricular rate when conduction occurs through the accessory pathway. Marked acceleration of the ventricular rate may be followed by ventricular fibrillation.

The combination of the typical set of ECG abnormalities and tachyarrhythmias constitutes the Wolff-Parkinson-White syndrome. While arrhythmias are common in patients with ventricular preexcitation, their frequency varies widely in individual patients. Thus, in many subjects, preexcitation is a benign disorder. It usually exists in otherwise normal hearts, but it also occurs in association with certain congenital lesions, notably Ebstein's anomaly of the tricuspid valve. The diagnosis is usually easily recognized using the conventional ECG if the typical short P–R interval and delta wave are present. In such cases, intracardiac electrography demonstrates a normal A–H interval and a short H–V interval. When the atria are paced at progressively more rapid rates, the A–H interval lengthens (a normal phenomenon), the H–V interval shortens, and the His bundle signal superimposes on or follows the ventricular signal. The QRS complex becomes progressively more aberrant (preexcited).

ECGs with a short P–R interval (<0.11 second) but no delta wave may be caused by an atrio-Hisian accessory pathway, and some subjects with this type of ECG do have episodes of paroxysmal tachycardia (Lown-Ganong-Levine syndrome). Evidence that this syndrome is due to preexcitation is equivocal. Some accessory pathways conduct in the retrograde direction only, delta waves are absent, and the diagnosis of accessory pathway conduction can be made only during electrophysiologic study of induced paroxysmal supraventricular tachycardia.

Ventricular preexcitation may cause difficulties in ECG differential diagnosis. Inverted delta waves in leads

II, III, and aVF may be mistaken for abnormal Q waves of inferior myocardial infarction. Upright delta waves in leads V_1 and V_2 may simulate true posterior wall infarction or right ventricular hypertrophy. QRS complex and repolarization abnormalities may suggest left ventricular hypertrophy or myocardial ischemia. As a general rule, if the ECG diagnosis of ventricular preexcitation is made, no other anatomic or physiologic diagnosis should be entertained.

THE FOLLOWING CRITERIA ARE REQUIRED FOR THE DIAGNOSIS OF VENTRICULAR PREEXCITATION.
1. **Short P–R interval and absent P–R segment.**
2. **Delta wave.**
3. **Varying degrees of QRS prolongation and ST–T abnormality.**
4. **Confirmatory intracardiac electrophysiologic data may be required.**

Disorders of Supravalvular, Valvular, or Subvalvular Function

AORTIC STENOSIS (SUPRAVALVULAR, VALVULAR, OR SUBVALVULAR OBSTRUCTION)

Obstruction of blood flow from the left ventricle can occur as the result of congenital anomalies or acquired disease and can involve the valve or regions above or below the valve (see also pages 84 and 157–159). Stenosis of the valve can result from calcific changes of unknown cause affecting a previously normal or bicuspid valve, from congenital abnormalities, and from changes induced by rheumatic fever. Supravalvular obstruction to blood flow can be caused by narrowing of the aorta induced by a fibromuscular membrane or hypoplasia of the aorta. Subaortic obstruction may result from a discrete fibrous diaphragm below a normal valve or from diffuse hypertrophy of the ventricular septum, which abuts the anterior leaflet of the mitral valve during systole.

When the area involved is considerably reduced, an increase in left ventricular systolic pressure ensues. A systolic pressure gradient is present between points proximal and distal to the obstruction. The left ventricle can hypertrophy, dilate, or fail as a consequence of the increased afterload imposed by the obstruction.

A paucity of symptoms characterizes lesser degrees of obstruction. Severe obstruction may be manifested by dizziness, syncope, anginal syndrome, left ventricular failure, or sudden death. Echocardiographic findings are discussed on page 84.

With obstruction due to valvular deformity or a subvalvular discrete fibrous membrane, the aortic component of the second sound can be reduced in intensity and delayed sufficiently to produce paradoxical splitting of the second sound. In the more severe degrees of obstruction, when hypertrophy of the left ventricle is marked, a fourth heart sound is audible. A harsh crescendo-decrescendo ejection systolic murmur of variable intensity is usually heard best to the right of the upper sternum and is also audible in the carotid arteries. The murmur is less well transmitted to the apical area, although sometimes this is the only site where it can be heard. A systolic thrill to the right of the sternum or over the carotid areas can accompany louder murmurs. Ejection clicks may occur. The pulse pressure in the systemic arteries may be small, and the pulse may rise slowly and have an anacrotic notch.

Supravalvular obstruction is almost always accompanied by other extracardiac anomalies. The aortic component of the second sound may be normal in intensity; the other physical findings resemble those encountered in valvular obstruction, except that ejection clicks are rare.

In patients with diffuse or focal subvalvular hypertrophy of the septum (see page 96), the aortic component of the second sound may be faint and delayed, with paradoxical splitting of the second sound. The systolic ejection murmur and thrill may be maximal along the left sternal border. The degree of obstruction and the intensity of the murmur are often increased by the Valsalva maneuver, inotropic agents, amyl nitrite, and premature beats. Echocardiographic evidence of dynamic obstruction may likewise be brought out by these procedures. Systolic clicks are common. The systemic arterial pulse rises and falls rapidly, with a secondary rise before the dicrotic notch. Characteristically, there are variations in the systolic pressure gradient between the left ventricular cavity and the subvalvular area. These variations result from changes in the force of left ventricular contraction, the size of the left ventricular cavity, and the transmural pressure that distends the outflow tract during systole. In addition, a systolic pressure gradient may exist across the right ventricular outflow tract caused by protrusion of the hypertrophied septum to the right. Mitral regurgitation is frequently present. Echocardiographic findings are discussed on page 96.

ONE OF THE FOLLOWING CRITERIA IS REQUIRED FOR THE DIAGNOSIS OF VALVULAR AORTIC STENOSIS.

Initial

The presence of a harsh, crescendo-decrescendo systolic murmur at the right base of the heart that radiates to the neck, with an absent or faint aortic component of the second sound and a small systemic arterial pulse pressure.

Definitive

Echocardiographic or angiocardiographic evidence of the stenotic area and of a pressure gradient estimated by Doppler flow study or demonstration by cardiac catheterization of a pressure gradient during systole.

ONE OF THE FOLLOWING CRITERIA IS REQUIRED FOR THE DIAGNOSIS OF SUBAORTIC STENOSIS DUE TO HYPERTROPHIC CARDIOMYOPATHY.

Initial

Presence of a harsh systolic murmur along the left sternal border that increases in intensity with the Valsalva maneuver or after administration of nitrites or inotropic agents.

Definitive

Echocardiographic evidence of dynamic left ventricular outflow tract obstruction.

AORTIC REGURGITATION

A wide variety of lesions can induce aortic regurgitation. The valve cusps may be deformed by congenital disease or by rheumatic fever, myxomatous degeneration, infective endocarditis, or degenerative disease. Lesions of the aorta capable of causing aortic regurgitation can be congenital or induced by syphilis, cystic medial necrosis, ankylosing spondylitis, or aortic dissection. Severe hypertension may also cause aortic regurgitation, which is usually hemodynamically trivial. (See also pages 85 and 155.)

Regurgitation causes an increase in left ventricular diastolic volume and wall stress; consequently, the left ventricle may dilate and hypertrophy. Dilatation of the ascending aorta is frequently present. Although regurgitation may be tolerated for long periods without symptoms, ultimately it may lead to left ventricular failure or anginal syndrome.

A blowing, decrescendo diastolic murmur starting with the aortic component of the second sound is characteristic of aortic regurgitation. The murmur is best heard in the third and fourth intercostal spaces to the left of the sternum with the patient leaning forward and with the breath expelled. It occasionally radiates to the cardiac apex. Because of the large stroke volume, there may be a systolic murmur heard over or cephalad to the aortic area. The pulse can be bounding, with an elevated systolic and a decreased diastolic pressure.

Echocardiography using Doppler flow techniques is the most sensitive and specific method for demonstrating transvalvular regurgitation from aorta to left ventricle.

ONE OF THE FOLLOWING CRITERIA IS REQUIRED FOR THE DIAGNOSIS OF AORTIC REGURGITATION.

Initial

A blowing, decrescendo diastolic murmur starting with the second heart sound, heard best in the third and fourth intercostal spaces close to the sternum, in the absence of causes for pulmonic regurgitation.

Definitive

1. **Echocardiographic evidence of blood flow from aorta to left ventricle.**
2. **Evidence of regurgitation into the left ventricle of angiocardiographic contrast medium or other suitable indicators following an aortic injection.**

MITRAL STENOSIS

Obstruction to the flow across the mitral valve most often results from valvular deformities following rheumatic fever. Rarely, congenital deformation of the valve or obstruction of the valve orifice by tumors can be encountered. Obstruction due to left atrial tumors may be intermittent and related to change in position as the tumor prolapses into the mitral orifice. (See also pages 86 and 162.)

When the area of the valve orifice is reduced considerably, the mean pressure in the left atrium exceeds that in the left ventricle during diastole. The increased pressure in the left atrium is reflected throughout the pulmonary vasculature. Left atrial, pulmonary arterial, and right ventricular enlargement ensue. Vascular changes may appear in the pulmonary arteries, further elevating pulmonary arterial pressure.

Patients usually present with symptoms of pulmonary congestion with or without concomitant evidence of right ventricular failure. The first heart sound and the pulmonic component of the second heart sound may be accentuated. Closely following the second heart sound, a short, high-pitched sound, the opening snap, is often audible in patients with valvular deformity. An early diastolic low-pitched, rumbling murmur that is localized to the apex, a presystolic crescendo murmur, or both are characteristic of mitral obstruction. Frequently, these murmurs can only be heard when the patient is placed in the left lateral decubitus position after exercise.

In patients with intermittent obstruction due to left atrial tumors, the abrupt fall in cardiac output may lead to dizziness or syncope with changes in position. The murmurs described above may be present. However, the first heart sound is often not accentuated and an early diastolic sound caused by movement of the tumor occurs later than an opening snap.

Echocardiography is the most sensitive and specific technique for detection and evaluation of mitral stenosis (see page 86). It can evaluate the amplitude of excursion and closing velocity of the anterior mitral leaflet, posterior leaflet motion, evidence of leaflet thickening and calcification, and mitral valve orifice size. Doppler flow techniques permit estimates of the pressure gradient across the mitral orifice. Left atrial tumors causing intermittent or fixed obstruction of the mitral orifice can also be seen by this technique.

ONE OF THE FOLLOWING CRITERIA IS REQUIRED FOR THE DIAGNOSIS OF MITRAL STENOSIS.

Initial

The characteristic murmur as previously described, with one of the following: accentuation of the first heart sound, an opening snap, radiologic evidence of enlargement of the left atrium, or calcification of the valve leaflets.

Definitive

1. **Doppler echocardiographic evidence of mitral stenosis, or**
2. **Demonstration by cardiac catheterization of a diastolic pressure gradient across the mitral valve.**

MITRAL REGURGITATION

Inability of mitral valve leaflets to appose precisely or to close completely may be caused by a wide variety of lesions. The valve leaflets may be damaged by myxomatous degeneration, rheumatic fever, or infective endocarditis. Rarely, extensive subannular calcification of the zone of attachment of the mitral valve to the left ventricular myocardium, with extension of the calcification to the mitral leaflets, can produce regurgitation. Regurgitation can also result from prolapse or congenital clefts in the mitral leaflets, rupture or fibrosis of the papillary muscles, or rupture of the chordae tendineae. Mitral regurgitation is common with hypertrophic cardiomyopathy. Hypertrophy of the ventricular septum such as may be encountered in idiopathic hypertrophic subaortic stenosis also may interfere with mitral valve closure. Regurgitation can also be produced by a variety of arrhythmias, particularly atrial fibrillation. (See also pages 87 and 160.)

The failure of the valve to achieve complete closure permits flow of blood from the ventricle into the left atrium during systole. This results in an added volume load on the left ventricle during diastole. Long-standing or severe mitral regurgitation may cause the left ventricle to dilate, hypertrophy, and ultimately fail. Left atrial enlargement usually is conspicuous with mitral regurgitation of long duration, especially when the onset is in childhood. Mitral regurgitation present for short periods of time is often not associated with enlargement of the left atrium.

The presenting symptoms may be those of easy fatigability or of pulmonary congestion. The first heart sound is usually diminished in intensity, and a third heart sound is commonly present. The timing, duration, and site of associated systolic murmurs and thrills vary and are dependent on the severity and the cause of the lesion. With regurgitation due to valvular deformity, a harsh, holosystolic, high-pitched murmur is present at the apex and is transmitted to the axilla. Regurgitation following rupture of the chordae tendineae predominantly involving the posterior mitral leaflet is associated with a holosystolic murmur best heard along the left sternal border, while rupture of the chordae tendineae of the anterior leaflet is often associated with a holosystolic murmur at the apex that radiates to the axilla or head.

Fibrosis of a papillary muscle may be associated with an apical systolic murmur that begins after the first heart sound and ends before the second. The finding of mid-systolic clicks and a late apical systolic murmur is frequently associated with a mild degree of regurgitation and is often found with myxomatous degeneration of the valve.

An early mid-diastolic murmur may result from the increased volume of blood flow across the mitral valve during diastole. Left atrial pressure curves characteristically show a loss of the X descent and a prominent V wave. Doppler echocardiography demonstrates flow from the left ventricle to the left atrium.

ONE OF THE FOLLOWING CRITERIA IS REQUIRED FOR THE DIAGNOSIS OF MITRAL REGURGITATION.

Initial

The characteristic systolic murmur.

Definitive

Evidence of mitral regurgitation by Doppler flow studies or contrast ventriculography.

PULMONIC STENOSIS (VALVULAR OR SUBVALVULAR OBSTRUCTION)

Obstruction to blood flow from the right ventricle is almost invariably the consequence of a congenital abnormality, either valvular stenosis or massive hypertrophy of the outflow tract of the right ventricle. Rarely, disseminated carcinoid tumor may affect the valve cusps, thereby producing stenosis. Right ventricular endocardial tumors may produce fixed or intermittent obstruction of the valve orifice. (See also pages 89 and 165.)

As a result of the obstruction, the right ventricular systolic pressure becomes elevated and exceeds that distal to the lesion, and right ventricular hypertrophy develops. Lesser degrees of obstruction may not produce symptoms. However, with severe obstruction, syncope is not unusual.

The pulmonic component of the second sound may be delayed and diminished in intensity. A characteristic loud, harsh, medium-pitched ejection systolic murmur, accompanied by a thrill, is best heard in the first and second left intercostal spaces but may be heard down the left sternal border, in the back, or in the neck. Ejection clicks are commonly present with valvular stenosis. Post-stenotic dilatation of the pulmonary artery, frequently restricted to the left main pulmonary artery, may be revealed by radiologic studies.

Echocardiography demonstrates thickened, immobile pulmonic valve leaflets. Doppler study demonstrates a transvalvular systolic pressure gradient. On M-mode echocardiography, an exaggerated "a" wave is noted.

ONE OF THE FOLLOWING CRITERIA IS REQUIRED FOR THE DIAGNOSIS OF PULMONIC STENOSIS.

Initial

The characteristic systolic murmur.

Definitive

1. **Echocardiographic evidence of pulmonic stenosis, or**
2. **Evidence by Doppler flow studies or cardiac catheterization of a systolic pressure gradient across the pulmonic valve.**

PULMONIC REGURGITATION

Pulmonic regurgitation is an uncommon physiologic abnormality that may result from congenital malformations of the cusps, infective endocarditis, surgical correction of pulmonary valvular stenosis, severe pulmonary hypertension of unknown cause or that following mitral obstruction, or the rarer forms of pulmonary heart disease. The pulmonary arterial diastolic pressure sometimes is reduced to the level of the elevated end-diastolic pressure of the enlarged right ventricle. (See also page 89.)

A high-pitched, blowing decrescendo diastolic murmur heard in the second, third, or fourth interspaces to the left of the sternum is characteristic of regurgitation through the pulmonic valve.

ONE OF THE FOLLOWING CRITERIA IS REQUIRED FOR THE DIAGNOSIS OF PULMONIC REGURGITATION.

Initial

The characteristic diastolic murmur.

Definitive

Evidence of pulmonary regurgitation by Doppler flow studies or of regurgitation into the right ventricle of contrast material injected into the pulmonary artery.

TRICUSPID STENOSIS

Tricuspid obstruction can result from scarring of the valve due to rheumatic fever, carcinoid tumor, occlusion of the valve orifice by tumors or thrombi, and, rarely, congenital anomalies (see also pages 88 and 169).

As a result of the obstruction, blood flow from the right ventricle is impeded during ventricular diastole, with a consequent rise in pressure in the right atrium and the appearance of a diastolic pressure gradient across the valve. Right atrial enlargement and systemic venous congestion ensue.

The diastolic or presystolic murmur associated with tricuspid obstruction is relatively low-pitched, blowing, and heard best to the right or left of the lower sternum. It frequently is accentuated during inspiration.

The echocardiogram demonstrates thickening and reduced excursion of the valve, a narrowed orifice, and a pressure gradient across the valve.

ONE OF THE FOLLOWING CRITERIA IS REQUIRED FOR THE DIAGNOSIS OF TRICUSPID STENOSIS.

Initial

Presence of the presystolic or diastolic murmur previously described.

Definitive

Evidence of a pressure gradient across the tricuspid valve during diastole demonstrated by Doppler flow studies or cardiac catheterization.

TRICUSPID REGURGITATION

The most common cause of tricuspid regurgitation is right ventricular hypertension with dilatation of the tricuspid annulus. It may also occur as a result of damage to the valves induced by rheumatic fever, carcinoid tumor, trauma, or infective endocarditis. Marked dilatation of the right ventricle can interfere with the function of the papillary muscle and chordae tendineae, so that valve closure is incomplete. Atrial fibrillation may also cause tricuspid regurgitation. (See also page 88.)

Regurgitation induces a rise in pressure during ventricular systole in the right atrium and consequently in the systemic veins. Right atrial enlargement and systemic venous congestion result, with loss of the X descent in the right atrial pressure curve and a prominent V wave.

The murmur associated with tricuspid regurgitation is pansystolic, blowing, of medium pitch, and best heard in the fourth and fifth intercostal spaces close to or over the sternum. The murmur is accentuated by inspiration. Echocardiography with Doppler flow study is an accurate technique for detection and evaluation of the degree of tricuspid regurgitation. When regurgitation is severe, reflux into the venae cavae and hepatic veins is manifest.

ONE OF THE FOLLOWING CRITERIA IS REQUIRED FOR THE DIAGNOSIS OF TRICUSPID REGURGITATION.

Initial

The characteristic systolic murmur.

Definitive

Evidence of tricuspid regurgitation by Doppler flow studies or contrast ventriculography.

MALFUNCTION OF PROSTHESES AND HOMOGRAFTS

Malfunction of intracardiac prostheses may be due to a paravalvular leak, degeneration of the leaflet portions of bioprostheses, mechanical failure of the valve disk, leaflet, poppet, or supportive structures, formation of a thrombus in and about the prosthesis, ingrowth of fibrous tissue, or vegetations following infection. Malfunction soon after implantation of the prosthesis suggests paravalvular leak rather than the other causes.

The manifestations of malfunction are those of valvular obstruction or regurgitation at the site of the prosthesis. Palpitations, syncope, ventricular failure, venous congestion, or new murmurs may suddenly appear. Hemolytic anemia may occur when trauma to the erythrocytes increases in the malfunctioning prosthesis. Rarely, the poppet, mechanical disk or leaflet may become dislodged from the cage and may embolize.

Prosthetic malfunction may be accompanied by diminution or absence of the prosthetic opening sound or variation in its intensity from beat to beat. Echocardiography or fluoroscopy may show restricted movement of a poppet, disk, or bioprosthetic valve leaflet, but Doppler study allows rapid and accurate determination of abnormal regurgitation or stenosis.

Malfunction of an aortic homograft or porcine xenograft in the aortic or mitral area is suggested by the onset of ventricular failure or progressive widening of the pulse pressure. Slight aortic regurgitation is often associated with tissue prostheses in the aortic position and does not necessarily indicate malfunction.

THE FOLLOWING CRITERIA ARE REQUIRED FOR THE DIAGNOSIS OF MALFUNCTION OF PROSTHESES AND HOMOGRAFTS.

Initial

Changes in the opening or closing sounds of valvular prostheses or the appearance of new murmurs.

Definitive

1. **Echocardiographic or fluoroscopic evidence of abnormal structure or motion of the valve prosthesis or its components.**
2. **Evidence for abnormal stenosis or regurgitation across a mechanical or tissue prosthesis demonstrated by Doppler echocardiographic studies or cardiac catheterization.**

PROLAPSE OF VALVES

Prolapse of the Aortic Valve

Prolapse of one or more cusps of the aortic valve may result from Marfan's syndrome, myxomatous degeneration, or aortic dissection. It may also develop in association with ventricular septal defects.

Aortic regurgitation may result. Echocardiography or aortography may demonstrate the abnormal displacement of a cusp.

THE FOLLOWING CRITERION IS REQUIRED FOR THE DIAGNOSIS OF PROLAPSE OF THE AORTIC VALVE.

Echocardiographic or aortographic demonstration of a cusp displaced downward toward the left ventricle.

Prolapse of the Mitral Valve

Marfan's syndrome or myxomatous degeneration of valve leaflets or the chordae tendineae may cause displacement of one or both mitral leaflets into the left atrium during ventricular systole. Barlow's syndrome, a common but relatively benign form of mitral prolapse, may be asymptomatic for long periods of time.

Prolapse is frequently associated with an apical midsystolic click and a late systolic murmur. Both click and murmur move earlier in systole with maneuvers that decrease left ventricular volume (sitting, standing) and become louder with increased arterial pressure (isometric exercise). Associated mitral regurgitation is common, and abnormalities in left ventricular contraction are sometimes present. Mitral valve prolapse can be diagnosed accurately by echocardiography when M-mode study reveals late systolic posterior displacement of one or both mitral leaflets at least 2 mm behind the mitral valve's C–D line or when two-dimensional long-axis views reveal clear-cut systolic protrusion of mitral leaflets into the left atrium.

THE FOLLOWING CRITERIA ARE REQUIRED FOR THE DIAGNOSIS OF PROLAPSE OF THE MITRAL VALVE.

Initial
The characteristic systolic click and murmur.

Definitive
Evidence of mitral valve prolapse and associated regurgitation by echocardiography or other imaging techniques.

Disorders of Myocardial Function

VENTRICULAR FAILURE AND CONGESTIVE HEART FAILURE

Ventricular failure is defined as impaired cardiac function resulting in reduction of effective cardiac output and inadequate perfusion of oxygenated blood to peripheral tissues. It may be caused by primary loss or malfunction of myocardial contractile elements or by augmented systolic or diastolic loading conditions. Either or both ventricles may be affected, and the principal ventricular dysfunction may occur in systole, diastole, or in both phases of the cardiac cycle. Commonly, ventricular failure is accompanied by adaptive or compensatory mechanisms such as ventricular hypertrophy, ventricular remodeling, and activation of neuroendocrine systems leading to circulatory congestion. The combination of ventricular failure and circulatory congestion defines congestive heart failure.

Ischemic and hypertensive heart disease, cardiomyopathies, and valvular deformities are the common causes of congestive heart failure in the adult population. The structural and functional abnormalities in the ventricles may be segmental or diffuse. A number of physiologic parameters have been evaluated as clinical measures of ventricular contractility (e.g., maximum rate of rise of pressure, maximum velocity of fiber shortening, fractional shortening, ejection fraction). All of them have specific advantages and limitations. The most widely used parameter in clinical medicine (despite its dependence on ventricular afterload) is the ejection fraction, the ratio of stroke volume to end-diastolic volume. Contrast ventriculography, radioisotope ventriculography, or echocardiography can be used to determine ejection fraction, and values below 55 percent represent impaired contractile function or ventricular failure.

Activation of the adrenergic, arginine vasopressin, and renin-angiotensin-aldosterone systems is an important consequence of cardiac muscle failure. Release of the vasoconstrictor hormones norepinephrine, vasopressin, and angiotensin II initially may improve end-organ perfusion and ventricular function, but in later stages of heart failure excessive vascular resistance increases ventricular afterload and reduces cardiac output. Retention of sodium and water induced by aldosterone and elevation of ventricular filling pressure caused by the increased end-systolic and end-diastolic volumes promote systemic and pulmonary congestion and constitute the fully developed syndrome of congestive heart failure. Failure of the left ventricle may be accompanied by manifestations of pulmonary hypertension and pulmonary circulatory congestion; failure of the right ventricle may lead to elevation of systemic venous pressure and to systemic circulatory congestion. Combined ventricular failure can occur; right ventricular failure often results from the pulmonary hypertension induced by left ventricular failure.

The diagnosis of ventricular failure in infants is often difficult but may be manifested by poor feeding, occasionally accompanied by sweating, irritability, a rapid respiratory rate, and failure to gain weight. An enlarged liver is difficult to evaluate unless it increases rapidly in size.

The diagnosis of ventricular failure cannot be made with certainty in the presence of pericardial disease severe enough to impair the filling of the heart.

Severe anemia, thyrotoxicosis, hypoxia, fever, and systemic arteriovenous fistula may aggravate or initiate congestive heart failure despite normal or increased blood flow (high-output failure).

Left Ventricular Failure

ONE OF THE FOLLOWING CRITERIA IS REQUIRED FOR THE DIAGNOSIS OF LEFT VENTRICULAR FAILURE.

1. A left ventricular ejection fraction measured by angiography, two-dimensional echocardiography, or radioisotope ventriculography less than 50 percent or greater than two standard deviations below normal where the normal is 55 percent for that laboratory. An M-mode echocardiographic fractional shortening of less than 25 percent can also be used.
2. In the absence of aortic or mitral valve disease, evidence of a dilated left ventricle accompanied by a cardiac index of less than 2.5 L/min/m^2 body surface area, the latter value measured at rest in the supine position and in the basal state.
3. In the absence of aortic or mitral valvular disease or left ventricular hypertrophy:
    a. Elevation at rest of the left ventricular end-diastolic pressure above 12 mm Hg, or mean left atrial or pulmonary capillary wedge pressure above 12 mm Hg (zero reference is 5 cm below the second costochondral junction with the patient supine) and a resting level of cardiac output less than 2.5 L/min/m^2; and/or
    b. Elevation of left ventricular end-diastolic pressure (or mean left atrial or pulmonary capillary wedge pressure) above 14 mm Hg on moderate supine leg exercise, and an inability either to increase cardiac output more than 800 ml for every 100-ml increase in oxygen consumption, to achieve a peak oxygen consumption of greater than 20 ml/kg/min, or to increase stroke volume; or
    c. Manifestations of pulmonary congestion or pulmonary edema in the presence of a large left ventricle. With a normal ejection fraction, this defines diastolic left ventricular failure.
4. In the presence of aortic obstruction or regurgitation, radiologic or echocardiographic evidence of a sudden or progressive increase in left ventricular size. This criterion reflects the fact that the valvular lesions themselves may reduce the level of systemic blood flow, both at rest and during exercise, and cause elevation of the end-diastolic pressure.

5. In the presence of mitral obstruction or regurgitation, evidence of an elevated left ventricular end-diastolic pressure. This criterion reflects the fact that elevation of the left atrial or pulmonary arterial wedge pressure and a reduced level of systemic blood flow both at rest and during exercise can result from the valvular lesions themselves. Similarly, in the presence of mitral obstruction, pulmonary congestion cannot be utilized as a criterion of left ventricular failure, even in the presence of a large left ventricle.

6. A third heart sound, or a summation gallop located over the left ventricle in adults in the absence of mitral regurgitation. Additional evidence is an increase in radiologic heart size.

Right Ventricular Failure

ONE OF THE FOLLOWING CRITERIA IS REQUIRED FOR THE DIAGNOSIS OF RIGHT VENTRICULAR FAILURE.

1. A right ventricular ejection fraction two standard deviations below normal for that laboratory using contrast or radioisotope angiography.

2. In the absence of pulmonary or tricuspid valvular lesions or massive right ventricular hypertrophy:

    a. Elevation of right ventricular end-diastolic (or mean right atrial) pressure above 8 mm Hg with a cardiac output greater than 2.5 L/min/m$_2$. These criteria apply when the patient is supine, at rest in a basal state, and with the zero reference level for measurement of pressure 5 cm below the second costochondral junction; or

    b. Elevation of right ventricular end-diastolic (or mean right atrial) pressure above 8 mm Hg on moderate supine exercise and an inability either to increase cardiac output more than 800 ml for every 100-ml increase in oxygen consumption, to achieve a peak oxygen consumption of greater than 20 ml/kg/min, or to increase stroke volume; or

    c. Evidence of systemic circulatory congestion in the presence of a large right ventricle.

3. In the presence of tricuspid obstruction or regurgitation, demonstration of an elevated right ventricular end-diastolic pressure. This criterion reflects the fact that elevation of right atrial pressure and a reduced level of blood flow at rest or during exercise may result from the valvular disturbances themselves.

4. In the presence of pulmonary obstruction or regurgitation, evidence of an enlarged right ventricle or a sudden increase in right ventricular size. This criterion reflects the fact that elevation of right ventricular end-diastolic pressure and a reduced level of pulmonary blood flow, both at rest and during exercise, may result solely from the valvular lesion and the ensuing myocardial hypertrophy and not from ventricular failure alone.
5. A third heart sound, or a summation gallop located over the right ventricle in adults that increases in intensity with inspiration.
6. Pulsus alternans in the pulmonary artery or right ventricle.

DIASTOLIC DYSFUNCTION

Ventricular diastolic dysfunction causes the diastolic portion of the pressure-volume loop to shift upward, so that pressures are high in relation to volumes. This results in increased impedance to diastolic ventricular filling.

Diastolic dysfunction is usually associated with overt systolic dysfunction but can occur when systolic function is normal. The causes are dynamic changes in ventricular relaxation, intrinsic changes in myocardial stiffness, or both. Ventricular relaxation involves an energy-dependent transfer of calcium from actin-myosin cross-bridges to the sarcoplasmic reticulum and can be impaired by myocardial ischemia. Intrinsic myocardial stiffness can be increased by hypertrophy or by infiltration with collagen, amyloid, or inflammatory cells. Extrinsic impedance to filling can be imposed by pericardial thickening or tamponade.

Diastolic dysfunction is common in hypertensive heart disease, atherosclerotic heart disease, hypertrophic cardiomyopathy, diabetic cardiomyopathy, and aged hearts. It may signal rejection of allografts. It can be unmasked when tachycardias encroach on ventricular filling time. The consequences of ventricular diastolic dysfunction may appear abruptly, with acute pulmonary edema, or gradually with chronic congestive failure. The alteration in ventricular compliance is clinically defined by an increased ventricular end-diastolic pressure, particularly when ventricular diastolic volume is normal, and by characteristic changes in the ventricular pressure-volume curve determined by cardiac catheterization. Typical changes in peak transmitral flow velocity can often be demonstrated by Doppler echocardiography or radio-nuclide ventriculography.

THE FOLLOWING CRITERIA ARE REQUIRED FOR A DIAGNOSIS OF ISOLATED VENTRICULAR DIASTOLIC DYSFUNCTION.

Initial

Symptoms and physical signs of congestive heart failure.

Definitive

Demonstration of increased end-diastolic pressure and characteristic changes in diastolic filling pattern in the presence of normal ventricular systolic function and ventricular volume associated with a disease known to cause altered myocardial compliance, with or without pulmonary or systemic circulatory congestion.

THE FOLLOWING CRITERIA ARE REQUIRED FOR A DIAGNOSIS OF VENTRICULAR DIASTOLIC DYSFUNCTION ASSOCIATED WITH DECREASED VENTRICULAR SYSTOLIC FUNCTION.

Initial

Symptoms and physical signs of congestive heart failure.

Definitive

Demonstration of increased ventricular end-diastolic pressure and characteristic changes in diastolic filling pattern, and reduced systolic function in the presence of a disease known to cause altered myocardial compliance, with or without pulmonary or circulatory congestion.

VENTRICULAR ASYNERGY

Localized areas of the ventricular wall may deviate from the coordinated pattern of contraction of the myocardium during systole. Such asynergic regions may show dyskinesis, or paradoxical expansion during systole; akinesis, or absence of motion; hypokinesis, or decreased motion; and asynchrony, or altered sequence of contraction. The type of asynergy reflects the number and contractility of the surviving myocardial fibers in a damaged or ischemic area, the elastic characteristics of inert scar tissue, and alterations in excitation or excitation-contraction coupling. Several patterns of regional asynergy can be present in the same heart.

Asynergic areas can decrease cardiac performance by

several mechanisms. The contribution of the asynergic region to force development is lost or decreased, and the surviving muscle must perform more work; blood may be displaced into a large dyskinetic or aneurysmal area; and the performance of adjacent myocardium may be affected by a change in the series elastic component contributed by the asynergic area. Cardiac output and the rate of force development will decrease, especially if the asynergic areas occupy more than 20 percent of the ventricular surface.

Asynergy is usually a consequence of myocardial infarction but can occur in cardiomyopathy. It is usually permanent but can be transient, as during anginal syndrome or ectopic beats.

Clinical findings usually include evidence of ventricular failure, an enlarged heart, and a double apical impulse. Echocardiography or ventriculography is needed to demonstrate the presence, size, and motion of asynergic areas.

THE FOLLOWING CRITERION IS REQUIRED FOR THE DIAGNOSIS OF VENTRICULAR ASYNERGY.

Demonstration of asynergy by echocardiography or ventriculography or by direct observation at surgery.

PERICARDIAL CONSTRICTION

A decrease in the compliance of the pericardium as a consequence of widespread fibrosis, calcification, neoplasia, or the accumulation of fluid in the pericardial sac may restrict filling of the heart during diastole. In these circumstances, the dissimilar compliance characteristics of the two ventricles are replaced by those of the effusion or the thickened pericardium. The end-diastolic pressures in the ventricles no longer reflect their individual compliances but that of the limiting fluid or pericardium. Hence the diastolic pressure in the two ventricles, their atria, and venous beds becomes elevated and virtually the same. The pulmonary arterial and right ventricular systolic pressures are only modestly elevated. The atrial curves show an accentuation of the Y descent, the X descent, or both. The ventricular pressure contours show an early diastolic dip at the time of rapid ventricular filling that is more prominent in the presence of pericardial thickening than with fluid accumulation. Evidence of pulmonary and systemic congestion appears, although the manifestations of the latter are dominant. Low voltage of the QRS complexes is often seen.

When the accumulation of fluid is abrupt (pericardial tamponade), not only is there a rise in ventricular, atrial, and venous pressures, but also the stroke volume and cardiac output fall, and ultimately so does the systemic arterial pressure. Dyspnea, orthopnea, engorged neck veins, and a syndrome resembling cardiogenic shock may ensue.

When restriction is due to a more gradual accumulation of fluid or to pericardial thickening, cardiac output and systemic blood pressure can be well preserved, and manifestations of circulatory congestion predominate.

Both excessive pericardial fluid and scar tissue can cause accentuation of the normal inspiratory fall in systolic pressure in the systemic arteries (pulsus paradoxus). The magnitude of this fall may be 10 to 20 mm Hg. Abnormal filling of the neck veins during inspiration can also be observed. Pericardial restriction due to thickening is usually associated with a heart sound early in diastole (pericardial knock). Removal of fluid and fall to normal of pericardial pressure with persistent elevation of right atrial pressure indicate that pericardial thickening rather than effusion is the cause of the restrictive phenomenon. In the presence of cardiac tamponade, the ECG can show electrical alternans, which is a regular alternation in the amplitude of either the P wave, the QRS complex, or both during normal sinus rhythm. Calcification of the pericardium is often, but not always, associated with pericardial restriction.

Echocardiography is the method of choice for the recognition of pericardial effusion and tamponade (see page 121).

ONE OF THE FOLLOWING CRITERIA IS REQUIRED FOR THE DIAGNOSIS OF PERICARDIAL CONSTRICTION.

Initial

Evidence of systemic venous circulatory congestion in the absence of myocardial or other causes of congestion.

Definitive

The characteristic abnormalities of the atrial and ventricular pressures and pressure pulses associated with pericardial calcification, thickening, or effusion.

MYOCARDIAL RESTRICTION

Decreased compliance of the ventricles may produce disordered ventricular filling. The underlying abnormality may be diffuse, extensive fibrosis, endocardial fibroelastosis, or diffuse infiltrative processes such as amyloidosis, progressive systemic sclerosis, hemochromatosis, or sarcoidosis.

As a consequence of the reduced compliance of the ventricular chamber, its diastolic pressure rises. This is accompanied by elevation of pressure in the corresponding atrium and venous beds. The ventricular pressure curves show an early diastolic dip, while the atrial pressure curves show an accentuation of the Y descent and a large A wave. A fourth heart sound is usually heard. Manifestations of pulmonary and peripheral congestion result from the elevated ventricular diastolic pressure. The physiologic consequences of dynamic ventricular diastolic dysfunction (see page 236) resemble those of myocardial restriction.

THE FOLLOWING CRITERIA ARE REQUIRED FOR THE DIAGNOSIS OF MYOCARDIAL RESTRICTION.

The presence of some infiltrative disease known to be associated with myocardial restriction with echocardiographic evidence of diastolic dysfunction or elevated end-diastolic pressure and early ventricular diastolic dip in the affected ventricle. Pericardial and endocardial disease should be excluded.

CARDIOGENIC SHOCK

The syndrome of cardiogenic shock is characterized by apprehension, cold wet skin, sustained systemic arterial hypotension, tachycardia, and decreased urine flow, all occurring as a consequence of a marked decrease in effective peripheral blood flow secondary to heart disease.

Cardiogenic shock most often follows acute myocardial infarction but can also be produced by tachycardias with rapid ventricular rates or acute left ventricular failure; it sometimes follows cardiac surgery. The cardiac output is severely reduced, and the systolic blood pressure in the systemic arteries in previously normotensive individuals is below 80 mm Hg.

THE FOLLOWING CRITERIA ARE REQUIRED FOR THE DIAGNOSIS OF CARDIOGENIC SHOCK.

Evidence of the syndrome of shock with increased intracardiac filling pressures, low cardiac output, and hypotension.

Disorders of Intravascular Pressure

PULMONARY ARTERIAL HYPERTENSION

At the moment of birth, pulmonary arterial pressure is approximately the same as systemic arterial pressure. Soon thereafter, pulmonary arterial pressure falls and continues to do so until, after the first 2 weeks of life, it lies at levels encountered in the normal adult.

After 2 weeks of age, pulmonary arterial hypertension exists when the pulmonary arterial pressure exceeds 30 mm Hg systolic, 10 mm Hg diastolic, and 15 mm Hg mean (zero reference is 5 cm below the second costochondral junction) at rest. Under the stress of moderate leg exercise, pulmonary arterial pressures do not normally exceed 30 mm Hg systolic, 14 mm Hg diastolic, and 20 mm Hg mean. Levels of pressure in excess of these limits indicate the presence of pulmonary hypertension, although strenuous exercise may normally be accompanied by higher levels of pressure.

Pulmonary arterial hypertension may develop solely as a consequence of pulmonary venous hypertension. It may also stem from an abnormal resistance to blood flow in the pulmonary arterial tree due to a variety of causes. Disturbances in respiratory gas exchange that lead to hypoxia and acidosis may produce pulmonary arterial vasoconstriction and hypertension. An anatomic curtailment of the pulmonary vascular bed as a result of disease processes either intrinsic or extrinsic to the vessels may also cause pulmonary hypertension. In certain patients, the cause of pulmonary hypertension has not been identified but has been attributed to vasoconstriction. Although pulmonary vascular lesions are associated with this form of hypertension, it is not known whether these lesions result from or cause the elevation in blood pressure.

Right ventricular hypertrophy, dilatation, and failure may ultimately result from pulmonary arterial hypertension.

Echocardiography of the pulmonic valve in patients with pulmonary hypertension demonstrates absence of the normal "a" wave, a flattening of the diastolic E–F slope, prolongation of the preejection period, and midsystolic notching.

ONE OF THE FOLLOWING CRITERIA IS REQUIRED FOR THE DIAGNOSIS OF PULMONARY ARTERIAL HYPERTENSION.

Initial

1. Radiologic evidence of enlargement of the main pulmonary artery and its major branches, with narrowing of the more distal segmental and subsegmental branches.
2. Evidence of right ventricular enlargement in the absence of pulmonary stenosis or left-to-right shunt at the atrial level.

Definitive

Elevation of pulmonary arterial pressures above 30 mm Hg systolic, 10 mm diastolic, and 15 mm mean at rest and moderate exercise.

PULMONARY VENOUS HYPERTENSION

Pulmonary venous hypertension exists when the mean pressure in the left venoatrial system exceeds 12 mm Hg at rest (zero reference level is 5 cm below the second costochondral junction) or 14 mm Hg on moderate supine leg exercise.

Pulmonary venous hypertension results from any disease that causes elevation of the left ventricular end-diastolic or mean left atrial pressure: left ventricular failure, massive hypertrophy of the left ventricle, mitral obstruction or regurgitation, or tumors or thrombi that obstruct the flow of blood from either the pulmonary veins or left atrium. Pericardial or myocardial lesions that affect filling of the left ventricle may also cause pulmonary venous hypertension.

Pulmonary congestion and pulmonary arterial hypertension frequently result from pulmonary venous hypertension.

ONE OF THE FOLLOWING CRITERIA IS REQUIRED FOR THE DIAGNOSIS OF PULMONARY VENOUS HYPERTENSION.

Initial

Evidence of pulmonary congestion or pulmonary arterial hypertension in the presence of left ventricular failure, left ventricular enlargement, or mitral valvular or pericardial disease.

Definitive

Elevation of mean left atrial or pulmonary arterial wedge pressure above 12 mm Hg or of the left ventricular end-diastolic pressure above 12 mm Hg at rest or 14 mm Hg on moderate leg exercise.

SYSTEMIC ARTERIAL HYPERTENSION

There is a progressive increment in cardiovascular morbidity and mortality from stroke, ischemic heart disease, and renal failure as the systemic arterial pressure increases. At every level of diastolic pressure, risks are greater with higher levels of systolic pressure. Table 3-2 is a classification of blood pressure values for adults aged 18 years and older. When systolic blood pressure and diastolic blood pressure fall into different categories, the higher category should be selected to classify the blood pressure status. For example, 165/95 mm Hg is stage 2 (moderate) and 175/115 mm Hg is stage 3 (severe). Isolated systolic hypertension is defined as systolic pressure greater than 140 mm Hg with diastolic pressure less than 90 mm Hg. Thus, a blood pressure of 175/85 mm Hg is defined as stage 2 (moderate) isolated systolic hypertension. All blood pressures should be based on the mean of two or more readings at each of two or more visits following an initial screening.

Measurements should be taken with a mercury sphygmomanometer, a properly and regularly calibrated aneroid manometer, or a calibrated electronic device. Blood pressure should be recorded with the patient seated and standing, with the arm bared and at heart level. The subject should not have smoked, ingested caffeine, or indulged in strenuous exercise within 30 minutes prior to measurement, and the measurement should begin after 5 minutes of rest. The appropriate cuff size should be used, an outsize cuff for patients with obese arms. Systolic blood pressure is recorded as the first appearance of Korotkoff sounds on deflation of the cuff, and diastolic pressure as the disappearance of sound (Korotkoff phase V).

Noninvasive 24-hour ambulatory blood pressure monitoring provides information about blood pressure over

Table 3-2. Classification of blood pressure for adults aged 18 years and older

Category	Systolic (mm Hg)	Diastolic (mm Hg)
Normal	<140	<90
Hypertension		
Stage 1 (mild)	140–159	90–99
Stage 2 (moderate)	160–179	100–109
Stage 3 (severe)	180–199	110–119
Stage 4 (very severe)	≤200	≥120

time, away from the clinic, and during circumstances not otherwise measurable. It is an important research tool, particularly for the evaluation of the efficacy of anti-hypertensive drugs over the whole 24-hour period. It is also useful in the assessment of "white coat" hypertension (i.e., blood pressure repeatedly elevated in an office setting but repeatedly normal out of the office), in the evaluation of drug resistance, in episodic hypertension, in the evaluation of blood pressure changes in nocturnal angina, and if carotid sinus syncope or pacemaker syndromes are suspected.

The distinction between essential (idiopathic, primary) hypertension and secondary hypertension remains useful. Most patients have essential hypertension, largely a diagnosis based on the exclusion of the rare but clearly definable causes of secondary hypertension listed in Table 3-3. While there has been intensive investigation of the pathogenesis of the increased peripheral arterial resistance of essential hypertension, and a number of hemodynamic, electrolyte, genetic, endocrine (particularly the renin-angiotensin system), autonomic and other factors and abnormalities have been described, none has sufficient clinical utility to make screening them mandatory, and the etiology of essential hypertension remains unknown.

Table 3-3. Etiologic classification of hypertension

Secondary hypertension
  Intrinsic renal disease
    Acute glomerulonephritis
    Chronic glomerulonephritis
    Polycystic disease
    Amyloidosis
    Chronic pyelonephritis
  Renovascular
    Atherosclerotic renal artery stenosis
    Fibromuscular dysplasia
  Coarctation of the aorta
  Adrenal disorders
    Primary aldosteronism (Conn's syndrome)
    Pheochromocytoma
    Cushing's syndrome
  Agents with mineralocorticoid or vasoconstrictor activity
    Oral contraceptives
    Licorice
    Cocaine
    Cyclosporine
    Erythropoietin
Essential hypertension

Generally, there will be clinical clues to the presence of causes of secondary hypertension. These include abdominal or flank masses (polycystic kidneys), abdominal bruits (renovascular disease), lower blood pressure in legs compared to arms and delayed or absent femoral pulses (aortic coarctation), truncal obesity and purple striae (Cushing's syndrome), and tachycardia, tremor, sweating, and pallor (pheochromocytoma). Specialized diagnostic procedures (in addition to routine laboratory tests) to determine the etiology of hypertension are not necessary for all patients but are required when clinical data, severity of hypertension, or initial laboratory results suggest secondary hypertension. Sudden onset of hypertension, especially if accelerated or malignant, and recurrence of hypertension previously well controlled should also prompt more detailed investigation.

The organs whose structure and function may be impaired as a consequence of hypertension are the eyes, heart, brain, and kidneys. Ocular funduscopic abnormalities include sclerosis and narrowing of retinal arteries with a decrease of the ratio of arterial to venous diameters, arteriovenous compression, flame-shaped hemorrhages and exudates, and papilledema. The coexistence of severe hypertension and papilledema is referred to as malignant or accelerated hypertension. It is often sudden in onset and accompanied by renal and cardiac dysfunction. Pathologically, necrotizing or fibrinoid arteriolitis is present, especially in the kidneys. The plasma renin concentration is usually elevated. Left ventricular hypertrophy and patchy myocardial fibrosis are the principal cardiac structural sequelae of hypertension.

Functional impairment of the left ventricle is manifested by prolonged diastolic relaxation and filling rate, reduced diastolic compliance, abnormal systolic ejection phase indices, and ultimately frank ventricular and congestive heart failure. Myocardial ischemia may also occur, secondary to the limitation in coronary reserve from myocardial hypertrophy as well as obstructive atherosclerotic coronary artery disease, which commonly complicates hypertensive disease. Hypertension is a major risk factor for stroke due to intracerebral hemorrhage or thrombosis and encephalopathy characterized by headache, confusion, somnolence, stupor, focal neurologic deficits, seizure, and coma. Renal disease may be a consequence as well as a cause of hypertension. In early hypertension, there may be an increase in glomerular filtration with microalbuminuria due to an increased efferent arteriolar resistance and rise in filtration pressure. This hyperfiltration may be the cause of the progressive glomerular sclerosis and nephron loss of hypertension. Later, there may be heavy proteinuria, a fall in glomerular filtration rate, and ultimately uremia.

Hypertension in children and adolescents is defined as average systolic or diastolic blood pressure, measured on at least three occasions, equal to or greater than the ninety-fifth percentile for age (Table 3-4).

In children, significant and severe hypertension may have an identifiable underlying cause. Children who have slight or periodic blood pressure elevation are at higher risk for future cardiovascular disease than normotensive children, often have a hypertensive parent, and often have other cardiovascular risk factors in early life, particularly obesity.

THE FOLLOWING CRITERIA ARE REQUIRED FOR THE DIAGNOSIS OF SYSTEMIC ARTERIAL HYPERTENSION.

Systolic and diastolic blood pressure in excess of 140/90 mm Hg staged according to values listed in Table 3-2.

PULMONARY OR SYSTEMIC CIRCULATORY CONGESTION

Circulatory congestion is defined as distention of systemic or pulmonary veins or capillaries by an abnormally large volume of blood. Pressures in these vessels may

Table 3-4. Classification of hypertension in children and adolescents

	Hypertension: 95–99th Percentile (mm Hg)		Severe Hypertension: >99th Percentile (mm Hg)	
Age	SBP	DBP	SBP	DBP
7 days	96–105		≥106	
8–30 days	104–109		≥110	
1 month–2 years	112–117	74–81	≥118	≥82
3–5 years	116–123	76–83	≥124	≥84
6–9 years	112–129	78–85	≥130	≥86
10–12 years	126–133	82–89	≥134	≥90
13–15 years	136–143	86–89	≥144	≥92
Adolescents	142–149	92–97	≥150	≥98

SBP = systolic blood pressure; DBP = diastolic blood pressure.

become elevated, and fluid can then shift from the vascular compartment to the adjacent interstitial spaces. The magnitude of such fluid shifts depends on the interplay of such factors as the level of intravascular pressures, tissue pressure, the vascularity of the organ or tissue involved, the presence and competence of venous valves, gravitational forces, oncotic pressures, and lymphatic drainage.

Congestion can result from ventricular failure, pericardial or myocardial restriction, lesions of the mitral or tricuspid valves, and venous or lymphatic occlusive disease. When hypervolemia develops in such conditions as cirrhosis of the liver and acute glomerulonephritis, congestion can arise. Furthermore, redistribution of the circulating blood volume, as in severe anemia, can cause regional congestion. It follows that congestion can involve single organs, regional circulations, or the greater part of the circulation.

ONE OF THE FOLLOWING CRITERIA IS REQUIRED FOR THE DIAGNOSIS OF PULMONARY CIRCULATORY CONGESTION.

Initial

Dyspnea, orthopnea, frothy pink sputum, or rales over the more dependent regions of the lungs in the presence of lesions that result in pulmonary venous hypertension.

Definitive

Radiologic evidence of enlargement of the hilar shadows (particularly in their upper portions), with dilatation of upper lung vessels and the occurrence of interstitial edema in the lower lung fields, particularly as manifested by horizontal, parallel septal lines (Kerley B lines), best seen in the costophrenic sinuses.

THE FOLLOWING CRITERION IS REQUIRED FOR THE DIAGNOSIS OF SYSTEMIC CIRCULATORY CONGESTION.

Edema, pleural effusion, ascites, or hepatomegaly constitutes acceptable evidence of congestion in the presence of either hypervolemia or elevation of right atrial or vena caval pressures (central venous pressure) above 5 mm Hg or 70 mm H_2O with the subject at rest (zero reference level is 5 cm below the second costochondral junction).

Abnormal Communications in the Heart or Great Vessels

Abnormal connections between the heart chambers, between the great vessels and the heart, or between the large arteries and veins permit direct transfer of blood from one vascular system to another without traversing capillaries. Such lesions are most often congenital in origin; rarely, they may be acquired.

Pressures in the left heart chambers and systemic arteries are normally greater than the pressures in the corresponding chambers or vessels of the right side of the circulation. Hence the flow of blood through such abnormal communications usually is from left to right. Only in the instance of abnormal connections between pulmonary arteries and veins is flow from right to left. The magnitude of blood flow depends both on the size of the defect and on the difference in pressures between the chambers or vessels it connects.

INTRACARDIAC SHUNTS

Left-to-Right Shunts

Left-to-right intracardiac flow of blood occurs in atrial septal defect, ventricular septal defects, and left ventricular–right atrial communications.

The physiologic consequences of a left-to-right intracardiac shunt are enlargement of the cardiac chambers traversed by the augmented blood flow and engorgement of the pulmonary circulation. With prolonged pulmonary overperfusion, secondary changes in the media and intima of the small pulmonary arteries may occur, resulting in the development of increased resistance to pulmonary blood flow and in pulmonary hypertension. As the pressures in the right ventricle, atrium, or both approach or exceed pressures in the corresponding left heart chamber, the magnitude of left-to-right shunt flow is reduced, and blood flow across the shunt may be reversed.

Right-to-Left Shunts

In the presence of pulmonary hypertension and the consequent rise in right ventricular and atrial pressures secondary to hypertrophy or ventricular failure, there may be right-to-left shunting of blood through an atrial defect, a foramen ovale, or ventricular septal defect (Eisenmenger's syndrome).

Right-to-left shunting may also occur in the absence of pulmonary hypertension if anatomic obstruction to blood flow through the right heart or lungs accompanies defects in the partitions between the right and left hearts.

Valvular or infundibular pulmonary stenosis or atresia, downward displacement of the tricuspid valve (Ebstein's malformation), and tricuspid stenosis or atresia may accompany a ventricular septal defect, an atrial septal defect, or a patent foramen ovale. In such instances, shunt flow may be from right to left.

The physiologic consequences of such a shunt are a reduction in pulmonary blood flow and in systemic arterial oxyhemoglobin saturation, at rest or at varying levels of exercise. Cyanosis, polycythemia, digital clubbing, exertional dyspnea, and fatigue may ensue.

EXTRACARDIAC SHUNTS

Left-to-Right Shunts

Abnormal communications may exist between the great vessels themselves or between the right heart and great vessels. Because of the usual differences between systemic and pulmonary (or right heart) pressures, the flow of blood is from left to right. Examples of such lesions are a congenital or acquired fistula between the aorta and right heart chambers, a fistula between a coronary artery and a right heart chamber, direct communication of one or more pulmonary veins to the right atrium, patent ductus arteriosus, aortopulmonary window, truncus arteriosus, and systemic arteriovenous fistula.

The physiologic consequences of these lesions are increased pulmonary blood flow and possible enlargement of the involved right-sided chambers or vessels. The various arteriovenous communications may produce enlargement of the left ventricle as well.

Right-to-Left Shunts

Venous blood may flow directly into the systemic circulation in the presence of complete or incomplete transposition of the great arteries. In the presence of total anomalous pulmonary venous drainage, the systemic circulation is perfused through a patent foramen ovale or atrial septal defect. With development of sufficiently severe pulmonary hypertension, the direction of flow through a patent ductus arteriosus or an aortopulmonary window may reverse. The physiologic consequences of such right-to-left shunts are the same as are encountered in intracardiac right-to-left shunts.

The diagnosis of shunts involving the heart and great vessels may be entertained on clinical grounds. The locations of such abnormal communications may be demonstrated by Doppler echocardiography or by a number of indicator dilution techniques that utilize oxygen, optically active or radiopaque dyes, and inert gases in conjunction with a wide variety of sensing devices.

ONE OF THE FOLLOWING CRITERIA IS REQUIRED FOR THE DIAGNOSIS OF A LEFT-TO-RIGHT SHUNT.

1. **Demonstration of an increase in blood oxygen content at the point of entry of the shunt and distal to it.**
2. **The early arrival of hydrogen or other indicator at the point of entry of the shunt.**
3. **Demonstration of a left-to-right shunt by Doppler echocardiography or angiocardiography.**

ONE OF THE FOLLOWING CRITERIA IS REQUIRED FOR THE DIAGNOSIS OF A RIGHT-TO-LEFT SHUNT.

1. **Demonstration of a right-to-left shunt by Doppler echocardiography or angiocardiography.**
2. **Demonstration of a right-to-left shunt by hydrogen or other indicator.**

Anginal Syndrome

The anginal syndrome consists of chest pain that is precipitated by effort, excitement, ingestion of a heavy meal, or exposure to cold and is relieved by rest. The pain is typically in the upper retrosternal area and most often radiates down the medial aspect of the left arm, but it may occur in other areas such as the anterior neck, the jaw, both shoulders, or the interscapular region. The quality of the pain is typically squeezing, but it may be pressing, burning, or choking and may vary in intensity from mild to severe. The pain is usually relieved by rest or use of nitrates. The duration of the sensation rarely exceeds 15 minutes. In some patients, pain may begin at rest or during sleep.

Although the actual mechanism that produces anginal pain is unknown, the discomfort is characteristically associated with episodic disproportion between the need of the myocardium for oxygen and the delivery of oxygen by the coronary arterial blood. The syndrome is most often caused by coronary atherosclerosis, and severe narrowing or occlusion of the coronary arteries can usually be demonstrated by arteriography. During episodes of anginal pain, there may be evidence of transient abnormalities in left ventricular function. Coronary venous blood obtained during an anginal attack often shows biochemical evidence of anaerobic metabolism in the involved segments of myocardium. ECGs obtained during anginal pain usually show S–T segment depression and T-wave inversion, which revert to normal when pain subsides. Transient ECG abnormalities indicative of myocardial ischemia may occur in the absence of chest pain ("silent ischemia"). Formal physiologic stress tests using ECG, radionuclide, pharmacologic, and echocardiographic methods are of value in establishing and refining the diagnosis of transient myocardial ischemia (see Section 6).

Anginal syndrome can appear abruptly or slowly, can precede or follow acute myocardial infarction, and can disappear following infarction. The pain of acute myocardial infarction may be qualitatively identical with the pain of the anginal syndrome but is usually of greater intensity and duration.

Unstable angina defines a subset of patients with ischemic heart disease who experience new-onset angina or angina at rest or an abrupt increase in frequency, intensity, and duration of chest pain, often with a sharp reduction in effort threshold for pain. Transient ventricular repolarization abnormalities are usually present. Atherosclerotic plaque disruption and fissuring, platelet aggregation, and coronary artery spasm are associated with this syndrome, and a distinctive, eccentric, scalloped appearance of the atherosclerotic lesions can be demonstrated angiographically. The clinical syndrome of unstable angina may closely resemble acute myocardial infarction, but enzymatic evidence of myocardial necrosis and the typical ECG evolution of myocardial infarction are not present. However, in a small minority of patients, unstable angina may progress to true myocardial infarction.

Anginal syndrome is not limited to patients with coronary atherosclerosis but may also be present with coronary arteritis, coronary ostial stenosis, or severe ventricular hypertrophy due to aortic stenosis or regurgitation. It can also be precipitated or aggravated by anemia in patients with those diseases.

Variant angina (Prinzmetal's angina) is a distinctive

form of transient myocardial ischemia caused by severe coronary artery spasm. The chest pain occurs at rest, usually during the early morning hours, and is associated with marked S–T segment elevation. Atherosclerotic lesions are often present at or near the site of spasm, and myocardial infarction, major ventricular arrhythmias, and sudden death may occur.

THE FOLLOWING CRITERIA ARE REQUIRED FOR THE DIAGNOSIS OF ANGINAL SYNDROME.

Pain in the chest (usually localized to the retrosternal area), neck, shoulder, or left arm that is usually caused by physical effort and relieved by rest or nitrates.

4

Functional Capacity and Objective Assessment

The need for some form of summary statement to describe the overall evaluation of a patient's cardiovascular status was recognized in previous editions of this publication as an important element of the complete cardiac diagnosis. The earliest editions used a two-component grading system labeled *Functional Capacity* and *Therapeutic Classification*. Functional Capacity was based entirely on the patient's subjective responses (dyspnea, anginal pain, fatigue, palpitation) to varying, loosely defined degrees of physical effort. Therapeutic Classification graded the expected results of treatment.

In the Seventh (1973) and Eighth (1979) Editions, *Functional Capacity* and *Therapeutic Classification* were replaced by the terms *Cardiac Status* and *Prognosis*. It was felt that an appraisal based on symptoms alone was clearly an incomplete and sometimes inaccurate representation of the severity of cardiovascular disease. Determination of Cardiac Status required evaluation of the composite etiologic, anatomic, and physiologic diagnoses including results of specific tests of cardiac structure and function as well as magnitude of symptoms. *Prognosis* was a paraphrase of the earlier *Therapeutic Classification*.

It is of interest, historically, that of the four proposed grading systems (Functional Capacity, Therapeutic Classification, Status, and Prognosis) only Functional Capacity has been regularly and continuously used by the medical profession. Despite the fact that this classification is based entirely on subjective symptoms, and despite the fact that it is often erroneously used as a classification of the degree of ventricular dysfunction or congestive heart failure, it remains the most widely used grading system of the group of common symptoms of cardiovascular disease. The Canadian Cardiovascular Society Grading Scale, another commonly used system, resembles and refines the original four-class New York Heart Association Classification of Functional Capacity but applies only to effort-induced angina pectoris.

The present Criteria Committee proposes modification of the previous classifications. The category Prognosis has been discontinued, since it is rarely used and like its predecessor, Therapeutic Classification, is an oversimplified expression of a complex interplay of multiple clinical and laboratory variables that cannot be summarized adequately as a brief generalization. Moreover, prognosis is not ordinarily part of a diagnostic formulation. Functional Capacity is retained as originally defined, since it is commonly used, and grading of symptoms is of some value as a component of the cardiac diagnosis.

The category Cardiac Status is replaced by Objective Assessment, which is based on and emphasizes the special importance of objective measures of cardiac structure and function (e.g., data obtained by physical examination, ECG, chest x-ray, cardiac catheterization, echocardiography, radiologic imaging, stress testing) to evaluate overall cardiac status. It is well-known that the severity of symptoms of cardiovascular disease is not necessarily matched by equivalent degrees of impaired structure and function. It is felt that Functional Capacity and Objective Assessment complement each other and provide a more complete and more realistic appraisal of overall cardiac status.

The following grading systems are recommended.

Functional Capacity

Class I. Patients with cardiac disease, but without resulting limitation of physical activity. Ordinary physical activity does not cause undue fatigue, palpitation, dyspnea, or anginal pain.

Class II. Patients with cardiac disease resulting in slight limitation of physical activity. They are comfortable at rest. Ordinary physical activity results in fatigue, palpitation, dyspnea, or anginal pain.

Class III. Patients with marked limitation of physical activity. They are comfortable at rest. Less than ordinary activity causes fatigue, palpitation, dyspnea, or anginal pain.

Class IV. Patients with cardiac disease resulting in inability to carry on any physical activity without discomfort. Symptoms of heart failure or of the anginal syndrome may be present even at rest. If any physical activity is undertaken, discomfort is increased.

Objective Assessment

  A. No objective evidence of cardiovascular disease.

  B. Objective evidence of minimal cardiovascular disease.

C. Objective evidence of moderately severe cardiovascular disease.
D. Objective evidence of severe cardiovascular disease.

Criteria for use of the terms *minimal, moderately severe,*
and *severe disease* cannot be precisely defined. Grading is
a judgmental process based on individual physicians'
estimates.

The following are examples of the use of Functional
Capacity and Objective Assessment.

A patient with no or minimal symptoms but a large
pressure gradient across the aortic valve or severe obstruction of the left main coronary artery would be classified:

Functional Capacity   I
Objective Assessment   D

A patient with a severe anginal syndrome but angiographically normal coronary arteries would be classified:

Functional Capacity   IV
Objective Assessment   A

A patient with acute myocardial infarction, shock, reduced cardiac output, and elevated pulmonary artery
wedge pressure would be classified:

Functional Capacity   IV
Objective Assessment   D

A patient with mitral stenosis, moderate exertional dyspnea, and moderate reduction in mitral valve area would
be classified:

Functional Capacity   II or III
Objective Assessment   C

A patient with cardiac disease who has not had specific
tests of cardiac structure or function would be classified:

Objective Assessment   Undetermined

5

Uncertain Diagnosis

NO HEART DISEASE: PREDISPOSING ETIOLOGIC FACTOR

The diagnostic category No Heart Disease: Predisposing Etiologic Factor includes patients in whom no cardiac disease is discovered, but whose course should be followed by periodic examinations because of the presence of a history of an etiologic factor that might cause heart disease. These should be recorded as No Heart Disease: History of (stating the etiologic factor).

NO HEART DISEASE: UNEXPLAINED MANIFESTATION

The diagnostic category No Heart Disease: Unexplained Manifestation includes patients with symptoms or signs referable to the heart, but in whom a diagnosis of cardiac disease is uncertain at the time of examination. These cases should be recorded as No Heart Disease: Unexplained Manifestation, with a further recommendation that reexamination be performed after a stated interval.

When there is a reasonable certainty that the symptoms or signs are not of cardiac origin, the diagnosis should be No Heart Disease.

6

Special Methods for Cardiovascular Diagnosis

Radiologic Imaging in Cardiovascular Diagnosis

THE PLAIN CHEST X-RAY

The heart configuration and size, the contours of the great vessels in the mediastinum, and the state of the lungs and pleural spaces are to be considered when examining the chest x-ray of patients with cardiovascular disease. While few radiologic features are pathognomonic, and specific details concerning chamber size, volume, contour, and spatial relationships are more accurately displayed by newer imaging techniques such as echocardiography, computed tomography and magnetic resonance imaging, the chest x-ray remains a useful initial diagnostic guide.

Heart Size

The overall heart size can be determined by plain film examination. However, the range of normal is wide and affected by a variety of extracardiac as well as cardiac factors including x-ray geometry of the image; body size, build, and weight; variations in the bony thorax (e.g., scoliosis, pectus excavatum, "straight spine"); size of lungs; abdominal organs; physiologic state (e.g., age, training, pregnancy, nutrition, metabolic rate); the phase of the heart cycle; heart rate; and phase of respiration. For these and other reasons, only approximate estimates of heart size are justified from the plain chest x-ray, and only qualitative expressions of normality are used (e.g., normal, significantly enlarged, borderline enlarged). Numerical parameters of increased heart size determined from the chest x-ray (e.g., cardiothoracic ratio greater than 0.5 and total cardiac volume greater than 500 to 550 ml/m^2 body surface area) have, for the most part, been replaced by the more accurate imaging technique mentioned above.

Heart Shape

The cardiomediastinal silhouette is conveniently analyzed in the frontal projection by considering the four segments of the left heart border: (1) The distal aortic arch, or aortic knob, which continues caudally as the descending aorta; (2) the main pulmonary arterial segment; (3) the left atrial appendage segment; and (4) the ventricular segment (usually the left ventricle). On the right side, two segments are considered: the upper one, in which the superior vena cava (or in older persons, the ascending aorta) forms the border, and the lower segment, in which the right atrium normally forms the border.

In the left lateral view, the posterior wall of the left ventricle is often seen contrasted against the lung. Opacification of the esophagus with barium can improve the outline of the dorsal margin of the left atrium. Commonly, a curved margin (concave dorsally), representing the back wall of the inferior vena cava, is seen intersecting the right dome of the diaphragm. The ventral and cephalad aspect of the heart is the usually indistinct margin of the right ventricular outflow tract, often obscured in older persons because of a prominent elongated ascending aorta. The left pulmonary artery can sometimes be recognized as it crosses over the left upper lobe bronchus.

Left Atrium

The outline of the left atrium can be quite accurately estimated on the frontal chest film using the medial margins of the right main and right intermediate bronchi and of the left main and left lower lobe bronchi; the second contour due to left atrium often seen close to the right heart border; and the region of the left atrial appendage on the left. There may be a general increase in heart density caused by the dorsal prominence of the left atrium. Mitral and aortic valve calcifications, when present, are also useful markers of the left atrial margins. The lateral view, especially with barium in the esophagus, is helpful in locating the posterior margins of the left atrium, particularly since slight left atrial enlargement is most impressive along its dorsal margin.

When left atrial contours deform the cardiac silhouette (by producing unusual bronchial displacement, straightening, or convexity of the left heart border or a prominent double contour on the right), disproportionate left atrial enlargement is present. In most patients with chronic left ventricular disease, the left atrial size parallels and is not disproportionate to that of the left ventricle. Occasionally, as is typical of atrial septal defect, the left atrium is exceptionally small.

Left Ventricle

In the frontal view, the ventricular region of the cardiac shadow can be considered to be that part inferior and to the left of a line connecting the right cardiophrenic angle with the pulmonary artery segment, or, more simply, that part to the left of the midline not accounted for by the left atrium. Enlargement of this region in adults is due to left ventricular enlargement in more than 90 percent of patients, but precisely the same appearance can be caused by right ventricular dilatation or pericardial effusion. Lengthening of the axis of the ventricular region toward the left costophrenic angle and increased prominence of the lower lateral ventricular border suggest left ventricular enlargement. Increased thickness of the heart on the lateral view at the level of the diaphragm, especially when the posterior left ventricular border overlaps the inferior vena caval margin, also suggests left ventricular enlargement. Again, calcifications in both aortic and mitral valves may help identify the margins of the left ventricle.

Right Ventricle

Since the right ventricle seldom contributes to the cardiac border in the frontal projection, its dilatation per se produces mainly nonspecific enlargement of the ventricular region. Enlargement of the right ventricle does, however, tend to displace the outflow tract and main pulmonary artery upward and to the left. The pulmonary artery segment becomes more prominent in the frontal projection, and in the lateral view, encroachment from below on the retrosternal clear space may be seen. This latter feature has limited value because of frequent obscuration by a large ascending aorta, thymus, or a narrow anteroposterior mediastinal dimension. With extreme dilatation of the right ventricle, this chamber often forms the left border of the cardiac silhouette and may produce a long convexity on the left heart border, which can be confused with prominence of the left atrial appendage.

Right Atrium

The length and prominence of the right heart border (lower segment) in the frontal projection is a rough indicator of right atrial size. The right atrium is most likely to be large when the right ventricle is large. Persistent prominence of the caval margins or of the azygos veins suggests elevation of right atrial pressure.

Great Vessels and the Lungs

Prominence of the right ventricular outflow tract and dilatation of the central pulmonary arteries are the most important, though indirect, indicators of right ventricular enlargement. Dilatation of the main pulmonary arteries indicates pulmonary hypertension (or post-stenotic dilatation) and therefore right ventricular hypertension, suggesting that right ventricular hypertrophy is likely to be present. The central pulmonary vessels (after discounting the effects of aging and normal variations) provide an extremely valuable index of pulmonary arterial pressure, or of turbulence, in the case of post-stenotic dilatation.

The appearance of the peripheral lung vessels also has great importance in diagnosis. *The lungs are the only organs in which the macroscopic vasculature is seen on plain x-rays*. The sizes of the more peripheral pulmonary vessels reflect pulmonary blood volume and flow (as well as acute pressure changes). Pulmonary edema (interstitial or alveolar) in heart disease usually implies pulmonary capillary and venous hypertension.

Characteristic patterns in the appearance of the pulmonary vasculature reflect different hemodynamic states. In normal subjects, the pulmonary vessels are more distended at the bases, sharply contrasted against the surrounding aerated lung. Increased pulmonary blood volume and flow at modestly increased pressures produces generally distended pulmonary vasculature (e.g., left-to-right shunts, severe anemia, pregnancy). Pulmonary artery hypertension due to pulmonary capillary and venous hypertension (e.g., left ventricular failure, mitral obstruction) causes relatively small-caliber arteries and veins in the lower lung fields, often with interstitial and pulmonary edema. Pulmonary hypertension induced by high peripheral pulmonary resistance causes tortuous central pulmonary arteries abruptly tapering toward the periphery.

MAGNETIC RESONANCE IMAGING AND COMPUTED TOMOGRAPHY OF THE HEART AND GREAT VESSELS

Noninvasive techniques have become increasingly important for the diagnosis, assessment, and follow-up of cardiovascular disease. In recent years, two different computer-based tomographic techniques have emerged that are applicable to cardiac and great vessel imaging: magnetic resonance imaging (MRI) and computed tomography (CT). They can both provide information about cardiac and great-vessel anatomy, regional myocardial perfusion, blood flow, regional and global myocardial function, and status of the coronary arteries. Although the information they can provide is in some cases similar, MRI and CT themselves have little in common.

Basic Principles of MRI

MRI does not use ionizing radiation. Rather, it employs a powerful magnetic field and radiofrequency pulses to create tomographic images of the body's hydrogen nuclei (protons) in any desired plane. Because it is completely noninvasive and because there is natural contrast between flowing blood and surrounding soft tissues, its role in cardiovascular diagnosis was recognized from the beginning. Perhaps no other single technique can provide as much information about the heart and vessels. For example, MRI makes it possible to image the coronary arteries, determine coronary artery blood flow, and show areas of hypoperfused myocardium with one quick, noninvasive examination.

Several features of MRI make it advantageous for the evaluation of the heart and great vessels.

First, there is natural contrast between the blood pool and the cardiovascular structures. Thus, internal structure of the heart and vessels can be visualized and an intravenous contrast agent is not needed for discrimination of the blood pool or assessment of cardiac or vascular morphology or function.

Second, MRI provides high spatial resolution in three dimensions, and tomographic imaging can be easily accomplished in any arbitrary plane, including those familiar to echocardiographers. As a result, an MRI data set, such as biventricular volumes, can be used to directly, accurately, and reproducibly measure cardiac mass and volumes without the use of assumed formulas or geometric models required by some other imaging methods. When compared with both contrast and radionuclide ventriculography, MRI has several advantages. MRI provides direct, dynamic visualization of the myocardium in tomographic planes. With other ventriculographic techniques, the myocardium is merely inferred from the motion of the chamber blood. Also, other techniques are planar rather than tomographic, and overlapping structures may conceal or diminish the appreciation of regional wall abnormalities. This is not a problem with MRI.

Third, using a variety of cine techniques, MRI has dynamic capabilities that can be used to assess global and regional ventricular contractile function.

Fourth, velocity-encoding techniques permit noninvasive measurement of blood velocity and flow.

Fifth, unlike echocardiography, MRI is not body habitus dependent. As long as the patient can fit in the magnet, obese or barrel-chested patients do not pose a problem.

Finally, MRI is noninvasive, and it can therefore be repeated safely and reproducibly.

MRI is a complex diagnostic tool. Although most clinical MRI systems are capable of very basic anatomic cardiac and vascular studies, more advanced equipment and a high level of expertise are required to implement more sophisticated studies successfully. With state-of-the-art techniques, MRI is versatile, relatively comprehensive, and time-effective, and it could provide all of the standard quantitative functional indices along with excellent anatomic discrimination. Nevertheless, it is important to realize that the techniques and tools for cardiovascular MRI are undergoing rapid advancement and that the applications will likely expand.

MRI Techniques

There are numerous techniques available for MRI of the cardiovascular system. Some require either prospective or retrospective cardiac gating (the synchronization of image acquisition to a consistent point in the cardiac cycle using the electrocardiogram [ECG] as a monitor) to minimize the effects of cardiac motion. Others, such as fast gradient echo techniques (e.g., turboFLASH) or echo planar imaging (EPI), have made it possible to acquire images so quickly (1 second or less) that gating is not needed. The appropriate techniques are determined by the clinical application and the equipment available.

Spin echo techniques represent flowing blood as a signal void, and flow abnormalities (or slow flow) may cause increased signal intensity. With gradient echo techniques, the continual entry of unsaturated spins into the imaging planes results in a very high signal, and flow abnormalities or absent flow is depicted as areas of flow void within the high signal intensity blood pool.

Multislice ECG Gated Spin Echo

Multiple static anatomic slices are acquired during a sequence. Typically, 6 to 12 slices are acquired in 8 to 12 minutes. The data for each slice are acquired at a different phase of the cardiac cycle. Thus, this sequence is most useful for anatomic assessment of the heart and great vessels, but it is generally not used for measuring cardiac dimensions and function.

Multiphasic Multislice ECG Gated Spin Echo

Each anatomic section is imaged at multiple equally spaced phases of the cardiac cycle. This technique is time-consuming and requires up to 30 minutes to acquire approximately five slices, each in five to eight different phases. From end-diastolic and end-systolic images of each anatomic level, diastolic and systolic volumes can be measured and can be used to compute stroke volume, ejection fraction, myocardial mass, and the extent of ventricular regional wall contractility.

Biphasic Multislice ECG Gated Spin Echo

Images are acquired at multiple anatomic locations in only two phases, end systole and end diastole. The entire ventricle can be imaged in about 10 minutes, and the data can be used to evaluate cardiac dimensions and function.

Cine Gradient Echo

The ECG is used to reference repetitive gradient echo sequences. This approach can produce approximately 16 to 30 images (sections, phases, or both) during the cardiac cycle. The images can be placed in a loop for dynamic cine display so that wall motion, valve motion, and blood flow pattern can be observed.

Magnetization Prepared Gradient Echo (TurboFLASH)

This method utilizes a preparation radiofrequency pulse prior to gradient echo data acquisition. Each image is acquired in 1 to 2 seconds. Although this technique has lower signal-to-noise and spatial resolution than spin echo and standard cine gradient echo techniques, the improved temporal resolution and contrast can be used to evaluate myocardial perfusion by monitoring the first-pass distribution of MR contrast media.

Echo Planar Imaging

In EPI, all of the image data are acquired during a single excitation. This is the fastest MRI technique and can acquire real-time images in as little as 40 msec. It is used to evaluate cardiac function. Specialized hardware and data acquisition capabilities are generally required to perform EPI optimally.

Magnetic Resonance Angiography

Magnetic resonance angiography (MRA) provides a local or global image of blood vessels in a two-dimensional or three-dimensional angiographic format. Two techniques are employed: time-of-flight (TOF) and phase contrast. Both may be implemented using two- or three-dimensional acquisition with maximum intensity projection (MIP) reconstruction algorithms. Arterial and venous structures may be delineated, and rotating displays of three-dimensional data sets allow separation of vessels that are superimposed.

Flow-Sensitive Imaging Techniques

These methods permit the measurement of blood flow expressed either as velocity or volume flow per unit time. The time-of-flight technique is based on tracking a volume of blood in which the signal is nulled by the application of a saturation pulse. The phase contrast technique is based on the principle that when protons in flowing blood move along a magnetic gradient, the phase of the signal changes in relation to stationary spins in direct proportion to the velocity. Flow-encoding gradient pulses are used to impart phase shifts to moving spins that are proportional to velocity. Instantaneous and integrated blood velocity measurements within vessels can be obtained over the cardiac cycle and permit determination of stroke volume, which can be used to calculate flow and cardiac output.

Magnetic Resonance Spectroscopy

Magnetic resonance spectroscopy (MRS) makes it possible to evaluate myocardial metabolism. MRS operates on the same principle as MRI in that after the radiofrequency energy is applied, certain nuclei resonate at a characteristic frequency, so that the presence of a particular atom within a chemical species (e.g., lactic acid or phosphocreatine) or living tissue can be identified. A map in the form of a magnetic resonance spectrum is created of the various sites where an atom exists. From this spectrum, the relative concentrations and properties of these nuclei can be determined. In general, MRS techniques are only applicable on higher magnetic field strength ($\geq$1.5 Tesla) MR systems.

Intravenous Contrast Agents

There are a number of intravenous MR contrast agents that may enhance the information available from cardiac MRI. These agents are not radioactive and are particularly valuable for evaluation of myocardial perfusion.

Tissue Tagging

MRI can document changes within specific locations in the heart wall either by the direct noninvasive placement of magnetic "tags" or using phase-contrast techniques for velocity wall mapping. These techniques permit noninvasive evaluations of left ventricular torsion, regional wall stress, and strain.

Indications for MRI

Thoracic Aorta

1. MRI can be used to establish the diagnosis and assess the extent and severity of nearly all diseases of the thoracic aorta, including dissections, aneurysms, occlusions, penetrating ulcers or pseudoaneurysm, and developmental anomalies, including coarctation. Compared with contrast angiography, MR is safer, since it does not involve the introduction of a catheter or potentially nephrotoxic contrast media. MR provides more information about the aortic wall and periaortic tissues than conventional angiography, facilitating the diagnosis of intramural hemorrhage ("dissection without intimal tear") and alternative diagnoses.
2. To monitor the course of thoracic aortic disease.
3. To define response to therapy and to monitor postoperative patients for symptomatic or asymptomatic complications.
4. Since MRI is noninvasive, it is especially useful in (a) patients with compromised renal or cardiovascular function who may not be candidates to receive intravenous iodinated contrast and (b) patients with Marfan's syndrome and family members of patients with Marfan's syndrome, who are at risk for thoracic aortic disease.
5. To differentiate between mediastinal mass and vascular abnormality in patients with abnormal chest x-rays.

Pulmonary Artery

1. MRI and CT can be used to evaluate intrinsic abnormalities of the pulmonary arteries, including central thrombi or tumors, aneurysms, stenoses, occlusions, and developmental anomalies.
2. Impingement on the pulmonary arteries by mediastinal tumors and bronchogenic carcinomas.
3. MRI techniques may be useful to evaluate patients for pulmonary emboli and other diseases involving the pulmonary arteries.

4. MR-determined flow measurements in the pulmonary arteries may be useful in patients with pulmonary hypertension.

Large Veins

1. Evaluation of congenital abnormalities of the superior and inferior vena cava and the pulmonary veins.
2. Diagnosis of vena cava thrombus, assessment of superior vena cava syndrome, and identification of superior vena cava invasion or encasement.

Acquired Heart Disease

1. Ischemic heart disease. MRI can be used to determine the presence, size, and location of previous myocardial infarction. It can also be used to demonstrate the complications of infarction, such as ventricular aneurysms, mural thrombi, and regional wall motion abnormalities. The demonstration of regional myocardial perfusion abnormalities requires the use of intravenous contrast media. Assessment of ventricular function can be performed with and without pharmacologic stress.
2. Cardiomyopathies. MRI can be used to diagnose and demonstrate the morphologic and functional abnormalities of congestive cardiomyopathy and restrictive cardiomyopathy. It is particularly useful for the evaluation of variant forms of hypertrophic cardiomyopathy.
3. Pericardial disease. MRI can be used to evaluate pericardial effusions, differentiate hemorrhagic from nonhemorrhagic effusions, differentiate between restrictive and constrictive pericarditis, detect pericardial metastases, identify direct extension of tumors through the pericardium, and evaluate pericardial masses such as cysts and tumors.
4. Paracardiac and intracardiac tumors. MRI can be used to demonstrate the presence, location, and extent of paracardiac and intracardiac masses and can help by confirming or failing to confirm equivocal findings on echocardiogram. Sometimes, the type of mass can be definitively determined, such as lipomatous hypertrophy of the right atrium. Use of an intravenous contrast agent can help differentiate between thrombus and tumor.
5. Valvular disease. Valvular incompetence can be assessed on cine MR images by identification and quan-

tification of a regurgitant jet. Estimation of the volume of valvular regurgitation can be achieved in patients with single-valve disease by determination of the difference in the stroke volumes between two ventricles. Velocity-encoded MRI can measure the velocity across stenotic valves, and peak velocity measurements enable calculation of the gradient across the valve. MRI should not be used to image details of valve morphology and vegetations.

6. Ventricular function. MRI provides accurate and reproducible measurements of dimensions (volumes and mass) and functional parameters of the ventricles, including measurements of systolic wall thickening and deformation dynamics, ejection fraction, stroke volume, and cardiac outputs. Since both the endocardial and epicardial borders are defined on MR images, it is possible to assess wall thickening during the cardiac cycle and detect regional myocardial dysfunction. The ability to assess right ventricular volume, dimension, mass, and function gives MRI an advantage over other techniques for assessing cardiac disease.

7. Coronary arteries. MRI can depict the major epicardial and branch vessels, which can be projected in a format similar to a conventional coronary angiogram. Coronary MRI has demonstrated a high sensitivity and specificity in identifying areas corresponding to stenoses on conventional angiograms. Because the current spatial resolution of coronary MRI is poorer than that of conventional angiography, it cannot completely supplant coronary angiography or be used to quantitate focal stenoses. MRI may prove useful as a noninvasive screening test for identification of significant disease in patients with clinical data suggestive of coronary artery disease as well as those with multiple risk factors for premature coronary artery disease. It could also prove valuable for patients with contraindications for coronary angiography such as allergic history, bleeding diatheses, and so on. It may offer a means for obtaining follow-up on patients after revascularization procedures.

Congenital Heart Disease

1. MRI is useful for the initial assessment of simple and complex congenital heart disease. It can define intra-

cardiac and extracardiac morphology, and it identifies cardiac, pulmonary, and systemic vascular connections.

2. MRI is useful for monitoring patients after operations for congenital heart diseases because repeated studies can be performed without concern for radiation exposure or adverse reactions to contrast media.

Magnetic Resonance Spectroscopy

The nuclei that have the greatest diagnostic potential for cardiovascular MRS in a clinical setting are hydrogen, ^{13}C, and ^{31}P. Hydrogen may be used to monitor lactate and lipid accumulation in ischemically injured tissue. ^{13}C MRS may be used to monitor the use of fat and glucose in normal and ischemic myocardium by the detection of metabolic substrates. ^{31}P MRS may provide a means to evaluate alterations in high-energy phosphate stores in myocardial diseases, therapeutic interventions, and transplants. MRS may make it possible to determine whether viable tissue remains in an area of reperfused myocardium and may be useful for assessment of ischemic heart disease and cardiac transplant rejection.

Safety Considerations for MRI

For the MRI examination, the patient is placed in a long and fairly narrow tunnel. Although almost all patients tolerate the procedure with little difficulty, some patients are anxious and may require light sedation. Occasionally patients are so claustrophobic that they are unable to undergo the study.

During the MRI examination, the patient is exposed to strong magnetic fields (static and dynamic) and radiofrequency pulses. The patient may experience a loud banging sound and feel some vibration. Surgical and vascular clips (with the exception of some cerebral aneurysm clips) and most other implanted metal devices do not pose any risk to the patient. Prosthetic heart valves are not considered to be contraindications for MRI, except in the case of questionable valve dehiscence. Cardiac pacemakers and other implanted electromagnetic devices are contraindications for MRI due to the possibility of electromagnetic interference and malfunction. Indwelling electrodes and wires are also felt to be contraindications due to the possibility of current induction.

Basic Principles of CT

In simplest terms, a CT scanner consists of a narrow beam of x-rays that traverses a patient. The nonabsorbed x-rays are detected by a radiation detector that scans synchronously with the beam. This linear scan sequence is repeated at multiple projections around the patient. The data then consist of a series of profiles of the attenuation properties of the object scanned at different angles. From these profiles, a complex mathematical algorithm is employed to reconstruct a tomographic section (slice) of the patient. This process is repeated until the anatomic region of interest is scanned. CT allows detection of minute differences in x-ray attenuation properties of tissues compared with conventional x-ray techniques, but for most cardiac or vascular examinations, intravenous injection of iodinated media is required to allow differentiation between the blood pool, myocardium, and other structures.

Despite the fact that CT has been widely available for many years and has been extremely useful for assessment of the thoracic aorta and a number of cardiac and paracardiac diseases, its role in cardiac diagnosis has been fairly limited. With the advent of new faster CT technologies, the role of CT in cardiovascular diagnosis is being redefined. Nevertheless, CT is still somewhat limited by the necessity to inject contrast dye for most applications, by the inability to scan in any desired plane, by the use of ionizing radiation, and by the limited soft tissue contrast available with x-ray.

CT Techniques

Conventional CT

In most commercially available CT scanners, the radiation detectors are arranged in a stationary ring encircling the patient, and the x-ray tube rotates around the patient within the detector array. With this type of technology, anatomic studies of the heart and major vessels are possible, but the scan time is in general too slow to accomplish functional studies.

Steerable Electron Beam CT

This technique permits 50- to 100-msec exposure per tomographic image, which "freezes" cardiac motion and allows the acquisition of images at end diastole and end systole. Real-time sequential imaging is accomplished within a single heartbeat at multiple levels, and these images can be displayed in a close-loop cine format. Alternatively, ECG triggering may be employed so that all images can be obtained at the same point of the cardiac cycle.

Spiral (Helical) CT

In this type of device, the gantry is continuously rotated while the patient table is continuously advanced. A volume data set is rapidly acquired that is free from discontinuities resulting from respiratory-induced misregistration. Three-dimensional representations of anatomy can be reconstructed at any view angle from a single scan.

Indications for CT

In general, the indications for CT are equivalent to those for MR when morphologic information is required concerning the thoracic aorta, pulmonary arteries, large veins, and paracardiac masses. In general, MRI is considered preferable for evaluation of intracardiac masses and congenital heart disease.

Acquired Heart Disease

1. Ischemic heart disease. CT can demonstrate the complications of myocardial infarction, such as true and false aneurysms of the left ventricle, mural thrombus, diastolic regional wall thinning, and the absence of systolic wall thickening at the site of a prior infarction.
2. Cardiomyopathies. The various forms of cardiomyopathy can be evaluated by quantification of myocardial mass and ventricular volumes.
3. Valvular disease. The severity of valvular regurgitation can only be assessed indirectly.
4. Ventricular function. CT can be used to assess regional myocardial abnormalities, quantify regional myocardial thickness, and evaluate left ventricular mass and wall thickening dynamics. Highly reproducible and accurate volume measurements can be performed for both the right and left ventricles.

5. Coronary arteries. CT can demonstrate coronary artery graft patency. Although assessment of graft stenosis or measurement of absolute graft blood flow cannot be accomplished, reduction of flow might be detectable by comparison of time density curves of aortic and graft flow or analysis of transit times in the graft. Ultrafast CT can be used to detect coronary artery calcifications. Since there is a positive relationship between coronary artery calcification and angiographically detectable coronary artery disease, ultrafast CT is proposed for screening of selected populations for the presence of atherosclerotic coronary disease. For this application, intravenous contrast media are used.

Safety Considerations for CT

The only major safety consideration for CT concerns the use of intravenous iodinated contrast agents, which can cause adverse reactions ranging from mild to severe. In younger patients and in women in the childbearing ages, the ionizing radiation exposure during CT examination is also a consideration, particularly if multiple studies are anticipated.

Echocardiography in Cardiovascular Diagnosis

BASIC PRINCIPLES OF ULTRASOUND

Cardiovascular applications of ultrasound rely on the fact that ultrasound, generated by the vibration of piezoelectric crystals at frequencies from 2 to 40 MHz or even higher, can be formed into a beam that (a) propagates at a uniform speed through most body tissues and (b) is reflected from structures in the body to return to strike the piezoelectric crystal from which it originated, which in turn generates an electrical signal. The time interval between transmission of a burst of ultrasound a few microseconds in duration and generation of an electrical signal by the returning "echo," taken together with the known velocity of ultrasound in the body, allows one to determine the distance along the ultrasound beam from the transducer to a reflecting structure, providing information that can be used to image the heart and large arteries and veins. Increases or decreases between the frequency of the emitted and reflected ultrasound can also be used, according to the Doppler principle, to determine the velocity of the reflecting structure's motion toward or away from the transducer. Use of the Doppler shift to determine the velocity along the ultrasound beam of red blood cells forms the basis of Doppler echocardiographic evaluation of blood flow.

Physical Properties of Ultrasound

An appreciation of the physical properties of ultrasound that determine the information that can be obtained is valuable to understand the strengths and limitations of various echocardiographic modalities. One of these is that the average speed of ultrasound (1540 m/sec in body tissues) determines the frequency with which the cycle of ultrasound transmission and echo reception can be repeated. This ranges from 1000 to 1500 times per second for echocardiograms in adults, in whom cardiac structures may be as far as 20 cm from body surface transducers, to higher frequencies for cardiac imaging in children or for evaluation of relatively superficial arteries or intravascular studies. Nearly instantaneous tracking of rapidly moving structures is obtained when the ultrasound beam interrogates the same portion of the heart or vessel through the cardiac cycle, as in M-mode echocardiography. Alternatively, the beam can be swept mechanically or electronically to create a tomographic slice. Because it is desirable to have at least 50 lines of primary information to produce a good quality 90-degree "sector scan," these can be obtained no more frequently than 20 to 30 times per second for cardiac imaging in adults. Thus, M-mode echocardiography has superior temporal resolution, whereas two-dimensional echocardiography provides superior spatial orientation but at a somewhat slow frame rate.

The spatial resolution of echocardiography is influenced by several additional factors. The ability to discriminate two nearby objects along the axis of the echocardiographic beam ("depth resolution") is directly related to the ultrasound wavelength and, hence, is inversely proportional to its frequency. The theoretic limit of depth resolution is about 1 mm at a frequency of 2.25 MHz and 0.5 mm at a frequency of 5 MHz. These limits may be achieved in vivo or even exceeded because of the effect of temporally (M-mode) or spatially (two-dimensional) adjacent lines of echoes to reduce ambiguity about the location of interfaces. High ultrasound frequency thus enhances depth resolution; however, the inverse relation between ultrasound frequency and depth penetration into the body has so far limited transthoracic echocardiography to maximum frequencies between 3 and 5 MHz, whereas frequencies between 7 and 15 MHz or even higher may be used for other applications such as imaging the carotid or other superficial arteries transcutaneously, evaluating coronary arteries during open heart surgery, or measuring arterial lumen and wall dimensions and characteristics by catheter-tip ultrasound transducers. The ability to discriminate two objects side-by-side and perpendicular to the ultrasound beam (lateral resolution) is determined by beam width and the extent to which it is focused. Even under ideal circumstances, lateral resolution is less good than depth resolution with all systems used for cardiovascular ultrasound studies. Difficulties with lateral resolution may cause echoes from solid structures to extend laterally into what should have been echo-free spaces containing blood, overstating the cross-sectional area of the left ventricular myocardium and understating that of the ventricular cavity.

Evaluation of blood flow by Doppler echocardiography is also influenced by several properties of ultrasound. The most important of these is that the maximum frequency shift—and, hence, velocity of blood flow that can be accurately detected—is proportional to the frequency with which pulses of ultrasound are repeated (the so-called Nyquist limit). This is no problem in continuous-wave Doppler, where ultrasound is continuously emitted from one transducer and the returning signal is received by another, but this modality has the limitation that the recorded velocity may be due to blood flow at any depth along the ultrasound beam ("range ambiguity"). Range ambiguity is eliminated by pulsed-mode Doppler, in which bursts of ultrasound are emitted intermittently and the returning signal is interrogated at an interval thereafter determined to allow the ultrasound to travel from transducer to target and back. However, the slow pulse repetition frequency this entails may, at greater depths within the heart, limit the maximum velocity that can be resolved to 1 m/sec or less, well within the physiologic range. Color flow Doppler recordings reduce spatial ambiguity even further by displaying blood flow patterns in two-dimensional tomographic slices but suffer from even more severe limitation of the maximum velocity that can be accurately detected.

Fundamentals of the Echocardiographic Examination

The most important primary measurements and derived variables for assessment of the most common forms of heart disease can be obtained from a relatively simple echocardiographic examination, provided that the ultrasound beam and imaging planes are correctly oriented to cardiac structures and blood flow. Because of the central importance of left ventricular structure and performance, the following discussion will focus on this chamber.

The left ventricle may be thought of as a prolate ellipsoid, relatively circular in short-axis views, with a long axis approximately twice its minor axis. To measure the left ventricular minor-axis dimension accurately, it is necessary to orient the two-dimensional echocardiographic tomographic plane from the parasternal (or less commonly the subcostal) window to pass through the interventricular septum and posterolateral left ventricular wall so that a cursor line through the chamber at the level of the junction of the papillary muscle tips and mitral chordae on the two-dimensional sector would be perpendicular to the walls. Rotation of the two-dimensional sector approximately 90 degrees to the short-axis projection allows one to measure the true maximum left ventricular diameter and correct wall thickness or to planimeter the area of the cavity and myocardium. If, as commonly occurs in older subjects, the best parasternal window is in a low interspace, left ventricular M-mode dimension and short-axis two-dimensional cross-sectional areas should not be measured in the usual fashion, although it may be possible to measure correctly other structures such as the aortic root and left atrium. Instead, a higher interspace should be used even though this may image only a narrow sector that includes the left ventricular minor axis.

A major advantage of two-dimensional echocardiographic imaging is its ability to visualize the left ventricular long axis and ventricular wall segments near the apex. To use these measurements to calculate variables such as left ventricular mass and ejection fraction, one must obtain the true (longest) long-axis dimension and visualize the ventricular walls in approximately orthogonal planes (e.g., apical four- and two-chamber views). The left ventricular long axis is commonly foreshortened in the four-chamber view, as may be seen when the transducer is rotated to the two-chamber view; the ventricular apex is observed to be out of the field of view. The transducer should then be moved inferolaterally until the left ventricular apex is centered as nearly at the top of the image "fan" in both views as possible. Accurate measurements are obtained when care is taken in recording two-dimensional images to visualize the short-axis views at an appropriate level (e.g., papillary muscle tips) that demonstrates the smallest cavity diameter or area and the smallest wall thickness, and to record parasternal or apical long-axis or two- or four-chamber views that display the largest cavity diameter and smallest wall thickness.

The accuracy of Doppler recordings depends on interrogating the flow of interest with the ultrasound beam parallel to the axis of flow. Because the direction of blood flow is not always exactly what it would seem to be from the imaging echocardiogram, Doppler recordings of flow through a particular orifice should be performed from several potentially appropriate chest wall locations. Variants of the apical four-chamber view should be used to sample left ventricular inflow at the levels of the mitral anulus or valve orifice, whereas the apical long-axis view is best to measure systolic flow across the aortic anulus for calculation of stroke volume and systemic hemodynamic parameters. Performance of color flow mapping in multiple planes and of pulsed and continuous wave recordings from additional acoustic windows (e.g., the right parasternal window to assess flow across possibly stenotic aortic valves) is needed to assess the presence and severity of valvular heart disease.

ECHOCARDIOGRAPHIC EVALUATION OF LEFT VENTRICULAR STRUCTURE AND PERFORMANCE

Extensive information about the structure and systolic function of a normally shaped left ventricle, such as occurs in patients with uncomplicated systemic hypertension, may be obtained by two-dimensionally guided M-mode echocardiography. Recordings with the M-mode beam oriented along the left ventricular minor axis by procedures described above permit visualization of the left ventricle's internal dimension (LVID) as well as inter-ventricular septal and posterior wall thickness (IVS and PWT, respectively). For accurate and reproducible measurement of these structures, dominant lines representing the necessary interfaces should exhibit continuous motion in the correct pattern for each structure for at least 0.10 second but should ideally do so throughout the entire cardiac cycle.

Evaluation of Left Ventricular Structure

Two methods of making M-mode echocardiographic left ventricular measurements are currently in widespread use. The first of these to be proposed, the Penn method, is commonly used to measure left ventricular mass. The thickness of the echocardiographic lines representing endocardial interfaces is excluded from wall thickness measurements and is included in chamber dimensions by the Penn convention. The more recent recommendations of the American Society of Echocardiography, in which all measurements are made from leading edge to leading edge, have been widely adopted and may be used for measurement of left ventricular mass and other variables. End-diastolic measurements (made at the peak of the R wave of the simultaneous ECG by the Penn convention and at the QRS onset according to the American Society of Echocardiography) can be used to calculate left ventricular mass by anatomically validated formulas and to estimate left ventricular chamber volumes. Measurement of left ventricular mass requires use of primary echocardiographic measurements in variants of the cube-function formula that have been regression-corrected by comparison with postmortem data.

Although left ventricular mass is, overall, the best measure of myocardial cell size (since the number of cardiac myocytes remains relatively constant after infancy in humans), valuable information about concentric hypertrophy due to hypertension or aortic stenosis can also be obtained by calculating "relative wall thickness" as 2PWT/LVID.

Left ventricular mass, wall thicknesses, and chamber volume may also be measured by two-dimensional echocardiography. Two methods for determination of left ventricular mass by two-dimensional echocardiography have been anatomically validated. The simpler of these methods employs an ellipsoid model that requires measurement of the left ventricular long axis and of the cross-sectional area (CSA) of left ventricular myocardium and cavity in short-axis projection. Left ventricular chamber volume is calculated by the long-axis length-short-axis area method as 5/6 (long-axis length × cavity CSA), and ventricular mass is derived from the difference between this volume and the total volume of the ventricular cavity plus myocardium calculated in the same way. The other method of two-dimensional echocardiographic determination of left ventricular mass utilizes a truncated ellipsoid formula that corresponds more precisely to the shape of this chamber but requires more complex computations.

Evaluation of Ventricular Performance

Systolic function of a symmetrically contracting ventricle, such as in patients with uncomplicated hypertension, can be easily assessed by measurement of the fractional shortening between end diastole and end systole of the left ventricular internal dimension. If ventricular wall motion is uniform, fractional shortening is closely correlated with global left ventricular ejection fraction and is a simple substitute for it. Left ventricular chamber volume at end diastole and end systole, calculated by the above methods or by several others, may be used to derive the left ventricular stroke volume and ejection fraction more directly, but with a greater time requirement. Regional left ventricular function can be assessed semiqualitatively from two-dimensional short-axis and long-axis views and apical two- and four-chamber views using the 14-segment classification of the Mayo Clinic or the 16-segment one recommended by the American Society of Echocardiography. In these systems, motion of each segment is graded as normal, hypokinetic, akinetic, or dyskinetic. A numerical score from 1 (normal) to 4 (dyskinetic) is assigned to each segment's motion, which when averaged provides a summary measure of left ventricular function that is inversely related to left ventricular ejection fraction.

The pattern of left ventricular diastolic filling can be assessed by measurement of transmitral blood flow during the early and late phases of ventricular filling. The normality of early diastolic ventricular relaxation may be assessed, albeit indirectly, by measuring the peak flow velocity in early diastole ("E" velocity) or the integral of early diastolic flow. Similarly, the peak flow velocity in late diastole ("A" velocity) and the integral of late diastolic flow will be increased by enhanced venous return or atrial Starling forces and diminished by impaired left ventricular compliance. Interpretation of Doppler findings as abnormal must be undertaken with caution because normal values are influenced by both subject age and echocardiographic technique (the E/A ratio declines with age in normal adults and is lower when measured at the mitral anular plane than at the level of the mitral orifice), whereas filling rates of diseased ventricles are affected by the level of atrial pressure.

Evaluation of Other Cardiac Structures and Parameters

Standardized transthoracic echocardiographic examination allows quantitative or semiquantitative assessment of other cardiac structures. Mitral and aortic valve morphology and motion are best assessed in long- and short-axis views. Aortic root size is determined by measuring its maximum diameter at the sinuses of Valsalva at end diastole in long-axis views; left atrial diameter or area is measured in the long-axis or apical four-chamber view at end systole. Apical four-chamber views, medially displaced parasternal long-axis recordings, and short-axis views are used to assess the right-sided chambers and tricuspid valve. Multiple views are needed to determine the presence, degree of loculation, and accessibility from the body surface of pericardial effusion. Use of suprasternal notch and subcostal windows allows additional assessment of the aortic arch and descending and upper abdominal aorta in many patients.

Doppler Evaluation

When detection and quantitation of valvular lesions, shunts, or other hemodynamic disturbances are needed, evaluation should include pulsed-mode or color flow (or both) examinations to localize disturbed flow and continuous wave recordings to determine peak velocity. Care in avoiding excessive or inadequate gain and in considering the duration and pattern of flow signals is necessary for correct recognition of abnormalities. Assessment of the area and width at the origin of regurgitant jets allows grading of the severity of regurgitant lesions, whereas calculation of peak and mean transvalvular gradients from *both* the upstream and downstream flow velocities and use of the continuity equation allows quantitation of the severity of stenoses.

Transesophageal Echocardiography

This semi-invasive technique uses closer proximity (especially to posterior cardiac structures), consequent ability to use higher-frequency ultrasound, and lack of interference from ribs and lungs to provide superior imaging and Doppler information for selected purposes. Indications for use of transesophageal echocardiography include evaluation of possible prosthetic valve dysfunction, detection of vegetations and complications of endocarditis, identification of clots in the left atrial appendage and other potential causes of thromboembolic events, evolution of aortic atherothrombotic lesions and descending aortic dissection, and detection of other cardiovascular conditions when needed in patients with inadequate transthoracic studies due to pulmonary disease, postoperative state, or other causes.

Stress Echocardiography

Echocardiographic imaging of the left ventricle before and after the imposition of several forms of stress may identify wall motion abnormalities that help identify the presence and distribution of large-vessel coronary artery disease. In addition to treadmill or bicycle exercise (with imaging immediately at the end of exercise), stress may be imposed pharmacologically by dipyridamole or dobutamine, which is especially advantageous for patients who are unable to exercise. Sensitivity and specificity of stress echocardiography are similar to those for radionuclide techniques.

Detection of Abnormal Structure and Function

Although measurements of cardiac structure and function are continuous variables that vary across the entire range of normal and abnormal values, it is often convenient—and, at times, necessary for clinical decision-making—to use partition values to separate abnormal from normal findings. This requires use of appropriate normal limits, derived from study of reasonably large, apparently normal populations, that take into account demographic and body habitus variables that influence normal findings. For instance, gender and a measure of body size (such as body surface area or height) need to be taken into account for left ventricular dimensions and mass and for aortic and left atrial diameter, whereas for relative wall thickness and Doppler flow velocities, no such adjustment is needed (Table 6-1).

Clinical Cardiac Electrophysiology in Cardiovascular Diagnosis

The techniques of intracardiac electrography that are used in clinical electrophysiology permit detailed and quantitative analysis of cardiac impulse formation and transmission. These direct measurements clarify and extend electrophysiologic conclusions derived from body surface electrocardiography, which depend heavily on inference and deductive reasoning. Summarized in this section are the basic instrumentation and methods of acquisition of electrophysiologic data, the clinical indications for electrophysiologic study in cardiovascular diagnosis, and the electrophysiologic characterization of the principal disorders of impulse formation and transmission. The important applications of electrophysiologic methods in the selection of treatment for cardiac arrhythmias will not be considered in this review.

METHODS AND EQUIPMENT

Electrophysiologic studies are conducted in cardiac catheterization laboratories and, in general, require the equipment, personnel, and disciplines of such laboratories. Specialized equipment includes multichannel amplifier and recording systems with sufficient channels to record multiple body surface and intracardiac electrograms, electrophysiologic stimulators capable of providing programmable extrastimuli that can be coupled to spontaneous or induced rhythms, temporary pacemakers capable of rate incremental, smooth ramp, and burst pacing as well as conventional VVI and dual-chamber units, and multipolar catheter electrodes. These and related equipment items allow acquisition of the basic types of data recorded in the electrophysiology laboratory — passive recording of cardiac rhythm during baseline states and ectopic rhythms, programmed extrastimulation for single impulse and tachycardia induction and termination, determination of refractory period duration and other

284

Table 6-1. Normal limits of echocardiographic measurements in adults

	Women		Men	
	Absolute	Indexed	Absolute	Indexed
Imaging parameters				
IVSd	≤1.1 cm		≤1.2 cm	
LVIDd	≤5.4 cm	≤3.2 cm/m²	≤5.9 cm	≤3.2 cm/m²
PWTd	≤1.1 cm		≤1.1 cm	
LVIDs	≤3.9 cm		≤4.3 cm	
Fractional shortening	≥26%		≥26%	
LVEDV		50–90 ml/m²		50–90 ml/m²
LVESV		15–35 ml/m²		15–35 ml/m²
LVSV		32–58 ml/m²		32–58 ml/m²
Ejection fraction	0.55–0.75		0.55–0.75	
Left ventricular mass		≤110 gm/m²		≤125 gm/m²
Relative wall thickness		<0.45		≤0.45
Aortic root		≤2.1 cm/m²		≤2.1 cm/m²
Left atrium	≤3.8 cm		≤4.2 cm	
Doppler measurements				
Peak aortic velocity	≤1.35 m/sec		≤1.35 m/sec	
Peak left ventricular outflow velocity	≤1.0 m/sec		≤1.0 m/sec	
Mitral E	≤0.9 m/sec		≤0.9 m/sec	
Mitral A	≤0.6 m/sec		≤0.6 m/sec	
Mitral P½T	<80 msec		<80 msec	
Mitral orifice	>3 cm²		>3 cm²	
Mean mitral gradient	<2 mm Hg		<2 mm Hg	
Peak aortic gradient	<10 mm Hg		<10 mm Hg	
Peak RV/RA gradient	<20 mm Hg		<20 mm Hg	

IVSd = interventricular septum thickness in diastole; LVIDd = left ventricular internal diameter in diastole; PWTd = posterior wall thickness in diastole; LVIDs = left ventricular internal diameter in systole; LVEDV = left ventricular end-diastolic volume; LVESV = left ventricular end-systolic volume; LVSV = left ventricular stroke volume; mitral E = peak velocity with early diastolic filling (E point); mitral A = peak velocity with late (atrial) diastolic filling; mitral P½T = half-time pressure in diastole; RV = right ventricle; RA = right atrium.

electrophysiologic parameters, and endocardial mapping to determine the sequences of depolarization in atria and ventricles and to localize the earliest sites of depolarization.

INDICATIONS FOR ELECTROPHYSIOLOGIC STUDY IN CARDIOVASCULAR DIAGNOSIS

Criteria for the selection of patients for electrophysiologic study have been summarized in guidelines published by the American Heart Association, the American College of Cardiology, and the North American Society of Pacing and Electrophysiology and divided into indications for study for which there is general agreement (class I); indications often used but not universally accepted (class II); and indications that should not be used by general agreement (class III). Limited forms of this classification will be used in this discussion, but the class III indications will be omitted and only selected class II indications will be mentioned. It is recognized that departures from these guidelines may be necessary for specific reasons related to individual patients.

Disorders of Sinus Node Function

The class I indication is symptoms consistent with sinus node dysfunction but a causal relation not proved. Class II indications include quantitative evaluation of sinus node dysfunction, response of the impaired sinus node to drugs, and evaluation for pacing.

Disorders of Atrial Function

There are no class I indications. Class II indications include evaluation of interatrial or intra-atrial conduction block as a cause for bradyarrhythmia and ruling out atrial tachycardia in symptomatic patients.

Disorders of Atrioventricular Nodal Function

While there are no specific indications for electrophysiologic study for known or suspected atrioventricular nodal disease, atrioventricular nodal function is commonly evaluated to determine the location of conduction delay within the atrioventricular junction in patients with acquired or congenital atrioventricular block and to characterize atrioventricular nodal physiology when atrioventricular nodal related tachycardias are suspected.

Dysfunction Within the His-Purkinje System

Disease of the His-Purkinje system is typically, but not uniformly, associated with an intraventricular conduction delay. Blocks within or distal to the His bundle are considered potentially malignant because syncope or death can result from an unstable slow or absent ventricular escape rhythm or from a bradycardia-related ventricular tachycardia or fibrillation. In patients with acquired atrioventricular block, class I indications include syncope or near syncope when His-Purkinje block is suspected but not established electrocardiographically, type I second-degree atrioventricular block in association with bundle branch block to differentiate atrioventricular nodal block from His-Purkinje block, persistent symptoms following pacemaker implantation for second- or third-degree atrioventricular block, fixed-ratio atrioventricular block with constant P–R interval to localize the site of block, and type II second-degree atrioventricular block with a normal QRS duration (suspected intra-Hisian block). Among class II indications for electrophysiologic study are symptomatic paroxysmal atrioventricular block, concealed atrioventricular junctional premature beats as a possible cause of atrioventricular block, and unexplained syncope or near syncope in the presence of first-degree atrioventricular block. In patients with intraventricular conduction delay, class I indications include suspicion of ventricular tachycardia and differentiation of aberrant ventricular conduction from ventricular tachycardia during tachyarrhythmias. During normal atrioventricular conduction, recurrent syncope or near syncope is a class I indication for electrophysiologic study if structural heart disease is present and noninvasive workup is nondiagnostic. Unexplained recurrent syncope in the absence of structural heart disease is considered a class II indication for study.

Indications for Electrophysiologic Study Following Acute Myocardial Infarction

Postinfarction study has been used for risk stratification and therapeutic guidance regarding the use of pacemakers and antiarrhythmic medication. The value of such studies remains under investigation. Specific objectives of electrophysiologic study following myocardial infarction include measurement of H–V intervals (the interval from the onset of the His signal to the beginning of ventricular depolarization), localization of persistent second-degree or third-degree atrioventricular block within the atrioventricular node or His-Purkinje system, and determination of ventricular tachycardia inducibility when ventricular tachycardia or fibrillation occurs more than 48 hours after infarction.

Supraventricular (Narrow Complex) Regular Tachycardias

The class I indication for electrophysiologic study is frequent or hemodynamically significant episodes of tachycardia, the mechanism of which (reentrant, automatic, accessory pathway) must be determined to select appropriate therapy.

Wide Complex Tachycardias

The class I indication for diagnostic electrophysiologic study is differentiation of ventricular tachycardia from supraventricular tachycardia with aberrant ventricular conduction or bundle branch block and antidromic atrioventricular reciprocating tachycardia using accessory bypass tracts.

Ventricular Preexcitation Syndromes

Demonstration of the presence of and accurate localization of accessory atrioventricular conduction pathways are the class I indications for electrophysiologic study when recurrent ectopic tachycardias require ablation therapy.

TESTS OF THE ELECTROPHYSIOLOGIC PROPERTIES OF SPECIALIZED TISSUES OF THE HEART

Sinus Node Function

The sinus node recovery time measures the length of time required for resumption of spontaneous impulse formation in the sinus node following cessation of rapid atrial pacing. Incremental atrial pacing is used at rates of 100 to 180 beats per minute each for 15 to 60 seconds. Overdrive suppression of the sinus node lengthens the sinus node recovery time, the upper limit of normal being 1500 msec. The corrected sinus node recovery time is calculated by subtracting the baseline pacing cycle from the recovery time, the normal value being less than 500 msec. Other methods of evaluating sinus node recovery time have been used. Sinoatrial conduction time evaluates impulse transmission between the sinus node and the atria. Atrial extrastimuli (A_2) with progressive short-ening of coupling intervals to sinus beats (A_1) are deliv-ered until the atrial refractory period is reached. When the coupling interval shortens enough to cause a less than fully compensatory pause after the extrastimulus, the sinus node has been depolarized and reset, and the interval between the extrastimulus (A_2) and the next sinus beat (A_3) is the sum of the sinus cycle plus the time occupied by atriosinus and sinoatrial conduction, and the sinoatrial conduction time is one-half of the difference between the A_2–A_3 interval and the A_1–A_1 interval. The reliability of this and similar methods is questionable. Sinoatrial conduction can be measured directly by a right atrial catheter electrode, which, when properly positioned and amplified, may record the low-frequency signal from the sinus node. The intrinsic rate of the sinus node is determined after chemical denervation of the node by propranolol and atropine.

Atrial Function

Intra-atrial conduction time is measured from the begin-ning of the P wave to the low medial atrial signal in the His bundle electrogram. This value (the P–A interval) ranges from 10 to 45 msec. Programmed electrical stimu-lation is used to measure the effective and functional refractory periods of the atria. The former is determined by sequential decremental atrial extrastimuli during sinus rhythm or atrial pacing and is the longest coupling interval that fails to excite the atria. The effective refrac-tory period varies with heart rate, averages 230 msec, and should be under 350 msec. The functional refractory period is measured between two sites in the atria (usu-ally the high right atrium and the His bundle electro-gram) and is the shortest A_1–A_2 interval in the His bundle electrogram in response to an A_1–A_2 interval in the high right atrium. The functional and effective re-fractory periods are almost identical. In addition to pro-longation of the refractory period, prolongation or frac-tionation of the atrial electrogram may indicate atrial dysfunction and disease.

Atrioventricular Nodal Function

The A–H interval of the His bundle electrogram repre-sents intranodal conduction and the H–V interval con-duction in the composite His-Purkinje system (His bundle, bundle branches, and Purkinje system). Prolongation of the A–H interval or failure of the His potential to succeed the atrial potential is caused by atrioventricular nodal block. Prolongation of the H–V interval or failure of the ventricular potential to succeed the His potential is referred to as infranodal block. Normal values for the A–H interval range from 50 to 140 msec. Rate incremental pacing of the atria in normal subjects causes smooth continuous prolongation of the A–H interval until more rapid prolongation is followed by Wenckebach periodicity. In adults, this occurs at an average rate of 150 beats per minute with a range of 100 to 200 beats per minute. Conduction periods within the atrioventricular node can be determined and are somewhat analogous to refractory periods. The effective refractory period of the atrioventricular node is measured in the His bundle electrogram using decremental coupled atrial extrastimuli and is the longest A_1–A_2 interval that does not result in a His signal. The average atrioventricular nodal effective refractory period is 300 msec. If, as is often true, the atrial refractory period is reached before the atrioventricular nodal refractory period, the latter cannot be determined. The atrioventricular nodal functional refractory period, also determined by the atrial extrastimulus technique, is the shortest H_1–H_2 interval resulting from any A_1–A_2 interval.

An abrupt increase in the A–H interval of more than 50 msec for an increase in heart rate of 10 beats per minute suggests the presence of two atrioventricular conduction pathways except at pacing rates just prior to Wenckebach periodicity. Similarly, during refractory period testing, prolongation of the A_2–H_2 interval by 50 msec or more in response to a decrement of 10 msec in the A_1–A_2 interval is indicative of two conduction pathways. Identification of dual atrioventricular node physiology is important, since it may be the substrate for atrioventricular nodal reentrant tachycardia. Enhanced atrioventricular node conduction is identified by a baseline A–H interval of 50 msec or less and if only minimal prolongation occurs when the atrial pacing rate increases. Enhanced atrioventricular nodal conduction may be associated with rapid ventricular rates during atrial flutter, fibrillation, or tachycardia.

His-Purkinje System Function

The His bundle potential may be multiphasic, but not fractionated, and is 25 msec or less in duration. The normal H–V interval is 30 to 55 msec and is recorded from the onset of the His signal to the earliest evidence of ventricular depolarization whether recorded in the His bundle lead or the surface ECG. The H–V interval remains constant at different pacing rates. A split His bundle signal is characterized by two distinct potentials. Using the extrastimulus technique, the effective refractory period of the His-Purkinje system is the longest H_1–H_2 interval that does not result in ventricular excitation. Average values range from 300 to 400 msec. The effective refractory periods of the right bundle branch and left bundle branch may also be measured in a similar way. The former is the longest H_1–H_2 interval that results in a right bundle branch block QRS configuration; the latter is the longest H_1–H_2 interval that results in a left bundle branch block configuration. The functional refractory period of the His-Purkinje system is the shortest V_1–V_2 interval generated by any H_1–H_2 interval. Phase 3 block (tachycardia-dependent block) occurs when a spontaneous impulse or extrastimulus reaches tissues that are still partially or completely refractory. The refractory period may be physiologic in duration or abnormally prolonged. Phase 4 block (bradycardia-dependent block) is due to conduction delay in tissues that are beyond their refractory periods, usually in late diastole.

Gap Phenomena

During assessment of refractory periods within the atrioventricular junction using the atrial extrastimulus technique, atrioventricular conduction may resume with further shortening of the coupling time of the extrastimulus after atrioventricular block occurred at a longer coupling interval. The interval during which conduction block persists is referred to as a gap. Several types of gap phenomena are recognized and reflect the interplay between conduction velocities and refractory periods of different parts of the conduction system. They are not abnormalities.

ELECTROPHYSIOLOGIC CHARACTERIZATION OF SELECTED ECTOPIC RHYTHMS

Ectopic rhythms constitute the class of disorders of impulse formation in which the site of origin of the pacemaker or pacing circuit lies outside the sinus node. These rhythms (which may be fast or slow) are thought to be due to three mechanisms—reentry, automaticity, and after-depolarizations. Reentrant rhythms depend on anatomically or functionally defined circuits that are composed of two or more conduction pathways with unidirectional block in one of the pathways and slow conduction in another. Common proximal and distal pathways may complete the circuit. Reentrant circuits may exist anywhere in atria, ventricles, or atrioventricular junction and may be relatively large in circumference (macro, e.g., accessory pathways in the preexcitation syndromes) or small (micro, e.g., atrioventricular nodal reentry, reentrant ventricular rhythms). Reentrant rhythms can typically be induced by critically timed extrastimuli or burst pacing. When initiated by extrastimuli, an induction zone can be identified with critical S_1–S_2 intervals (S_1 is the spontaneous or baseline beat, S_2 is the extrastimulus). During this interval, as the S_1–S_2 interval decreases, the interval from S_2 to the first beat of the ectopic rhythm prolongs. Reentrant rhythms can be typically terminated by properly timed extrastimuli or rapid pacing. Automatic rhythms arise in normal pacemaker cells or in cells that have acquired the property of automaticity (abnormal automaticity) and depend on phase 4 depolarization reaching threshold and initiating a propagated impulse. Automatic rhythms cannot be induced or terminated by programmed extrastimuli. However, rapid pacing may overdrive and temporarily suppress automatic rhythms. Ectopic rhythms due to afterdepolarizations, occurring during repolarization (early afterdepolarizations) or in early diastole (delayed afterdepolarizations), have been studied primarily in tissue preparations in basic science laboratories. They are difficult to study in clinical electrophysiology laboratories because afterdepolarizations and the triggered rhythms due to them are difficult to identify. Early afterdepolarizations have been associated with the torsades de pointes form of polymorphous ventricular tachycardia.

Atrial Tachycardias

Atrial tachyarrhythmias (and abnormal sinus rhythms) arise and are perpetuated within the atria and may be reentrant or automatic. Electrophysiologic study demonstrates earliest electrograms in the atria. The atrial rhythm is not dependent on the atrioventricular node or ventricle, and H–V intervals are the same as during sinus rhythm. Reentrant (but not automatic) rhythms may be induced and terminated by extrastimuli. During both types of atrial tachycardia, V–A intervals usually exceed A–V intervals.

Atrioventricular Nodal Reentrant Tachycardia

This is the most common form of paroxysmal supraventricular tachycardia. Dual atrioventricular node physiology can usually be demonstrated. The reentrant circuit within the atrioventricular node typically conducts slowly antegrade to the ventricles and rapidly retrograde to the atria. This slow-fast sequence causes atrial and ventricular excitation to occur almost simultaneously. In the less common form of fast-slow atrioventricular nodal reentrant tachycardia, the fast pathway conducts antegrade and the slow pathway retrograde, and the atrial signal precedes the ventricular. Critically timed atrial extrastimuli can initiate and terminate this arrhythmia.

Atrioventricular Reciprocating Tachycardia (Wolff-Parkinson-White Syndrome)

These reentrant rhythms utilize the normal atrioventricular junction and accessory atrioventricular conduction pathways that bypass all or part of the atrioventricular junction (see also pages 218–221). There are many accessory pathways. The more important ones are those that bypass the entire atrioventricular junction and conduct both antegrade and retrograde (atrioventricular fibers, Kent bundles); those that bypass the entire atrioventricular junction but conduct only retrograde; those that bypass all or part of the atrioventricular node but reconnect to the distal atrioventricular node or bundle of His (atrionodal, James fibers or atrio-His, Brechenmacher fibers); and those that bypass only the distal His-Purkinje system (fasciculoventricular, Mahaim fibers). The classic arrhythmias related to accessory bypass tracts are orthodromic atrioventricular reciprocating tachycardia, in which antegrade conduction is via the normal atrioventricular junction and retrograde conduction via the accessory pathway, and antidromic atrioventricular reciprocating tachycardia, in which the antegrade and retrograde pathways are reversed. Rapid conduction via the accessory pathway during atrial tachycardia, flutter, or fibrillation may cause very rapid ventricular rates and ventricular fibrillation. A variety of electrophysiologic observations may be used to identify functioning accessory pathways. Atrioventricular bypass tracts (Kent bundles) result in shortened A–V and H–V intervals because of ventricular preexcitation. When the atria are paced rapidly, prolongation of the A–H interval causes the H–V interval to shorten and the His potential to shift closer to the ventricular potential or to superimpose on it. Atrionodal or atrio-His bypass tracts are associated with short H–V intervals, with little or no change during rapid atrial pacing. The demonstration of atrioventricular or ventriculoatrial conduction outside of the normal atrioventricular junction is strong evidence for an accessory pathway. This may be accomplished by mapping the arrival of electrograms at different atrial and atrioventricular junctional sites and demonstrating an "eccentric" or abnormal sequence of impulse transmission. Also in support of accessory pathway conduction is evidence of atrioventricular or ventriculoatrial conduction when the normal atrioventricular junction is refractory.

Ventricular Tachycardias

The major forms of ventricular tachycardia are sustained monomorphic ventricular tachycardia, nonsustained monomorphic or polymorphic ventricular tachycardia, sustained polymorphic ventricular tachycardia, torsades de pointes ventricular tachycardia, and bundle branch reentry tachycardia. These arrhythmias are described in Section 3. Bundle branch reentrant tachycardia is an unusual reentrant tachycardia involving antegrade conduction over the right bundle branch and retrograde conduction over the left bundle branch. The electrophysiologic hallmark of the ventricular tachycardias is the absence of a His bundle potential preceding the ventricular potential. Some tachycardias, including bundle branch reentry, can be initiated and terminated by appropriately timed ventricular extrastimuli or rapid pacing. Specialized intracardiac electrophysiologic mapping methods permit accurate localization of the sites of origin of some forms of ventricular tachycardia.

Stress Physiology in Cardiovascular Diagnosis

EXERCISE STRESS TESTS

The resting state is often not ideal for the optimal evaluation of the individual with known or suspected cardiac disease. Diseases of the heart frequently are best evaluated during an altered state of physiologic stress of the cardiovascular system. The most common method of creating that altered cardiovascular state is an exercise stress test. The cardiovascular exercise test can lead to a more definite cardiac diagnosis, a more accurate assessment of functional capacity, a more effective therapeutic regimen, and a more precise prognosis.

Indications

Three criteria are to be considered before performing an exercise test: The test should answer a specific clinical question, the answer should modify patient management or therapy, and the answer should not be obtainable by alternate means that involve less risk, discomfort, or expense for the patient.

The American Heart Association has codified the indications for the performance of exercise stress tests into three classes. In class I are found the indications for which there is general agreement that an exercise test is justified. In class II are the indications for which an exercise test is regularly performed, but for which there is some divergence of opinion with respect to the value or appropriateness of the test. In class III are the indications for which there is general agreement that an exercise stress test is of little or no value.

The class I indications are (1) the diagnosis of coronary artery disease in men with symptoms that are atypical of myocardial ischemia; (2) the assessment of the functional capacity and prognosis of patients with known coronary artery disease or of selected patients with congenital heart disease; and (3) the evaluation of patients after an uncomplicated myocardial infarction or after coronary artery revascularization, those with symptoms consistent with recurrent exercise-induced arrhythmias, or those with rate-responsive pacemakers.

The class II indications are (1) the diagnosis of coronary disease in women or in asymptomatic individuals with risk factors for coronary artery disease; (2) the assessment of the functional capacity of selected patients with valvular disease and of the efficacy of medical therapy in patients with coronary artery disease, congestive heart failure, hypertension, or arrhythmias; and (3) the evaluation of the ventricular response of patients with atrial fibrillation or of asymptomatic individuals who wish to start a vigorous exercise program.

The class III indications are (1) the diagnosis of coronary disease in asymptomatic individuals with no risk factors for coronary artery disease, (2) the assessment of individuals with benign arrhythmias (such as single premature ventricular contractions), and (3) the evaluation of individuals whose chest pain is not of cardiac origin.

Contraindications

A complete medical history and a directed physical examination should prevent the performance of an exercise stress test on individuals who may be placed at undue risk by the test. A contraindication to the test exists if at the time of its expected performance, a patient has (1) a recent myocardial infarction (within 5 days); (2) recent unstable angina (within 3 days); (3) severe left ventricular dysfunction (that results in either marked hypotension or congestive failure); (4) complex arrhythmias at rest or a history of potential lethal arrhythmias with exertion; (5) severe arterial hypertension (200 mm Hg systolic or 120 mm Hg diastolic); (6) severe valvular heart disease (specifically aortic, subaortic, and mitral stenosis); (7) acute cardiac inflammation (endocarditis, myocarditis, or pericarditis); (8) a history of severe exercise-induced bronchospasm; (9) an arthritic, muscular, neurologic, or orthopedic condition that interferes with exercise; or (10) any acute or general illness that may be adversely affected by exercise.

Methods and Equipment

Monitoring

Present standards of exercise stress testing require the continuous oscilloscopic monitoring of a 12-lead ECG. Also standard is a separate amplified display of three leads reflecting disparate electrical vectors (usually V_1,

V_5, and aVF) to allow easy detection of arrhythmias and rapid identification of their origin as either ventricular or supraventricular. Essential numerical screen displays are heart rate, blood pressure, and the exercise workload (the grade of incline of the treadmill in percent and the speed of the belt in miles per hour). Another useful feature is a magnified display of the ECG lead that shows the greatest magnitude of S–T segment shift at any time during the test. These visual features add to the safety of the exercise stress test.

Paper tracings of the 12-lead ECG are to be recorded in a standardized fashion:

1. Before exercise: with the patient in the standing and sitting positions and at times, if postural ECG changes are present, also in the supine position.
2. During exercise: every third minute or at the end of a particular exercise level stage; when relevant clinical, electrophysiologic, or hemodynamic events occur; and always at peak effort.
3. During the recovery period: at 3-minute intervals until that time when the ECG reverts to its preexercise morphology or for a total time of 10 minutes, whichever time is longer.

Both systolic and diastolic blood pressures are to be measured and recorded frequently, usually every 3 minutes, and optimally at the same time that the ECG paper tracings are recorded.

Equipment

At present, exercise stress tests are most commonly performed on a motorized treadmill. Used less often are leg (bicycle) ergometers and arm ergometers. Exercise properly performed on a treadmill involves the musculature of both legs, of both arms, and of the torso as well. This involvement of large muscles and several muscle groups results in the greatest total oxygen consumption of any method of exercise stress testing. High heart rates and blood pressure responses are generated, which translate into a high work double product and a high myocardial oxygen demand.

Ergometry usually involves only one group of muscles, either those of the arms or of the legs. Such exercise usually results in comparatively lower peak heart rates, lower work double products, and lower myocardial oxygen demand than does treadmill exercise. In some subjects, the lower heart rate with ergometry is compensated by a higher systolic blood pressure that can result from tight gripping of the bicycle ergometer handles or of the upper ergometer pedals. For the successful completion of the exercise stress test, very little conscious cooperation is required of a subject exercising on a treadmill. The speed of the belt and the incline of the machine are controlled by the medical personnel supervising the test. However, in both bicycle and upper extremity ergometry exercise, the performance is limited by a subject who has full control of the pedals.

Protocols

Many different exercise stress test protocols have been developed over the years for clinical testing and investigative work. They all include (1) an initial lower exercise intensity or warm-up phase, (2) a continuous noninterrupted exercise phase with progressive increases in workload, (3) the expectation that the individual's maximal effort level will be achieved within 20 minutes of exercise, and (4) a recovery or cool-down phase.

The Bruce treadmill protocol is the most common protocol in use for clinical and investigative work. It is excellent for the diagnosis of exercise-induced myocardial ischemia and arrhythmias. It calls for the simultaneous increase in both the speed and incline of the treadmill at the beginning of each successive 3-minute stage. These changes cause abrupt and marked increase in effort for the exercising subject with a significant average increment in workload of 50 percent over each prior stage. METs achieved at the end of each stage of the Bruce protocol are roughly: stage I, 5 METs; stage II, 7 METs; and stage III, 10 METs. (One MET is the energy requirement of an individual at rest. One MET = 3.6 cc of oxygen consumption per kilogram of tissue per minute.)

The performance of the Bruce protocol is difficult for the elderly, for persons of any age with chronic physical deconditioning, and especially for those with recent prolonged bed rest. Its performance should be avoided in the recent postinfarction period. Gentler protocols are used for these population groups. Such protocols include (1) the Modified Bruce, which precedes the regular Bruce protocol with a 6-minute warm-up period of slower speed and lower incline; (2) the Bensen, whose stages alternate the increases in speed and incline, resulting in workload increments of only 25 percent over each prior stage; and (3) the Naughton, which keeps a constant speed of 3 mph and increases the treadmill incline by 2.5 percent every 2 minutes, resulting in a workload increment of about only 1 MET with each stage.

Ergometer protocols, whether enlisting leg or arm exercise, call for a constant rate of pedaling, usually at 60 rpm. The ergometer protocols in most common use require an initial power output by the exercising subject of about 50 W or 200 Kpms (kilopound-meters per minute or kilogram-weight force × meters per minute). The increased resistance to pedaling is set by the examiner to result in increments of 25 W or 200 Kpms at each 3-minute stage. The workload achieved by an individual with exercise ergometry should be expressed in METs for ready comparison with treadmill workloads and with daily life activities.

Interpretation of Exercise Tests

Electrocardiographic Changes

Exercise results in increased metabolic demands on the myocardium that cannot be met if its perfusion is compromised by a diminished blood flow through a physiologically significant atherosclerotic coronary artery stenosis. The exercise-induced ischemia is confined primarily to the endocardium.

Subendocardial ischemia is expressed by surface subendocardial ECG as S–T segment depression in ECG leads with dominant R waves. In the normal 12-lead ECG, the leads with the greatest R-wave amplitude are usually the lateral precordial leads (V_4, V_5, and V_6), followed in amplitude by the inferior leads. These leads, with their greatest sensitivity for detection of a subendocardial ischemic response with exercise, will be the ones to manifest S–T segment depressions regardless of the location of the specific ischemic myocardial segment. S–T segment depression in the lateral leads or in the inferior leads does not necessarily localize ischemia in the corresponding lateral and inferior myocardial segments. Thus, the exercise ECG is not useful in determining the location of ischemia. This lack of regional localization of ischemia by ECG is a particular limitation of stress testing in assessing the effectiveness of revascularization of specific zones of myocardium.

The generally accepted ECG manifestation of exercise-induced myocardial ischemia is 0.10 mV (or 1 mm) flat or downsloping S–T segment depression 0.08 second after the J point. This standard achieves the best test sensitivity and specificity.

The normal ECG response to exercise is depression of the junction of the QRS complex and S–T segment, or J-point depression. This may be as much as 2 mm and results in upsloping S–T segment depression. This deviation should not be confused with true ischemic horizontal S–T segment depression. However, the upsloping type may also be the first phase of a true ischemic response. If the exercise test is terminated prematurely, before complete evolution of the S–T segment shift, a false-negative interpretation may be made. If there is deviation of the S–T segment in the resting ECG because of bundle branch block, left ventricular hypertrophy, digitalis effects, or other causes, additional S–T changes with exercise lack specificity and predictive accuracy for myocardial ischemia.

Several stress test ECG parameters are directly related to the severity of coronary atherosclerosis and myocardial ischemia: (1) the magnitude of S–T segment depression, (2) the duration of S–T segment depression during recovery, and (3) the number of ECG leads showing S–T segment depression. Inversely related are (1) the duration of exercise, (2) the workload, and (3) the work double product achieved at the onset of S–T depression. Thus, marked (> 3 mm) S–T segment depression in six ECG leads that occurs with less than 3 minutes of exercise, at a low work double product (< 15,000), and at a low workload (<5 METs) and do not resolve until after 10 minutes of recovery are usually caused by severe multivessel coronary artery disease. In contrast, depressions of about 1 mm in less than three ECG leads, after vigorous exercise and with a rapid postexercise resolution, correlate best with single-vessel disease of only moderate severity.

In about 5 percent of positive exercise stress tests, the S–T segment shift is an elevation rather than a depression. This S–T segment elevation expresses transmural ischemia secondary either to very severe chronic fixed coronary artery stenosis or to acute coronary lumen reduction from exercise-induced coronary artery spasm. A nonischemic S–T segment elevation may occur in ECG leads with Q waves in patients who have experienced a recent myocardial infarction. This ECG response is thought to occur because of an exercise-induced abnormal ventricular wall motion of the partially scarred myocardium or of the adjacent myocardial area. This S–T segment elevation with exercise may persist in patients who later develop a left ventricular aneurysm.

Depressions of the S–T segment that occur only in the recovery period but not during exercise were long deemed to be nonspecific and to have no diagnostic value. Recent investigations show, however, that recovery-only changes do reflect exercise-induced ischemia. If the S–T changes occur after vigorous exercise, at a high workload, and at a high work double product, they are usually associated with single-vessel coronary disease. If they occur after an exercise level of less than 7 METs, they are often associated with multivessel disease.

Physiologic Changes

In the evaluation of exercise test results, it is important to consider changes in heart rate and blood pressure as well as symptoms and total duration of exercise. If these physiologic responses are evaluated in addition to the ECG, the sensitivity and specificity of the stress test for atherosclerotic coronary artery disease are increased.

HEART RATE RESPONSE. In sinus rhythm, the heart rate is usually linearly related to exercise duration and exercise intensity. The age-adjusted target heart rate is usually accurately determined by subtracting the subject's age from the number 220. With the crossover from aerobic to anaerobic metabolism with increasing exercise, the total body oxygen consumption reaches a plateau, as does the heart rate response. The normal response is thus a steady acceleration of heart rate with a plateau at the attainment of the anaerobic threshold and a return to the preexercise baseline heart rate within 5 minutes of the termination of exercise. Two types of abnormal heart rate responses may be observed in exercise stress testing: a bradycardic response or a tachycardic response.

A bradycardic or blunted heart rate response occurs naturally in older individuals, in those with intrinsic sinoatrial nodal disease, and in those experiencing the effects of therapeutic levels of beta-adrenoreceptor blocking agents. It is also seen in well-trained athletes who engage in regular vigorous aerobic exercise. They have on average a heart rate response of 10 beats per minute lower than age-matched sedentary controls for comparable effort levels. The inability to reach 85 percent of age-adjusted predicted heart rates results in a less-sensitive stress test with a greater number of false-negative results. Thus, the exercise stress test has a lower positive predictive value for the diagnosis of obstructive coronary artery disease in this population.

A tachycardic heart rate response with exercise is more common than a bradycardic response. This response is most commonly seen in individuals free of cardiac disease but who are physically deconditioned. It is also demonstrated by patients with severe ventricular dysfunction—those who have a greater dependence on heart rate increases rather than on stroke volume increments to generate increased cardiac output. Both deconditioned individuals and decompensated cardiac patients have increased circulating catecholamines at rest and with any level of effort relative to their well-conditioned counterparts with normal cardiac function. The elevated catecholamines result in a fast rate or even sinus tachycardia at rest, a rapid acceleration of heart rate with exercise, an earlier achievement of anaerobic threshold and of target heart rates, and a persistent postexercise tachycardia. These individuals exhibit prompt development of effort dyspnea and fatigue. They may have palpitations and are generally prone to premature atrial and ventricular ectopic beats and tachyarrhythmias with their usual daily exercise activities and specifically with stress testing.

Atrial fibrillation is a common arrhythmia in patients undergoing stress testing. In these patients, the routine use of digitalis alters the refractoriness of the atrioventricular node and lowers the ventricular rate at rest. However, the high circulating catecholamine levels provoked by exercise usually negate the effect of digitalis on atrioventricular nodal conduction. Most patients with atrial fibrillation will exceed heart rates of 150 beats per minute in the early stages of an exercise stress test, unless they also receive concomitant beta-blocker therapy. Exercise stress testing of patients with atrial flutter should be avoided. Useful information is usually not garnered, and the individual may be placed at risk. Assuming the usual atrial rate of 300 beats per minute, patients often quickly convert from a 4 : 1 atrioventricular block (with a ventricular rate of 75 beats per minute) at rest to a 2 : 1 atrioventricular block (with a ventricular rate of 150 beats per minute or faster) with minimal exercise.

Diagnostic information is not usually obtained from the stress tests of patients with permanent pacemakers without rate-responsive features. The intrinsic sinus rhythm seldom overrides the paced rhythm. The fixed heart rate while performing exercise limits the cardiac output, resulting in rapid fatigue and a very short test duration. Furthermore, the stress ECG does not accurately detect an ischemic response. The ECG is potentially both less specific because of the pacing-related abnormal S–T segments at rest and less sensitive because of the lack of rate change caused by a fixed pacing rate.

BLOOD PRESSURE RESPONSE. The normal systolic blood pressure response to an exercise stress test is a progressive increment of about 20 mm Hg with each stage of the standard Bruce protocol, with a normal total increase of about 50 ± 30 mm Hg and a peak exercise pressure ranging between 160 and 210 mm Hg, depending on the baseline preexercise blood pressure.

A blunted systolic blood pressure response, less than a 20 mm Hg rise at peak exercise, is seen in patients with an impaired cardiac output secondary to ischemic disease, valvular disease, or cardiomyopathies; those with fixed-rate pacemakers; those receiving therapy with beta blockers; and those who cannot generate an adequate exercise effort. A hypertensive systolic blood pressure response (> an 80 mm Hg rise at peak exercise) is seen in inadequately treated hypertensive patients; some patients who may have a prehypertensive state (normal resting pressure at present that will become abnormal at a future date); those with autonomic nervous system disorders, such as some diabetics; and otherwise healthy but physically deconditioned individuals.

A fall in systolic blood pressure with exercise is highly correlated with exercise-induced global ventricular ischemia from multivessel coronary stenosis or left main coronary artery disease. Such an abnormal pressure response is usually associated with marked ischemic ECG changes and with symptoms of angina, dyspnea, and dizziness. Another abnormal response blood pressure, that of a modest fall (≤20 mm Hg) with progressive exercise (below a previously higher exercise pressure but still above the preexercise level), is a less specific response for the detection of ischemia, and it is usually not accompanied by ischemic ECG changes. It is most often seen in patients receiving therapy with nitrate compounds, dehydrated individuals with orthostatic hypertension, or healthy elderly individuals.

The normal diastolic blood pressure response is a drop of about 10 mm Hg in normal young individuals. A modest rise (<20 mm Hg) occurs in the elderly, the physically deconditioned, and patients with an abnormal cardiac output. An abnormal rise (>20 mm Hg) may occur in those with a prehypertensive state or in inadequately treated hypertensive patients.

SYMPTOMS. At present, most exercise stress testing is symptom limited. That is, general or specific sensations are induced with exercise that motivate the test subject or direct the supervising physician to terminate the test. Less commonly, an exercise stress test is ended in an asymptomatic subject because of the development of excessive S–T segment shifts (especially S–T depressions greater than 3 mm or any S–T elevations), supraventricular or ventricular tachycardia, or any conduction block.

The most common symptom provoked by stress testing is fatigue. It is also the most common reason for the termination of symptom-limited exercise tests. Fatigue usually occurs about the time that anaerobic threshold is crossed, and its time of onset is dependent on the physical conditioning of the individual.

Dyspnea, also a common symptom with exercise, is usually the subjective correlate to the physiologic tachypneic response to increasing carbon dioxide levels, which are a product of anaerobic metabolism. Dyspnea is also seen in patients with intrinsic pulmonary disease. Most importantly, it may be a sign of exercise-induced excessively elevated pressures within the heart and the pulmonary capillary beds of the patient with severe cardiac disease. Peripheral vascular atherosclerosis is common in patients with coronary artery atherosclerosis, and claudication is often the limiting symptom with exercise. It is most easily provoked by treadmill protocols that call for steep incline increments.

Chest discomfort is a common, yet often nonspecific symptom, provoked by exercise stress tests. Usually this discomfort is bronchial or pleuritic in origin and reflects the conscious awareness of labored breathing with vigorous exercise. The provocation of the typical anginal syndrome by the exercise test obviously increases the sensitivity of the test for the detection of coronary disease to nearly 100 percent. Angina pectoris induced by an exercise stress test is usually a self-limited event and resolves within 5 minutes after the termination of exercise without the need of antianginal medication.

EXERCISE DURATION. By itself, the duration of exercise in a stress test is an important predictor of prognosis, not only in patients with coronary disease but also in those with other cardiac conditions such as left ventricular dysfunction. Individuals who complete three stages of the standard Bruce protocol, or achieve a 10-MET workload, have an excellent prognosis (a 5-year survival > 90% in some studies), regardless of the ECG abnormalities they may have developed during the exercise test. In contrast, cardiac patients who cannot complete stage I of the standard Bruce protocol, or achieve a 5-MET workload, have a poorer prognosis (a fourfold increase in mortality in some studies), even in the context of a normal exercise ECG.

Limitations of Exercise Testing

There are limitations to the use of the exercise stress test as a diagnostic tool. Those individuals who cannot exercise cannot be evaluated. Both the sensitivity and the specificity of exercise stress testing for the detection of coronary artery disease in a general population are at best no greater than 85 percent. Indeed, its diagnostic value in some population groups, such as women, remains uncertain.

However, many of the limitations of exercise stress testing have been overcome by the development of pharmacologic stress tests and nuclear cardiac imaging.

NUCLEAR CARDIOLOGY

Methods and Equipment

The development of nuclear cardiology over the last three decades has led to the improved evaluation of the cardiovascular system at rest and with exercise. Moreover, it has made possible the development of pharmacologic stress testing for the cardiac assessment of patients who cannot perform physical exercise. Nuclear cardiology, when combined with stress testing, results in a more definite diagnosis and a more precise prognosis in patients with cardiac disease than does the stress test alone.

Instrumentation

The essential tool of nuclear cardiology is the gamma or scintillation camera. It consists of three basic components: a lead collimator, a crystal detector, and a computer.

The collimator, akin to the lens of a camera, absorbs gamma rays that do not originate from the target organ or that strike it at a nonuseful angle. In nuclear cardiology, a parallel hole collimator is most frequently used. Thousands of parallel holes perpendicular to the crystal allow only the appropriate photons to strike the crystal detector. The wide, short holes of a high-sensitivity collimator achieve high count rates and increase sensitivity at the expense of spatial resolution, while the narrow, longest holes of a high-resolution collimator maximize spatial resolution but reduce overall sensitivity. In nuclear cardiology, high-sensitivity collimators are often used in studies where accurate quantitation of photon flux is required, such as first-pass angiocardiography. Higher-resolution collimators are used in other studies such as myocardial perfusion imaging or gated blood pool scanning, where delineation of the spatial distribution of the radiopharmaceutical is paramount. General-purpose collimators, which combine features of both high-resolution and high-sensitivity collimators, are often used for these applications.

The crystal detector is usually composed of sodium-iodide material that is photon sensitive and converts a portion of the incident gamma or x-ray photon into light photons—a process called scintillation. A scintigram, the proper name for a nuclear scan, is thus an image of the distribution of radioactivity in an individual subject or in a particular organ.

These light photons are subsequently detected by an array of photomultiplier tubes that produce converted electrical signals that identify the precise location and intensity of the incident energy photon. Two types of electrogeometries are used in cardiology: the multicrystal camera, consisting of a rectangular matrix of individual crystals (14 × 21 crystals is the most common configuration), and the more popular Anger gamma camera, consisting of a single, relatively large crystal.

The digital computer is essential in nuclear cardiology to record and organize the electrical signals produced by the gamma camera into interpretable time-activity curves or visual images. Important parameters to be considered in the selection of such a computer include the matrix size of the displayed image (64 × 64 pixels is the minimum acceptable dimension) and the rapidity with which these images can be acquired, at least 40 frames per second. As the demands placed on camera-computer configurations increase (e.g., for single-photon emission computed tomography [SPECT]), the tighter integration possible between a camera and computer provided by a single vendor becomes more important.

Radiopharmaceuticals

Radiopharmaceuticals are agents used in nuclear medicine for diagnostic purposes. They all contain a radioactive atom combined with another moiety that renders the agent either organ specific or gives it some other useful property for anatomic or physiologic imaging. A radionuclide is an atom with an unstable nucleus that will transform in a spontaneous fashion to a more stable state. During the transformation, radiation is emitted that is available for detection by the gamma camera or other imaging device.

In nuclear cardiology, the potassium-analog thallium 201 (as the injectable radiopharmaceutical thallous chloride 201) has emerged as the radionuclide of choice for myocardial perfusion and viability imaging. This is due to the many favorable biologic properties of [201]Tl: a high correlation of myocardial uptake with myocardial blood flow at rest and with exercise, a high myocardial extraction fraction of about 90 percent at rest and even higher with exercise, and a maximal heart-to-blood ratio generally achieved within 10 minutes of injection. These characteristics, along with the slow myocardial washout and redistribution rates of thallium, make it an excellent agent for the identification of myocardial ischemia, scar, and viability.

On the other hand, the physical properties of ^{201}Tl are less than ideal for its use as a diagnostic imaging agent. Its relatively long physical half-life of 73.2 hours makes unfeasible serial re-injection imaging studies of the myocardium within a short time interval and requires that only a relatively low amount be injected to keep patient irradiation to an acceptable level. Its low-energy x-ray emissions of 70 to 80 keV result in soft tissue attenuation and in false-positive interpretations that reduce the specificity of the ^{201}Tl scintigrams for the detection of myocardial ischemia. Moreover, it is not always readily available because its production requires a cyclotron, although this has recently become less of a problem.

The radionuclide technetium 99m is used in several different radiopharmaceutical preparations for gated equilibrium ventriculograms, first-pass angiocardiogram studies, and myocardial perfusion studies. The physical properties of ^{99m}Tc make it an excellent radionuclide for nuclear cardiology imaging. Its short physical half-life of 6 hours allows relatively larger amounts to be injected due to the correspondingly more favorable dosimetry. Its relatively high-energy gamma emission of 140 keV results in less soft tissue attenuation and better spatial resolution and may increase both the sensitivity of the scans and their specificity. Moreover, ^{99m}Tc is generally available because its production requires only a small, inexpensive on-site generator.

One of the greatest assets of ^{99m}Tc is its versatility. It readily combines with other agents to result in a wide array of radiopharmaceuticals. As ^{99m}Tc pertechnetate, it can be used for the labeling of red blood cells by a variety of methods for first-pass or gated equilibrium radioventriculograms. In vivo labeling, the most common labeling method, calls for the pretagging of the red blood cells by the injection of stannous chloride containing between 550 mg and 1 gm of stannous ion approximately 20 minutes before the administration of the ^{99m}Tc pertechnetate. In the form of ^{99m}Tc pyrophosphate, it is used in infarct-avid scans for the diagnosis of a recent myocardial infarction, necrosis, or contusion.

In the form of isonitrile radiopharmaceuticals, ^{99m}Tc is often used in myocardial perfusion imaging for the detection of ischemia and scarring. Their comparative value to ^{201}Tl for the identification of myocardial viability remains controversial at the present time. ^{99m}Tc-sestamibi (methoxyisobutyl isonitrile) and ^{99m}Tc-teboroxime (carbomethoxyisopropyl isonitrile) are both currently available for this indication. Both of these radiopharmaceuticals, for different reasons, distribute proportionally with myocardial blood flow, have high initial myocardial uptake, and show little evidence of redistribution into zones of ischemia. The sestamibi preparation behaves like a chemical microsphere and thus is slow to wash out from the myocardium. This property renders it particularly useful in clinical situations that call for imaging studies hours after the initial injection. An example is the comparison of the myocardial area at risk of necrosis in a patient with an acute myocardial infarction before and after reperfusion with coronary angioplasty or thrombolytic agents. Teboroxime is a large lipophilic molecule that probably does not enter the myocyte but remains within its membrane and thus rapidly washes out of the myocardium with a myocardial half-time of less than 10 minutes. This property renders it useful in clinical situations that call for the performance of serial studies at relatively frequent intervals. An example is the serial assessment of myocardial perfusion in a patient undergoing multivessel coronary angioplasty.

Tomographic Imaging

Planar imaging of myocardial perfusion, viability, or metabolism has been largely replaced in the last decade by tomographic imaging: single-photon emission computed tomography (SPECT) or positron emission tomography (PET). The tomographic method is superior to the planar method for the more accurate identification and quantification of photon sources. The technique requires the acquisition of images, or projections, of the distribution of radiopharmaceutical within the heart either 180 or 360 degrees around the patient's chest. These images may be acquired by a rotating gamma camera consisting of one or more individual imaging heads or by a stationary ring-type detector in which an annular array of detectors surrounds the patient. The multiheaded gamma camera facilitates proportionately greater photon sensitivities relative to single-headed cameras, allowing for faster acquisitions or higher spatial resolutions. Ring-type detectors afford the highest photon sensitivities but generally limit the size of the volume that can be imaged during a single scan. In any case, the acquired projections are processed by computer to produce a set of standardized orthogonal slices through the chest in the transaxial, sagittal, and coronal planes. This method is superior to planar imaging in that it produces better target-to-background ratios and thus results in improved edge detection and image contrast.

When properly used, these newer tomographic techniques increase the sensitivity and specificity of nuclear cardiology studies. However, without strict quality control, artifacts may be introduced into the reconstruction images, reducing the specificity of the technique. The popular bull's-eye format of displaying SPECT myocardial scan data and its automatic quantitative computer analysis can allow such reconstruction or soft tissue attenuation artifacts to go undetected or even to be amplified. Thus, this display and analysis method can further compromise the positive predictive accuracy of SPECT myocardial perfusion imaging when poorly utilized.

The American Heart Association has recommended a standardized nomenclature and display mode to facilitate the interpretation and comparison of cardiac tomographic studies. The SPECT cardiac images should be displayed in a left-to-right or top-to-bottom format in three different axes: (1) short-axis tomograms with serial slices beginning at the apex and progressing to the cardiac base, (2) vertical long-axis tomograms with serial slices beginning at the septum and progressing to the lateral wall of the left ventricle, and (3) horizontal long-axis tomograms with serial slices beginning at the inferior surface and progressing to the superior surface. These recommendations also apply to PET, MRI, and cine CT imaging.

Myocardial Perfusion Tests

Indications

The main indication for the use of myocardial perfusion tests is to increase the sensitivity and specificity of exercise stress testing for the diagnosis of coronary artery disease to as high as 95 percent. The sensitivity is increased by the fact that the scintigraphic technique allows direct visualization of perfusion of all left ventricular myocardial segments, while the ECG technique is a derivative at best. The specificity is greater because of the potentially fewer sources of false-positive results in scintigrams when compared to the exercise ECG of the many patients who have abnormal resting ECGs.

An unfortunate common practice that is to be avoided is the referral for myocardial perfusion exercise testing of persons who belong to a population group with a low prevalence of coronary artery disease, namely young women and asymptomatic individuals of either gender. Even after all possible factors that would lead to a false-positive interpretation are assiduously eliminated, a positive result in a population with a pretest prevalence of coronary disease of less than 15 percent is still more likely to be a false-positive rather than a true-positive result.

The American Heart Association indications for the performance of exercise stress testing also generally apply to myocardial perfusion tests. However, nuclear cardiology tests should not be performed when the main reason for the exercise test is the evaluation of an individual's functional capacity or the measurement of some specific physiologic response such as blood pressure or heart rate.

A distinct advantage of myocardial perfusion scans over the nonnuclear exercise tests is the inherent ability of the scans to detect the location and extent of myocardial ischemia or scar. This ability renders the perfusion scans particularly useful in (1) the assessment of the success of coronary revascularization with angioplasty or bypass surgery and (2) the risk stratification of presurgical and postinfarction patients.

Methods

In exercise myocardial perfusion scans, 2 mCi of ^{201}Tl is injected at peak exercise (a slightly greater dose may be administered for heavier or taller subjects or if tomographic views are being obtained). A heart rate that is at least 85 percent of target heart rate is considered optimal for injection; a lower exercise heart rate may result in lower test sensitivity. The subject is to continue exercise for an additional minute to maintain the increased myocardial flow and thereby maximize ^{201}Tl extraction from the blood.

Imaging should begin about 10 to 20 minutes after injections. This interval is the time-window between a maximal thallium target-to-background ratio and the beginning of its net redistribution into myocardial areas with decreased isotope concentration. With planar imaging, three standard views are usually obtained: a 45-degree left anterior oblique (LAO) view, an anterior view, and a 70-degree LAO or left lateral view. Since the orientation of the heart is variable, adjustment of the LAO view must be made to obtain the best septal and posterolateral wall views. The 70-degree LAO or left lateral view is generally obtained with the patient in the right lateral decubitus position, minimizing overlap of the left hemidiaphragm with the inferobasal myocardium, while the other images are obtained with the patient supine.

Redistribution images, more popularly known as rest or equilibrium images, are nominally obtained about 4 hours after the initial injection. The positioning of the subject and the camera angulation during the equilibrium scans must be as close as possible to those of the postexercise scans to permit proper analysis and interpretation.

Re-injection protocols have been developed to maximize the detection of ischemic yet viable myocardium. The re-injection techniques increase the ^{201}Tl concentration in some myocardial segments that were traditionally deemed as being scarred or dead tissue. These are segments that remained ischemic for prolonged periods postexercise or are those that are chronically underperfused because of a severely compromised blood supply through a nearly totally occlusive coronary artery stenosis. It is estimated that the re-injection protocols identify viability in about 10 percent of the myocardial segments that were previously considered dead. An alternate technique to the re-injection protocols is delayed imaging, as late as 24 hours after the initial injection. However, these delayed protocols are not optimal. The effective ^{201}Tl half-life (a combination of its biologic clearance and its physical half-life) results in very low myocardial photon flux a day later and often leads to poor quality scans that are uninterpretable.

Interpretation

The normal postexercise reperfusion scans and the redistribution scans should show a uniform or homogeneous isotope distribution in the myocardium of the left ventricle. The typical horseshoe-shaped image is due to the lower concentration of the isotope in (1) the thinner basilar myocardium, (2) the membranous basal portion of the septum, (3) the fibrous valvular rings, and (4) both atria.

The right ventricle, being thinner walled than the left, is also not usually visualized unless it is pathologically hypertrophied. There is also less isotope uptake in the left ventricular apex, which reflects its thinness relative to the other myocardial segments. This finding is reported as the normal variant of apical thinning and occurs in about half of all imaged subjects.

Analysis of the images takes place by a visual qualitative evaluation and, optionally, by a computer quantitative assessment of the isotope activity or image pixel intensity in all the myocardial segments of the three images obtained in planar studies or in all the tomographic cuts in SPECT studies. Each segment is compared to (1) anatomically adjacent segments in the same image or plane, (2) its anatomic counterparts in the same set of images, and (3) its corresponding segment from postexercise to redistribution views.

A reversible perfusion defect is a myocardial segment exhibiting relatively or absolutely less radiopharmaceutical uptake on the stress images that disappears, or normalizes, on the redistribution images. This is commonly believed to be due to transient, exercise-induced myocardial ischemia, which takes place when vigorous exercise increases myocardial oxygen demand that cannot be met by a physiologically significant coronary artery stenosis. (Such a stenosis is usually defined as an angiographically determined coronary artery lumen occlusion of 70% or more.) The ischemia temporarily and partially impedes the active Na-K-ATPase pump–mediated transport through the myocyte membrane of ^{201}Tl, a potassium analog.

However, the transient perfusion defects are probably most commonly caused not by ischemia but by the physiologic phenomenon of differential flow distribution. Vigorous exercise results in an increased coronary blood flow through normal vessels—up to fivefold in some instances. The flow through a significant lesion is fixed. Since the relative flow of ^{201}Tl is dependent on and proportional to the relative flow of blood, myocardial segments supplied by normal arteries will show relatively greater concentrations of thallium than those segments supplied by stenotic vessels.

Therefore, the greater sensitivity for the detection of coronary disease of ^{201}Tl scintigraphy as compared to the stress test alone may be secondary to this differential flow distribution. To detect coronary disease in the ECG, exercise must cause ischemia; however, the scintigram need not cross the ischemic threshold. Transient perfusion defects are thus probably caused by differential flow distribution, without ischemia, in (1) most dipyrida-mole pharmacologic stress tests and (2) most exercise stress tests where the subject develops neither symptoms nor ischemic S–T segment ECG changes.

A nonreversible or fixed perfusion defect is a wall segment exhibiting relatively or absolutely diminished myocardial uptake on stress imaging that persists un-changed on redistribution images. This is usually due to myocardial death, although "stunned" or "hibernating" myocardium may present with a similar pattern. A scar is almost always a result of infarction but can be second-ary to other etiologies of myocardial necrosis. Fixed perfusion defects may be artifacts of soft tissue attenua-tion, especially if ^{201}Tl is the injected isotope. In women, most common are apparent septum and anterior wall perfusion defects—from overlying breast tissue; in men, most common are apparent inferior or inferobasal wall perfusion defects—from intervening hemidiaphragm. In the evaluation of these defects, a false-positive inter-pretation can be avoided and a greater specificity achieved if the nuclear scan findings are considered in the context of (1) the pretest Bayesian likelihood of coronary artery disease, (2) the lack of a clinical history of an infarction, and (3) the lack of pathologic Q waves in the ECG. Some nu-clear cardiology laboratories relate the imaging of ECG-gated wall motion to the perfusion scintigram, whether it be a planar or SPECT study. A patient with no ECG evidence or clinical history of myocardial infarction, with a normal wall motion in a segment with a fixed perfusion defect, is more likely to have an attenuation artifact rather than a true scar.

Interpretation of the perfusion scintigrams requires knowledge of coronary artery anatomy. Atherosclerotic disease of the left anterior descending artery causes perfusion defects of the septum and of the anterior and lateral segments. Because of variable anatomy, perfusion defects of the inferior wall and posterior wall segments can be caused by disease of either the right coronary or the circumflex coronary arteries. Apical defects can be the result of disease of any of the three vessels, since this is a watershed area that can be supplied by any and all coronary vessels.

In addition to the analysis of segmental defects, proper interpretation of scintigrams requires the evaluation of apparent chamber size. Enlargement of the left ventricle seen only in the stress scans with a normalization of cavity diameter in the redistribution scans is termed transient ischemic dilatation. It correlates highly with multivessel disease and the development of exercise-induced global ischemia with resultant decreases in cardiac output and in stroke volume and a corresponding increase in end-diastolic volumes and pressures. This scintigram finding is often accompanied by the symptom of dyspnea and an abnormal blood pressure response with exercise, and the auscultatory finding of a new transient gallop after exercise.

The pulmonary uptake of ^{201}Tl in the stress and redistribution scintigrams should be assessed because of its important diagnostic and prognostic implications. Increased lung activity on the exercise scans reflects increased pulmonary blood volume resulting from elevated intracardiac pressures. These elevations are the consequence of decreased myocardial compliance produced by exercise-induced global myocardial ischemia. Both the qualitative visual finding and the computer-derived quantitative lung-heart activity ratio are highly specific for the presence of multivessel coronary disease and highly predictive of a poor prognosis. Suboptimal exercise effort and an excessive smoking history may also enhance pulmonary uptake, unrelated to any underlying cardiac disease.

Ventricular Function Tests

Indications

Ventricular function is the major determinant of cardiovascular morbidity and mortality. The evaluation of myocardial performance is therefore essential to establish a proper therapeutic plan for the patient with cardiac disease. Ventricular function studies at rest and with exercise often guide the choice of specific medical or surgical treatment of individuals with heart disorders of any etiology. By providing qualitative and quantitative information of ventricular ejection fraction and wall motion, these studies play a central role in the assessment of patients with coronary, myocardial, valvular, or congenital heart disease.

The indications and contraindications for ventricular function studies are similar to those for myocardial perfusion studies and for exercise stress tests without nuclear scans. For diagnosis of coronary disease, either test is excellent. Myocardial perfusion scans are preferred for the assessment of the success of a revascularization procedure. Ventricular function studies are preferred for the evaluation of the effects of a particular cardiac disease on myocardial performance, and they are also preferred in the workup of the patient whose main symptom is exertional dyspnea. Some nuclear cardiology laboratories prefer to perform one study almost to the exclusion of the other. Most laboratories use them interchangeably. The choice of test often merely reflects the preference of the individual referring physician, or expertise with one procedure over the other.

Under optimal conditions, the sensitivity and specificity of radionuclide ventricular function scans are probably similar to those of myocardial perfusion scans for the detection of coronary artery disease. However, it is commonly assumed that the ventricular function studies have a lower sensitivity but a higher specificity than the perfusion studies. These differences may be secondary to two factors:

1. Ventricular function studies are performed in conjunction with bicycle ergometer exercise rather than with treadmill exercise. While the bicycle ergometer protocols allow for the torso to remain relatively immobile for image acquisition during exercise, bicycle exercise provokes a slower heart rate response and a lower myocardial oxygen demand at peak effort and therefore a lower likelihood of ischemia. More false-negative tests and a lower sensitivity may result.
2. Ventricular function studies with exercise depend on the development of a new wall motion abnormality as the marker of ischemia. Myocardial perfusion studies with exercise do not require the causation of actual ischemia for the development of a transient perfusion defect. Differential flow distribution of the isotope, below an ischemic threshold, suffices to indicate disease. In addition, several factors other than ischemia can cause an apparent perfusion defect, but few cause a new wall motion abnormality. Therefore, bicycle ergometry may produce fewer false-positive tests and hence may provide greater specificity.

Methods

The methods and techniques of nuclear ventricular scans are used to evaluate the ejection fraction, wall motion, diastolic function, and end-diastolic and end-systolic volumes of the left ventricle (and less frequently of the right ventricle). In addition, these methods can also assess valvular regurgitation, intracardiac shunts, and circulation transit time. There are two principal methods for the performance of nuclear ventricular function scans: equilibrium studies and first-pass studies.

EQUILIBRIUM STUDIES. The performance of an equilibrium ventricular function study requires the radiopharmaceutical to be administered in such a fashion as to allow the achievement of an equilibrium distribution within all the cardiac chambers before imaging takes place. The imaging agent is usually ^{99m}Tc pertechnetate as either an in vitro or an in vivo preparation, with the prior injection of stannous chloride to ensure better binding of the radionuclide to the red blood cells.

In equilibrium studies, imaging is performed in multiple projections to allow for the better separation of overlapping cardiac structures. Standard projections of rest studies are similar to those of planar myocardial perfusion studies. These are an anterior view, a 45-degree LAO view, and a 70-degree LAO or left lateral view. It is imperative when positioning for the shallower LAO view to consider the variability of orientation of the heart. The projection must result in the best possible septal delineation, or best separation of the left and right ventricular chambers, and also in the least supra-imposition of the left atrium over the left ventricle. This "best septal" view maximizes the accuracy and reproducibility of the determination of left ventricular ejection fraction.

The camera orientation for the exercise imaging generally should be identical to the "best septal" LAO view obtained at rest. This positioning ensures the most valid comparison of ejection fraction and ventricular segmental wall motion during exercise with rest. At most nuclear cardiology laboratories, the exercise scans are obtained only during peak effort. For an optimal study that gives the greatest physiologic information, scans should also be obtained at each 3-minute stage of bicycle ergometer exercise and also during the recovery phase, specifically at about the fifth minute postexercise. The positioning of the patient on the bicycle ergometer is essentially a compromise between a vertical or upright position, which allows for the most physiologic exercise, and a horizontal or supine position, which allows for the closest positioning of the camera against the chest of the patient.

Equilibrium ventriculography requires synchronization, or gating of image acquisition with the patient's cardiac rhythm. Each image set comprises a series of images of the patient's heart, each one covering a short time-slice of the cardiac cycle. The duration of each time-slice is selected to match the heart rate. In addition, slower frame rates of about 8 to 16 frames per cycle are adequate for accurate measurement of ejection fraction, while more rapid frame rates on the order of 64 frames per cycle are recommended if accurate diastolic function curves are required. As the dose of administered radioactivity is quite low, it is necessary to acquire hundreds of heart beats of data to result in a study with sufficient statistic validity. Each of these hundreds of heartbeats must be superimposed accurately over one another as they add together in the computer's memory. Electronic detection of each QRS complex allows this registration process to occur. The regularity of the cardiac rhythm is an important determinant of the quality of the final study, although advanced computer processing techniques may be employed to filter out undesirable beats from the final product.

FIRST-PASS STUDIES. The performance of a first-pass ventricular function study requires the radiopharmaceutical to be rapidly injected as a small bolus (<3 ml) into a large antecubital vein. The imaging agent is either ^{99m}Tc DTPA or an in vitro preparation of ^{99m}Tc pertechnetate and usually carries 25 to 30 mCi of activity. The transit, or first-pass, of the radioactive bolus is followed from the peripheral circulation, to the right side of the heart, to the pulmonary vasculature, to the left side of the heart, and to the aorta.

In first-pass studies, imaging is done with the camera in the anterior or shallow (<15 degrees) right anterior oblique projection. This angulation permits the optimal separation of the left atrium and the left ventricle. The spatial overlap of the ventricles that occurs with this positioning is not an issue because the sequential arrival of the bolus in each chamber separates them temporally rather than spatially. Rapid, dynamic images are obtained with a temporal resolution suited to the intent of the study. For example, to evaluate left-to-right shunts, two frames per second is adequate, while a much higher frame rate would be necessary to evaluate exercise ejection fraction (on the order of 50–100 frames per second). Digitization and capture of the patient's cardiac rhythm are optional.

Interpretation

VENTRICULAR EJECTION FRACTION. The determination of ventricular ejection fraction is based on the fact that radioactive counts detected in systole and diastole are proportional to systolic and diastolic volumes. In first-pass studies, systolic and diastolic counts are determined from time-activity curves obtained from a sequence of usually less than 10 cardiac cycles. In equilibrium studies, systolic and diastolic counts are determined by manual or computer-generated edge detection methods. In both methods, the background radioactivity is first determined and subtracted. A ventricular ejection fraction is then derived using the following formula:

Ejection fraction = diastolic counts − systolic counts/diastolic counts

Both methods provide a highly accurate determination of left ventricular ejection fraction. The results obtained with either procedure highly correlate with each other and with those obtained with invasive ventriculography in the cardiac catheterization laboratory.

The normal left ventricular ejection fraction at rest is about 50 percent. With exercise, the ejection fraction increases, resulting in a smaller end-systolic volume in the context of a relatively unchanged end-diastolic volume. The increase in stroke volume together with an increased heart rate augments the cardiac output needed to meet the increasing metabolic needs of exercising peripheral skeletal muscles.

A decrease in ejection fraction or an absolute increase of less than 5 percent, with moderate exercise, is considered an abnormal response and is highly specific for the detection of exercise-induced ischemia and significant coronary artery disease. The specificity further increases when the abnormal ejection fraction response is accompanied by new wall motion abnormalities. Very few conditions other than ischemia can cause both of these abnormal responses with exercise. A wall motion abnormality with exercise, without a corresponding drop in ejection fraction, implies milder, less extensive, or single-vessel disease and carries a better prognosis. A drop in ejection fraction with exercise implies severe, extensive, or multivessel disease and carries a poor prognosis.

VENTRICULAR WALL MOTION. The analysis of wall motion abnormalities at rest and with exercise in nuclear ventricular function tests is similar to that of perfusion defects in nuclear myocardial scans. A segmental wall motion abnormality at rest most commonly signifies myocardial scarring from infarction. Abnormal septal wall motion can also be seen in patients who are free of coronary disease but have an intraventricular electrical conduction defect such as left bundle branch block, recent open-heart surgery, or right ventricular volume overload states. An abnormal apical wall motion can be seen in patients with valvular disease.

Descriptive terms describing wall motion are hyperkinetic, normokinetic, hypokinetic, akinetic, and dyskinetic. Wall motion analysis should always address whether the wall motion abnormalities are segmental or global. Coronary artery disease is the predominant cause of segmental wall motion abnormalities and usually spares the left ventricular basal and upper posterolateral wall segments. A pattern of global wall motion abnormalities, where all myocardial segments are hypokinetic, does not often correlate with ischemic heart disease. Global wall motion abnormalities correlate best with the dilated cardiomyopathies caused by alcohol, diabetes, chemotherapy, or viral myocarditis or those of unknown cause.

The normal wall motion response to exercise is a more vigorous, or hyperkinetic, motion. A segmental wall motion abnormality (hypokinesis, akinesis, or dyskinesis) not present at rest that develops with exercise highly correlates with and is extremely specific for exercise-induced myocardial ischemia. As with myocardial perfusion scans, the particular pattern of wall motion abnormalities identifies the location of physiologically significant coronary artery stenosis. Atherosclerotic disease of the left anterior descending coronary artery causes wall motion abnormalities of the septum and of the anterior and lateral segments. Because of variable anatomy, wall motion abnormalities of the inferior wall and posterior wall segments can be caused by disease of either the right coronary or the circumflex coronary arteries. Apical wall motion defects can be the result of disease of any of the three vessels, since this is a watershed area that can be supplied by any and all coronary vessels.

Index